Skills for Practice in Occupational Therapy

Second Edition

Skills for Practice in Occupational Therapy

Second Edition

Edited by

Edward A.S. Duncan PhD BSc(Hons) DipCBT

Professor of Applied Health Research, Nursing, Midwifery and
Allied Health Professions Research Unit,
The University of Stirling,
Stirling, Scotland, UK

ELSEVIER

Notices

Practitioners and researchers must always rely on their own experience and knowledge in evaluating and using any information, methods, compounds or experiments described herein. Because of rapid advances in the medical sciences, in particular, independent verification of diagnoses and drug dosages should be made. To the fullest extent of the law, no responsibility is assumed by Elsevier, authors, editors or contributors for any injury and/or damage to persons or property as a matter of products liability, negligence or otherwise, or from any use or operation of any methods, products, instructions, or ideas contained in the material herein.

ISBN: 978-0-702-07752-4

Content Strategist: Trinity Hutton
Project Manager: Shruti Raj
Designer: Patrick Ferguson
Marketing Manager: Belinda Tudin

Printed in Bell & Bain (LTD), Scotland

Last digit is the print number: 9 8 7 6 5 4 3 2

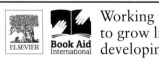

In memory of my brother David Duncan (1965–2022) and Professor Emeritus Averil Stewart FRCOT (1943–2022), both of whom have left the world a poorer place.

LIST OF CONTRIBUTORS

The editor(s) would like to acknowledge and offer grateful thanks for the input of all previous edition contributors, without whom this new edition would not have been possible.

Katrina Bannigan, BD BSc PhD
Professor of Occupational Therapy and Head of Department of Occupational Therapy, and Human Nutrition and Dietetics,
Glasgow Caledonian University
Glasgow, UK

Mary Alicia Barnes, OTD
Lecturer,
Department of Occupational Therapy,
Tufts University
Medford, Massachusetts, USA

Thomas Bevitt, B.AppSc(OT) PhD candidate
Lecturer and Professional Practice Convener for Occupational Therapy
Faculty of Health, University of Canberra
Bruce, Australian Capital Territory, Australia

Sally Boa, PhD BSc CertMRCSLT
Head of Palliative Care Education, Research and Practice Development and Honorary Senior
Research Fellow, University of Stirling
Strathcarron Hospice
Denny, UK

Ted Brown, PhD MSc MPA BScOT(Hons) GCHPE OT(C) OTR MRCOT FOTARA FAOTA
Professor and Undergraduate Course Coordinator
Department of Occupational Therapy
School of Primary and Allied Health Care
Faculty of Medicine, Nursing and Health Sciences
Monash University - Peninsula Campus
Frankston, Victoria, Australia

Charles H. Christiansen, EdD MA BS OTR FAOTA
Professor Emeritus
Department of Occupational Therapy
School of Health Professions
The University of Texas Medical Branch
Galveston, Texas, USA

Nichola Duffy, BSc (Hons), PGDip
Advanced Practice Occupational Therapist,
NHS Lothian,
Midlothian Health and Social Care Partnership
Edinburgh, UK

Edward A.S. Duncan, PhD BSc(Hons) DipCBT
Professor of Applied Health Research
Nursing, Midwifery and Allied
Health Professions Research Unit,
The University of Stirling,
Stirling, UK

Kirsty Forsyth, PhD MSc OTR
Professor
Department of Occupational Therapy
and Art Therapy, Queen Margaret
University College
Edinburgh, UK

Jane Grant, MSc, BA (Hons), BSc
Specialist Occupational Therapist,
NHS Lothian, UK

Priscilla Harries, PhD MSc DipCOT FHEA FRCOT
Professor of Occupational Therapy
Director, Centre for Applied Health and Social Care
Head of Graduate Research School and Researcher Development
Directorate of Research and Impact
Kingston University London
London, UK

Stephen Isbel, HScD MOT MHA GCTE B.AppSc(OT)
Associate Professor and Discipline Lead of Occupational Therapy
Faculty of Health, The University of Canberra Hospital
Bruce, Australian Capital Territory, Australia

Alister C. Landrock, BDSDip BA PGDip[†]
Formerly Lecturer, Department of Occupational Therapy and Art Therapy, Queen Margaret
University College, Edinburgh, UK

[†]Deceased

Anne Landrock
Formerly Principal Teacher of Art and Design,
Glenwood High School, Fife, UK

Lisa McCaw, BSc (Hons), MSc Occupational Therapy
Occupational Therapy Team Lead,
North Edinburgh CAMHS Team
NHS Lothian, Scotland, UK

Lianne McInally
Senior Manager AHP,
East Ayrshire Health and Social Care Partnership,
Scotland, UK

Elizabeth Anne McKay, PhD
Head, Department of Occupational
Therapy, Faculty of Education and
Health Sciences, University of Limerick,
Limerick, Ireland

Amy McKenzie, GCertHealthScience (Health Services Innovation) BOccThy
Clinical Education Support Officer,
Royal Brisbane & Women's Hospital,
Metro North Hospital and Health Service,
Brisbane, Queensland Australia

Jane Melton, MSc DipCOT
Consultant Occupational Therapist,
Gloucestershire Partnership NHS
Foundation Trust, UK

Susan Prior, D Health Soc Sci BSc
Senior Lecturer Occupational Therapy
Queen Margaret University
Musselburgh, UK

Sharan L. Schwartzberg, EdD FAOTA, FAGPA, CGP
Professor of Occupational Therapy Emerita
School of Arts & Sciences,
Tufts University,
Department of Occupational Therapy,
Medford, Massachusetts, USA

Lesley Scobbie, PhD MSc BScOT
Clinical Research Fellow
Department of Occupational Therapy, Human Nutrition and
Dietetics
Glasgow Caledonian University & NHS Lanarkshire
Glasgow, UK

Jenny Strong, PhD MOccThy BOccThy
Emeritus Professor of Occupational Therapy,
School of Health & Rehabilitation Sciences,
The University of Queensland,
Queensland, Australia
and
Occupational Therapy Research Coordinator,
Royal Brisbane & Women's Hospital,
Metro North Hospital and Health Service,
Brisbane, Queensland Australia

M. Clare Taylor, DipCOT BA(Hons) MA(Distinc) PGCE PhD FHEA MRCOT
Freelance occupational therapist

Renee R. Taylor, PhD
Professor, Licenced Clinical Psychologist;
Department of Occupational Therapy,
University of Illinois, Chicago, USA

Mong-Lin Yu, PhD MOccTh BSc(OT) GCHPE
Senior Lecturer and Practice Education Coordinator (Clinical Placement)
Department of Occupational Therapy
School of Primary and Allied Health Care
Faculty of Medicine, Nursing and Health Sciences
Monash University - Peninsula Campus
Frankston, Victoria, Australia

Skills for Practice in Occupational Therapy is all about what occupational therapists do and the skills they require to have to excel in contemporary practice. These skills have evolved considerably in recent years and are continually developing. Now more than ever, practitioners are required to draw on different types of thinking and evidence-based ways of working, as well as using their leadership and management expertise. Practitioners are also expected to be competent in the professional use of social media and in multiple means of dissemination. This text provides essential information on all these topics and is an essential resource for practitioners working in contemporary health and social care and other settings.

Throughout my years as a practitioner, I was always struck by how poorly connected the theory and practice of occupational therapy were from the real world of many practitioners' lives. This largely remains as true today as it did over 25 years ago. To many, the idea of truly connecting research and practice remains a utopian concept: Theories are often taught in university but for many are rarely fully implemented in practice. This need not be the case. *Foundations* was written to emphasise the practical implications of the theory base being discussed. *Skills* has been developed to do the same in reverse: linking practice with theory and research wherever possible. Clearly, this is achievable more in some chapters than others, which are perhaps by their nature inherently pragmatic. This second edition of *Skills* has involved updating all chapters and introducing new chapters required for the competent practice of occupational therapy.

All such texts are influenced by the experiences and perspectives of the editor. Understanding these influences can help to understand the structure and content of the book. I was very fortunate to have an extremely rich undergraduate experience. This had a lasting impact on my development both as a practitioner and more latterly as an academic. For 10 years after qualifying, I worked as an occupational therapist in a variety of mental health settings. My earliest professional experiences were in community mental health teams in various areas of urban deprivation in Glasgow, Scotland, UK. Here I became aware of the impact of social deprivation on people's well-being and the importance of the social determinants of health (such as income, housing, and education) on people's functioning. After a few years, I changed jobs to help establish a new occupational therapy service in a high-security forensic psychiatric hospital. Both community mental health and forensic mental health settings provided excellent opportunities to develop and enhance my practice as an occupational therapist. During this time, I was deeply (but not exclusively) influenced by two central theories for occupational therapy practice: the Model of Human Occupation and the cognitive behavioural frame of reference. Since that time, I have become more convinced of the importance of understanding and judiciously employing a wide range of theoretical perspectives, including evidence-based theoretical occupational therapy models and non-profession-specific theories and frames of reference, according to the context in which they are required. I have spent the last 25 years leading and collaborating in research studies that have been variously profession specific, multidisciplinary, and increasingly interdisciplinary. Each of these studies has reinforced the need and importance of having a wide range of *Skills* not only as a practitioner but also as a researcher and academic.

This second edition of *Skills* is the result of an international collaboration with eminent contributors from across the world. As with all edited texts, the voice and style of each chapter change according to the authors. These differences have, by and large, been left unaltered in the editing process. Through the various chapters of this book, I aimed to provide an engaging, useful, and practical introduction to the essential skills required by occupational therapists for contemporary practice. I hope it's found to be valuable to students and practitioners alike.

Edward A.S. Duncan
United Kingdom

ACKNOWLEDGEMENTS

While authors (or editors) of a book have their names on the cover, it is rarely, if ever, truly their work alone—even less so with an edited text. The second edition of *Skills for Practice in Occupational Therapy* would not have been achieved without the considerable contribution of many people, some of whom merit particular mention:

THE CONTRIBUTORS

This book has been contributed to by a range of exceptional therapists (both practitioners and academics) each of whom brought a wealth of personal and professional experience to this work. It has been extremely enjoyable to work with established and new collaborators. Each of them has my greatest respect and thanks for the contributions they have made.

The second edition of *Skills* was developed during the Covid-19 pandemic, and this inevitably led to some delays in its production. The patience of the contributors throughout this process is greatly appreciated.

THE PUBLISHERS

Elsevier, as always, has been extremely supportive in this book's development and production. My thanks are due to them for their patience, wisdom, and support throughout the publication process.

NURSING MIDWIFERY AND ALLIED HEALTH PROFESSIONS RESEARCH UNIT, UNIVERSITY OF STIRLING

I'm fortunate to have spent almost 20 years working in this interdisciplinary research environment where high-quality impact-focused research is undertaken for the greater good of health and social care services and society. My thinking has been strongly influenced by colleagues, which in turn has impacted this second edition as much as it did the first.

MY FAMILY

Anne, Catherine, Eleanor, and Joseph continue to support and encourage me in all my work. Without their continued love, understanding, and patience this book would never have been realised.

CONTENTS

Introduction

Edward A.S. Duncan

THE PURPOSE AND STRUCTURE OF THIS BOOK

Skills for Practice in Occupational Therapy introduces the reader to the wide range of skills that occupational therapists require to have so to practice effectively in contemporary health and social care environments. Each chapter is written with a practice skills focus in mind, but wherever possible this is directly linked to theory and existing evidence. The book is clearly targeted at and relevant for occupational therapy students who are developing these skills. The direct practice relevance of the chapters also makes it a resource that should not be left on the student shelf, never to be opened after graduation, but become used as a resource for new and experienced practitioners alike.

While this chapter provides a useful orientation to the book's purpose and contents as a whole, it is not necessary to read the text from cover to cover in chronologic order. Readers will access different chapters at different stages depending on what they wish to know. However, chapters have been extensively cross referenced so the reader opening this book at one chapter may find oneself journeying through each section as the reading builds up a bigger picture of what is required to deliver effective skills for practice.

The structure of each chapter, in the main sections of the book, is consistent. Chapters begin with a brief overview of the subject and chapter content, a highlight box is located at the front of each chapter to provide an even briefer and punchier synopsis. The body of the chapter then follows. Wherever possible, case vignettes are included to illuminate and illustrate the points being made. Each chapter concludes with a summary to bring together the key issues that have been presented and discussed. A reflective learning box is included at the end of each chapter to help you think about the relevance of what has been discussed to your own practice experience.

WHAT EXACTLY DO OCCUPATIONAL THERAPISTS DO?

The venue may differ (e.g., a student house party, a family get-together, a meeting with a professional colleague, an interdisciplinary conference, or a multidisciplinary team meeting), but invariably the question is asked: "What do you do?" or "What is occupational therapy, anyway?" One way of responding could be to recite a definition of the profession; telling the interested inquirer that occupational therapy:

- Is concerned with the key elements of occupational performance and identity: how people identify themselves and their future aspirations, their roles and relationships, together with their personal capacity for fulfilling these within their physical and social environment.
- Aims to enable and empower people to be competent and confident in their daily lives, and thereby to enhance well-being and minimise the effects of dysfunction or environmental barriers.
- Uses everyday occupations and tasks creatively and therapeutically to achieve goals that are meaningful to people and relevant to their daily life.
- Encourages people to collaborate in the therapeutic process to become partners with the therapist in the designing and directing of therapy (Duncan 2021a, p. 3).

Such an approach, however, is not recommended: It would likely lead to bemused stares, a polite thanks, and a quick exit by the person concerned! So how can one appropriately respond to such questions? What is your 2-minute elevator pitch about the profession? Why can such a straightforward question be so challenging to answer?

Often when asked, "What do you do?" it is tempting to respond by saying what you *are*, rather than what you *do*. Even when occupational therapists respond by saying what they do, their description can belie the true depth and breadth of practice. Hagedorn (2000) discussed the challenges associated with being seen as doing simple things. Occupational therapy, Hagedorn stated, is by and large a low-tech intervention in a high-tech health care environment. When compared to high-tech interventions, such as three-dimensional imaging or vaccinations, occupational therapy may be viewed as merely common sense. Therefore describing the depth and breadth of what occupational therapists do is challenging. Part of the reason for this is the visible portion of practice is only a small percentage of what actually occurs. Hagedorn (2000) presented two differing images to illustrate this. First, occupational therapy was compared to an iceberg, where only the tip of the vast mass is visible. Hagedorn felt that this was an unattractive analogy as icebergs appear clumsy. Second, and more favourably, Hagedorn compared occupational therapy to a computer; each has an easy-to-use interface but is highly complex beneath the surface interface. However, this image too could be criticised as being excessively mechanistic. Of course, because visual analogies are subjective, different people will find them more or less helpful. They can be useful strategies, however, to convey the message that the totality of what occupational therapists do is not immediately apparent. As an aside, I quite like the analogy of occupational therapy being like the common garden mint plant: highly useful and very adaptable, deeply rooted, fast spreading, and very difficult to remove once embedded!

SKILLS FOR PRACTICE

This book is about what occupational therapists actually do: the skills they bring to practice. Skills are "the aptitudes and competencies appropriate for a particular job" (*Chambers Dictionary*, 1994, p. 1617). Occupational therapists are now required to have and use a complex range of skills (Vignette 1.1) to maintain their competence in a swiftly developing health care environment (Ryan et al., 2003). It is for this reason that this book has been developed in four key sections that outline the broad range of skills required by practitioners to deliver best practice: thinking, judgement, and decision-making skills; professional skills; evidence-based and research skills; and leadership, supervision, and management skills.

Skills for Practice in Occupational Therapy addresses the aptitudes and competencies required by today's practitioners, introducing these in a way that is accessible, relevant, closely linked to theory, and wherever possible evidence based. If Duncan's (2021b) *Foundations for Practice in Occupational Therapy* aims to link theory with practice, then *Skills for Practice in Occupational Therapy* aims to link practice with theory!

Although this book contains practical advice and guidance on a range of issues, it is not designed to be a how-to textbook that will take you step by step through an intervention or theoretical approach. Similarly, it does not claim to cover every necessary skill. Instead, the book covers a broad range of skills that are essential for today's practitioner. The chapters vary in theoretical and academic depth. Several of the chapters present complex areas of study that have been subject to research and theoretical development for many years: These chapters aim to introduce the topic to readers, provide them with a foundation of knowledge in the area, and signpost them to other resources to develop their knowledge further. Other chapters are inherently pragmatic. This diversity of depth and focus is appropriate as it reflects the differing types of skills that occupational therapists use in their everyday practice. This second edition brings each chapter up to date and includes new chapters that address contemporary issues.

Thinking, Judgement, and Decision-Making Skills for Practice

Practitioners spend a lot of time thinking, judging/ assessing, collaborating with clients, making decisions, and reflecting on what they have done. Yet how often, and for how long, do people spend time to stop and consider why they made certain decisions, on what evidence they based their decisions, how successful their strategy of collaborating with clients is, and how evidence based their judgements in practice are? These skills are central, yet largely invisible to competent and successful practice. Section 1 untangles the vast literature of this field and introduces the reader to a range of ideas, theories, and evidence that highlight ways in which practitioners' thinking, judgements, decisions, and reflections are influenced and can be enhanced.

Professional Skills for Practice

Section 2 focuses on the everyday skills practitioners use when intervening with clients. The chapters in this section focus on the core skills (Creek, 2003) that occupational therapists use in practice:

- Assessment
- Use of activity/activity analysis (which includes environmental analysis)
- The therapeutic use of self
- Problem solving
- Group work

Each of these skills assists practitioners to enable their clients to develop, maintain, or explore their daily lives, enhance their well-being, and minimise the effects of occupational dysfunction or environmental barriers. Additionally, this section includes chapters on goal setting and report writing and recordkeeping—neglected but essential components of skilled practice. Each chapter, though practice

VIGNETTE 1.1   A Day in the Life of an Occupational Therapist

Beth is an advanced clinical occupational therapist in an acute mental health inpatient service. She arrives at work at 8.30 a.m. and is immediately greeted by a client who has been on the ward for a week. The client is worried about a visit that she will be receiving from her parents in the afternoon and wants to share her concerns with Beth, asking her what she should do. Beth spends some time listening to the client and arranges to see her later. Beth then attends the ward handover meeting with the nursing and psychiatric staff and discusses the relevance and urgency of several clients whom the team have referred and wish to be assessed. The turnover on the ward is fast, so she may not have time to see them all and needs to judge which referrals are highest priority. Having completed the handover meeting, Beth then prepares and runs an open creative arts group for clients on the ward. This is always a challenging session as the needs of the group are varied, but the creative medium is popular throughout the ward and the group enables Beth to observe clients' range of functioning in a group setting. Once the group is completed and the notes are written up, Beth returns to the client she met first thing. The client shares some more details with Beth who decides to take a problem-solving approach to help the client generate her own solutions to the difficulties she foresees will arise when her parents visit.

Beth's next task is to carry out an initial assessment with a 26-year-old man (Chris), who was recently readmitted to the ward. Beth has heard that Chris is unhappy at being on the ward once again and is also aware that he is viewed by the nursing staff as being noncompliant with his medication and the ward routine. Beth's first aim is to engage with Chris and communicate with him that she wished to understand what he thought his difficulties were, and that she wanted to discover if there was anything he felt he wished to address. Her hope was that together they would be able to agree on what his functional problems were and develop an intervention plan they could both agree with and work toward.

Having spent longer than anticipated with Chris, it was time to rush to her lunchtime journal club meeting. The journal club is a monthly interdisciplinary event that Beth had initially set up with a clinical psychologist. The club has now

been attended by staff from various professional groups for over a year, and some changes to practice have occurred due to discussions that have taken place. Beth had recently carried out an audit of the club and it was found to be well attended and highly valued. The findings of the audit had been submitted to a clinical effectiveness conference, and her abstract was accepted for a poster presentation at a virtual conference. Beth has now developed a draft poster using PowerPoint. She wants to show it to the journal club members to get some feedback before it is finalised.

Beth's afternoon begins with a clinical supervision session with her junior occupational therapist. This is quickly followed by a kitchen session with another client who is preparing to go home after an unusually lengthy admission (by this ward's standards). After this she attends the ward development meeting. This is a staff meeting for the senior staff members on the ward and plans new developments to its structure and routine. Beth is concerned about the level of therapeutic engagement as a whole and wants to encourage all staff to be more interactive with clients. However, she is very aware of ward politics and draws on all her leadership and personal management skills to communicate these issues with the rest of the team. After the meeting, Beth returns to her ward office. This is the first chance she has had to read her emails. Amongst the usual stuff, two messages stick out: One of them is from the hospital's practice education facilitator to ask Beth if she would mind having an occupational therapy student, for 6 weeks, starting the following week? Another email is from a colleague in the local university with whom Beth is a co-grant applicant on a research study application to conduct a feasibility study of an activity scheduling intervention they have developed for clients with eating disorders. Beth needs to review the procedure that her colleague has suggested they use for recruiting participants. Half an hour before home time, Beth makes herself a well-deserved coffee and opens Twitter on her phone to see what other colleagues in #occupationaltherapy are saying. There is a buzz about a recently published paper, so she clicks on the hyperlink and reads the abstract to see if it is of any relevance. If it looks good she will bookmark it and read it in full later.

focused, is closely linked to developments in evidence, theory, and policy.

Evidence-Based and Research Skills for Practice

Section 3 addresses the importance of evidence-based and research skills in practice. Research is now the business of

every practitioner (Bannigan et al., 2007). In the United Kingdom, the Royal College of Occupational Therapists has stated, "Occupational therapists have a responsibility to contribute to the continuing development of the profession by utilising critical evaluation, and participating in audit and research" (Creek, 2003, p. 17). A contemporary textbook on skills for practice in occupational therapy cannot be without a section to guide practitioners in finding relevant research and appraising it for quality, examining how to implement the recommendations of research into practice, and evaluating how successful this has been. Further, occupational therapists now have to examine how they can undertake and implement research in practice. Despite the very real challenges that face practitioners who wish to undertake research, it can be done. This section outlines various approaches that have been successful in undertaking and implementing clinically relevant research in practice and discusses the strengths and limitations of each. The section concludes with a chapter that contains important information on the skills that are required by practitioners to successfully present or publish their work.

LEADERSHIP, SUPERVISION, AND MANAGEMENT SKILLS FOR PRACTICE

Making good clinical judgements, having expert professional skills, finding and using the best evidence, and engaging with research are essential skills for practice. Yet, if a practitioner does not have high-quality personal and interpersonal skills, the work will not reach its full potential. Section 4 addresses precisely these issues for practice. Every practitioner can be a leader; it is not an attribute that is solely attributed to people in authority, and being in authority does not mean that a person will be able to lead. First and foremost, skilled leadership requires leadership of self. Among other attributes, effective practitioners need to be authentic, have integrity, and be trusted by others. Even with these positive attributes (and others are necessary, too), there is no escaping the demands of working in health and social care environments where practitioners frequently face challenging situations and people, and clients too! Therefore positive self-management (looking after one's personal resources) is also vital for the individual who wishes to be an effective and skilled practitioner. When able to self-manage, practitioners' influence on others will grow and so too will the range of issues they have an impact on and their influence in the work environment. Sometimes this will evidence itself through practitioners leading changes in a wider circle than their immediate professional discipline (as seen in Vignette 1.1). At other times it will be observable through the influence they have with their colleagues within their professional discipline—either informally or through formal structures such as student or clinical supervision. Contemporary occupational therapists exist in an increasingly digital world. Most practitioners are involved in social media in one form or another. This can be a professional asset, but it also poses some risks and requires careful consideration to responsibly engage to maximum effect.

SUMMARY

So, what do occupational therapists do? Perhaps this question cannot be satisfactorily answered in a catchy strap line. Competent occupational therapists are required to have a startling depth and breadth of knowledge, practical skills, and personal and professional attributes. *Skills for Practice in Occupational Therapy* provides students and practitioners with an introduction and overview of the key skills for practice that are required for contemporary practice.

REFERENCES

Bannigan, K., Hughes, S., & Booth, M. (2007). Research is now every occupational therapists' business. *The British Journal of Occupational Therapy*, *70*(3), 95.

Chambers Dictionary. (1994). Skills. Chambers Harrap.

Creek, J. (2003). *Occupational therapy defined as a complex intervention*. College of Occupational Therapists, London.

Duncan, E. A. S. (2021a). Introduction. In E. A. S. Duncan (Ed.), *Foundations for practice in occupational therapy* (5th ed., pp. 2–5). Elsevier/Churchill Livingstone.

Duncan, E. A. S. (Ed.). (2021b). *Foundations for practice in occupational therapy* (5th ed.). Elsevier.

Hagedorn, R. (2000). *Tools for practice in occupational therapy*. Churchill Livingstone.

Ryan, S. E., Esdaile, S. A., & Brown, G. (2003). Appreciating the big picture: You are part of it! The socio-political influences on health practice in the public and private sphere. In G. Brown, S. A. Esdaile, & S. E. Ryan (Eds.), *Becoming an advanced health care practitioner* (pp. 1–29). Butterworth Heinemann.

Thinking, Judgement and Decision Skills for Practice

Judgement and Decision-Making Skills for Practice

Priscilla Harries

HIGHLIGHTS

- Practitioners form judgements and make decisions in everyday practice.
- Making judgements and decisions are two of the key cognitive tasks used in professional thinking.
- These judgements and decisions can have a considerable impact on the quality of client care.

- It is important that students and practitioners understand the different manners in which judgements and decisions can be understood in practice.
- Practical examples are included to help the reader consider the different factors involved in judgement and decision making.

OVERVIEW

Why is judgement and decision making important and worthy of inclusion in a book that focuses on skills for practice? Few practitioners would contest the notion that they possess knowledge upon which they base their decisions in practice. What the basis of this knowledge is and how they use it in practice is, however, much less clear. Making judgements and decisions are two of the key cognitive tasks used in professional thinking. This chapter teases out how practitioners think in practice, form judgements, and make decisions; each of these, when made well, enables people to take wise action and ultimately enhance the effectiveness of a service's provision.

The chapter begins by looking at definitions for key terms in the area. It then continues by presenting some of the early occupational therapy studies of clinical reasoning, discussing what this research has told us about the way occupational therapists think and the limitations of the research methods they used. Two related but differing theories of judgement and decision making that have developed from cognitive psychology are then presented: cognitive continuum theory and dual process theory. The contribution of each of these theories to practice is examined.

The chapter then considers how practitioners can apply judgement and decision-making skills in practice, and exercises are provided to illustrate the challenges and processes of judgement and decision-making tasks. To conclude, the chapter discusses the impact of practitioners' personal and professional values on judgement and decision making in practice.

DEFINITIONS

Researchers studying different cognitive tasks have used a wide variety of terms to describe different types of thinking such as reasoning, judgement, problem solving, and decision making (Gale & Marsden, 1985). Reasoning implies the drawing of conclusions. Reasoning may be deductive, when the conclusion is logically drawn based on factual information, or inductive, when the conclusion drawn is only possible and needs to be tested in light of further information (Eysenck, 1993). A judgement requires a person to consider an item of information or an option and to assign a weight based on the perceived level of importance. Problem solving involves generating alternatives to select from. Decision making occurs when a person makes a selection from possible alternatives that have been considered. In occupational therapy the term clinical reasoning tends to be used to cover all these thinking processes, but each term can be defined independently and can be used with a distinct meaning.

What tends to clarify the meaning of the terms is understanding the theoretical and methodological orientation of the researcher. Those most interested in the outcome of thinking tend to compare how information has been used with the decision that has been taken. They are most interested in judgement and decision making. Such researchers tend to use quantitative methodologies characteristic of the schools of judgement analysis and decision analysis. They are interested in identification of statistical weightings of judgements or the calculation of the probability that a particular decision has been, or will be, made. Research using judgement analysis has been conducted in occupational therapy by, for example, Unsworth (1996, 2001), Harries and Harries (2001a, 2001b), Harries and Gilhooly (2003a, 2003b), and Rassafiani et al. (2008). To date decision analysis research has not been published in occupational therapy literature.

Researchers more interested in describing the actual processes of thinking, as opposed to the decision outcome, tend to focus their attention on reasoning and problem solving. These latter researchers tend to use qualitative methods such as those informed by phenomenological and ethnographic theories. To date, these have accounted for the majority of occupational therapy clinical reasoning research studies.

THE EARLY STUDIES[1]

Joan Rogers used her Eleanor Clark Slagle lecture of 1983 to talk about the ethics, science, and art of clinical reasoning. Rogers (1983) defined clinical reasoning as "...the scientific, ethical and artistic dimensions" of practice (p. 616), emphasising that these are inextricably linked.

Later, Mattingly and Fleming (1994) conducted an influential research project of American occupational therapists' clinical reasoning. It was the first major study to explore the reasoning strategies used by occupational therapists and used an ethnographic and action research approach: interviewing, observing, and videoing 17 occupational therapists over a 2-year period. The researchers identified reasoning tracks or styles and linked these to reasoning strategies. Their findings emphasised that occupational therapists' reasoning was "largely tacit, highly imagistic and deeply phenomenological" (Mattingly, 1991, p. 797).

Since the work of Mattingly and Fleming (1994), there has been a burgeoning of research in occupational therapy examining the clinical reasoning of occupational therapists (see, for example, Alnervik & Sviden, 1996; Chapparo, 1999; Crabtree & Lyons, 1997; Creighton et al., 1995; Crennan & MacRae, 2010; Doyle et al., 2013; Fleming, 1991a; Fondiller et al., 1990; Fortune & Ryan, 1996; Fossey, 1996; Hagedorn, 1996; Hooper, 1997; Kuipers & Grice, 2009; McKay, 1999; Mitchell & Unsworth, 2005; Munroe, 1996; Murphy & Stav, 2018; Paterson, 2003; Paterson et al., 2002; Stephens et al., 2018; Stark et al., 2015; Taylor et al., 2007; Tempest & McIntyre, 2006; Unsworth, 2011; Wainwright & McGinnis, 2008).

Despite a few exceptions, the defining characteristics of this body of research are that the methods are qualitative, the sample sizes are generally small, and the participant populations are predominantly North American.

A few key points can be generalised from these and other studies of a similar format in nursing and other professions (Fawcett et al., 2001; Rycroft-Malone et al., 2004; Sefton, 2001; Upshur et al., 2001). Generally, these studies view clinical reasoning (or decision making) as being formed of several components, including the use of knowledge, self-reflection by the clinician (a component of metacognition), clients' needs, expectations, or desires, and shared decision making. Crucially, the vast majority of these studies view the components of clinical reasoning as being of equal value—like pieces of a jigsaw that are each as important as the other.

Although qualitative approaches were chosen to try to give a holistic understanding of thinking in terms of context, they appear to be limited in terms of their ability to represent the holism of actual thinking. Their lack of validity relates specifically to the difficulty the approaches have in reliably accessing experts' well-practiced intuitive thinking.

Analytical Versus Intuitive Thinking

The first major study of thinking processes in clinical situations was the study of medical problem solving by Elstein et al. (1978). Their study used three methods of data collection: direct observation of problem solving using simulated clinical problems, concurrent think aloud, and retrospection (while viewing video footage). Elstein et al. (1978) identified hypothetico-deductive reasoning as the strategy for diagnosis formation in medicine. Occupational therapists also identified hypothetico-deductive reasoning through the occupational dysfunction diagnosis (Fleming, 1991b). However, when comparing differences between novices and experienced practitioners' diagnosis formation strategies, Elstein et al. (1990) found there were other forms of thinking. As experts had the advantage of previous experience, they had developed a store of scripts (Abernathy & Hamm, 1994). If a client had a familiar problem practitioners used pattern matching to trigger the direct automatic retrieval of an appropriate script. Therefore experts confronted with a familiar problem used a rapid and automatic form of processing that was acknowledged as intuitive reasoning (Abernathy & Hamm, 1994).

---

[1]From Harries and Harries (2001a), with permission of the College of Occupational Therapists.

The more practiced in a thinking process a practitioner is, the more intuitive it may become. People are aware of how a motor task such as driving can become partially subconscious; in the same way cognitive tasks can become partially automatic when they have been well practiced. It is therefore difficult to verbalise thinking pertaining to a high level of expertise; and post hoc rationalisation can reduce the verbalisation to a report of a lower quality thinking process.

Ethnographic and Information-Processing Methods

Ethnographic and information-processing methods appear to have had difficulty in establishing thoughts used in clinicians' intuitive thinking. These methods have to rely heavily on the reasoner's awareness of how information has been used to make judgements; they have been limited in their ability to access the more unconscious, rapid, and unrecoverable reasoning at the intuitive end of the continuum (Ericsson & Simon, 1980). In the early studies intuitive reasoning was not given much attention; for example, in the occupational therapists' study, intuitive reasoning was only nominally identified and described as "difficult to map" (Fleming, 1991a).

While these studies were being conducted, other theorists were concurrently drawing into question the efficacy of using verbal reports to access thinking. If intuitive thought was nonrecoverable the issue of whether decision makers would have any access into their thinking became apparent (Nisbett & Wilson, 1977). With regard to accessing the thinking of experts in particular, verbal reports were recognised by some as inefficient and misrepresentative (Hoffman, 1987). Concurrent verbalisations, at best, only got to the content of working memory, or the information attended to (but not necessarily how it is used), and retrospective verbalisations were prone to forgetting and post hoc rationalisation (Ericsson & Simon, 1980). However, it is not clear cut. Some recall can be valuable, and measures are being taken to maximise the accuracy of recall methods. Unsworth (2004) has begun to use head-mounted video cameras to record occupational therapists' interventions. This approach has been shown to enhance the accuracy of memory during retrospective recall.

Roberts (1996) and Robertson (1996) recognised the influence of expertise on occupational therapists' reasoning. The AOFT/AOTA study had focused on hypothetico-deductive strategies in problem identification tasks. These can be verbalised more easily and hence are reported more effectively. Roberts (1996), however, demonstrated that reasoning varied according to the level of expertise and the nature of the task. In her research, 38 practitioners wrote down their thoughts immediately after reading three referral letters. Although some of the reasoning may have been lost before the participant began to write down their thoughts, interesting findings were made. Some practitioners initially used rapid formulations of the issues involved (pattern matchers/heuristic reasoners). They mentioned their recognition of the scenario and recalled previous cases. Others searched for cues and reasoned using various hypotheses, sometimes not reaching any specific formulation. They appeared to have less experience to draw on. The rapid formulators did not show intuitive reasoning exclusively. Evidence of hypothetico-deductive reasoning was also seen when considering some aspects of the case. In these instances participants were thought to have been less familiar with the information. This would concur with the view that reasoning strategies result from interaction between both the experience of the practitioner and the nature of the task.

THE VALUE OF EXPERIENCE

In Elstein's 1978 study, differences between novice and expert thinking were explored. They identified that it was the extent of clinical experience in a particular domain that was key to expert thinking. Experts were able to interpret data more accurately when testing hypotheses than novices. This finding had implications for medical education, as contrary to what had been thought, it was not the reasoning strategies themselves that can improve clinicians' problem solving but the domain-specific knowledge that is important. Preregistration problem-solving training would therefore not create experts: Lifelong learning would be necessary to achieve mastery of knowledge domains. Education subsequently made a move away from problem-solving training and towards problem-based learning (Norman & Schmidt, 1992). This new method of education increased clinical knowledge through facilitating exposure to clinical case scenarios.

COGNITIVE CONTINUUM THEORY

To better understand why certain thoughts are difficult to access, it is necessary to gain a deeper understanding of how and why differing modes of thought occur. Hammond and Brehmer's (1973) cognitive continuum theory (CCT) can be valuable in understanding these issues.

Hammond and Brehmer's CCT described a range of cognitive modes from intuitive to analytic with quasi-experimental processing as a midpoint. Hammond and Brehmer felt that in more intuitive reasoning, strategies such as pattern recognition and heuristics (rules of thumb) were used: Information available (cues) is immediately linked to known patterns (Larkin, 1979). This is therefore a largely subconscious, rapid, automated process and is essentially nonrecoverable (Hammond & Brehmer, 1973). At the other end of the continuum, analytic thought occurs. In this mode of thought, hypothetico-deductive reasoning is used: a slower, step-by-step method of thinking that is highly conscious. In hypothetico-deductive thinking, cues are used to generate possible hypotheses and further cues used to test these hypotheses.

Many theorists have agreed that when less practiced in a cognitive task, analytic processing is more likely to be used, but when more practiced in a task, and the information is familiar, intuitive strategies are more likely (Benner, 1984; Elstein et al., 1990; Norman et al., 1994). In addition to the role of expertise, the cognitive continuum identified the influence of task characteristics on reasoning strategy. Task characteristics, such as stability and availability of task information, are thought to have a strong influence on the possible types of cognitive processing (Shanteau, 1992). Therefore the mode of cognitive processing (i.e., thinking) used tends to be a result of the combined effect of level of experience of the practitioner and the characteristics of the task.

DUAL-PROCESS THEORIES OF THINKING

Dual-processing theory (Stanovich & West, 2003) is a more recent decision-making theory that has developed from cognitive psychology. Although bearing similarities to CCT (as both differentiate between intuitive and analytic thinking), there is an important difference in approach. Dual-processing theory posits that the two cognitive systems (the intuitive, which is automatic, holistic, and fast; and the analytic, which is deliberate, rational, explicit, and slow) are in fact two different systems; they are not a single continuum as proposed in Hammond and Brehmer's CCT. Functional magnetic resonance imaging has indicated that these systems are in fact neurologically different (Goel et al., 2000). In dual-processing theory, the fast, automatic form of processing is referred to as System 1 (S1) and the slow, deliberate form as System 2 (S2).

Dual-processing theory can be understood in the following way: S1 delivers judgements through largely subconscious reasoning (tacit knowledge), and only the outcome is conscious; S2, conversely, is a highly conscious and logical reasoning process. S2 type reasoning enables practitioners to think about hypothetical situations and analyse potential future possibilities and other features of a situation that are not immediately apparent. S2 type thinking uses central working memory (Gathercole, 2003), focuses on one task at a time, and is correlated with general intelligence (Stanovich & West, 2000). S2 type reasoning is viewed as having evolved more recently than S1 and, interestingly, is a faculty that only humans have (Evans, 2003).

Parallels between the components of clinical reasoning, for instance the work of Mattingly and Fleming (1994), and dual-process theory are easy to make. Concepts such as tacit knowledge and intuitive reasoning appear closely linked to the holistic nature of S1, whereas knowledge and research drawn from an objective basis are more closely associated with the objective reasoning of S2.

Paley et al. (2007) drew comparisons between clinical reasoning and empirical knowledge using dual-process theory. Although their paper focused on nursing research, the arguments are valid for other areas of health care research, including occupational therapy. To draw comparisons with dual-processing theory they referred to the type of reasoning associated with intuitive reasoning and artful practice as N1 and objective knowledge drawn from quantitative research as N2.

Paley et al. (2007), however, highlight one major difference between the N1/N2 distinction and the S1/S2 distinction, whereas the majority of occupational therapy clinical reasoning literature regards N1 and N2 as equal partners. Cognitive dual-processing theory, on the other hand, emphasises that the principal function of S2 is to override, monitor, and suppress the invalid inferences of S1 (Evans, 2003; Evens & Over, 2004; Kahneman & Frederick, 2002). Therefore, while occupational therapy literature to date generally views N1 and N2 as equally valid ways of thinking, it is clear that S2 ways of thinking are epistemologically superior.

HEURISTICS AND BIASES

The heuristics and biases research literature explains why there is a disparity between S1 and S2 ways of thinking (Gilovich et al., 2002; Kahneman et al., 1982). This research shows that people often make mistakes when the clinical experience (S1) is not controlled by measurable objective evidence (S2). The reasons behind this are outlined in greater detail by Paley et al. (2007).

Interestingly S1 type thinking is not only responsible for clinical errors in thinking but can also explain some academic errors. For example, how people view and understand scientific research can be compromised by their prior beliefs about its findings (Koehler, 1993). Resch et al. (2000) and Kaptchuk (2003) have both established that well-designed studies can be dismissed because they indicate either an unconventional intervention is effective or a well-respected intervention is ineffective. Conversely, poorly designed studies can sometimes be accepted as they appear to support widely held beliefs. This principle is not only restricted to experimental research. Generally any method will be regarded as valid if its conclusions are believable and as invalid if its conclusions are disagreeable

(Fugelsang & Thompson, 2000; Fugelsang et al., 2004; Roberts & Sykes, 2003).

So what does knowledge of S1 and S2 tell us about N1 and N2 types of thinking in occupational therapy? It means that intuitive clinical reasoning is likely to make mistakes (due to S1 type weaknesses in thinking) when it is not corrected by the more structured and objective approach of S2 thinking processes. The impact of thinking errors associated to S1 type thinking are not limited to occupational therapy or nursing. Stanovich (2003) has stated that through such errors "physicians choose less effective medical treatments; people fail to accurately assess risks in their environment; information is misused in legal proceedings; millions of dollars are spent on unneeded projects by government and private industry; parents fail to vaccinate their children; unnecessary surgery is performed; animals are hunted to extinction; billions of dollars are wasted on quack medical remedies; and costly financial misjudgements are made" (p. 292). Dual-processing theory demonstrates that tacit knowledge and experience (S1/N1) cannot be viewed equally to knowledge that is rigorously researched and empirically based (S2/N2). To continue to view N1 and N2 forms of knowledge as equal, Paley et al. (2007) state, is to celebrate the possibility of error in practice.

It could be said that the notion that we should base our practice on "generalisable evidence demolishes our traditional practice. Such worldviews urge us to swap our ideas of crafting care around the unique complexity of the individual, for a generalisation about what worked for most people in a study" (Barker, 2000, p. 332). This is an argument that has proven popular in health care literature in general, and occupational therapy is no exception. The structure of this argument is as follows:

> "Quantitative studies refer to populations; practitioners care for individuals; therefore, quantitative studies are irrelevant to clinical practice. This is similar in form to: epidemiological studies of cancer refer to populations; individuals make decisions; therefore, epidemiological studies are irrelevant to my decision to smoke. Both of these arguments dismiss the concepts of probability and risk, and would make a nonsense of actuarial procedures and insurance. In any case, the experience on which the nurse, [or occupational therapist] draws when working with an individual is also population-based: the population of clients she or her colleagues have previously seen. If the population defined by a research study is irrelevant to the unique individual, so is the population defined by clinical experience"
>
> **(Paley et al., 2007, p. 697).**

So, how can we use our knowledge of dual-processing theory in practice? S1 is how most practitioners reason, most of the time. But if practitioners use S2 type thinking it will monitor and improve this intuitive form of reasoning (Degani et al., 2006). It is this rationale that supports evidence-based practice, helps practitioners to question their judgements about practice, and encourages the search for more evidence-based ways of thinking and working.

Three factors, however, inhibit the use of S2 thinking in clinical practice. First, there appears to be a natural resistance to the use of S2 type thinking and a general reluctance to accept the idea that practitioners make S1 type errors in reasoning. Second, evidence-based decision making and S2 type thinking do not come naturally. Third, S2 type thinking requires time and space—something that challenges everyone (Paley et al., 2007).

The idea that intuitive reasoning and holistic practice (S1/N1) are equal in weight and status to scientific evidence (S2/N2) is persuasive, but this should not get in the way of delivering the highest quality services to clients. To achieve this, practitioners must use S2 type strategies. There is of course no single answer to this issue, but there is one possibility that may offer a solution: the use of conceptual models of practice.

Conceptual Models of Practice

Within occupational therapy, structured use of conceptual models of practice such as the Canadian Model of Occupational Performance and Engagement (CMOP-E; Townsend & Polatjko, 2007) or the Model of Human Occupation (MOHO; Kielhofner, 2007) could be viewed as approaches that adopt S2 supervisory functions in practice. Their conscious use ensures that all necessary factors have been considered and given due priority when working with a client. When viewed in light of the evidence that supports the supervisory nature of S2 over S1, conceptual models such as MOHO and CMOP-E, which have evolved through rigorous research, do not provide an illusion of safety, as Smith (2006) suggested. They are not a panacea for perfect practice. They do, however, ensure that the inherent biases and mental shortcuts of practitioners, masquerading under the guise of artful practice or clinical reasoning (and typify S1 type thinking), cannot be carried away unabated, drawing clients into decisions that are ill considered and lacking in reliable evidence to support their validity.

Conceptual models of practice, as an answer to the dual-processing dilemma, are only one option, and their endorsement here should not be taken to suggest that these models are viewed as perfect or infallible. Some do provide an evidence-based structure to follow, though, which limits the possibilities for personal S1 type biases, and conceptual models continue to be researched and refined.

APPLYING JUDGEMENT AND DECISION-MAKING SKILLS IN PRACTICE

Judgement and decision skills have to be learnt for every stage of the occupational therapy process from referral through to evaluation. Through the use of scenarios as well as real-life experience, reasoning skills can be exercised in relation to specific domains. The following examples are designed to improve your reasoning in practice.

Imagine you are an occupational therapist on an adult community mental health team. You may consider taking some general referrals that have been sent to both your team and directly to you. These referrals fall into the second category: They have been sent directly to you. Look at the referral in Fig. 2.1 and indicate the degree of priority you feel the referral warrants. In practice you would also likely see the client before making a fully informed judgement; however, for this task use your initial impressions of whether you would work with the client. How much priority would you give it? Put a cross on the line at the bottom of the referral to give your decision.

In doing this task you will have decided how much attention to give to the differing types of information. You will have judged how important those types of information are to the decision of prioritisation. You will have used

your skills of judgement and decision making. If you have experience of this field the referral may have reminded you of someone similar whom you, or a colleague, have worked with. In that case you may have been influenced by your previous experience. Has any knowledge of current government policy influenced your thinking? For example, some governments require services to focus on clients with severe enduring mental health needs. If you do this task with colleagues or fellow students discuss:

- Did you know what to look for?
- What types of referral information were most important and why?
- Was any type of information irrelevant and why?
- How well did you agree in relation to your judgements?
- Were any types of information used in relation to each other (nonlinear cue use)?
- How closely did you agree in relation to your final prioritisation rating (decision making)?
- Have you drawn on any prior experience of a client who was similar (use of scripts)?

A common comment is that it is difficult to make a decision without knowing what other referrals might look like. This is linked to the phenomenon of calibration. Experience is needed to know how to appropriately calibrate judgements and decisions. Now look at a second referral (Fig. 2.2).

FIG. 2.1 An example of a community occupational therapy mental health referral.

Adult Mental Health Services   ⊠

Community Occupational Therapy Mental Health Referral Form (Adult Mental Health Services)

Client's name	Mr xx	Address	Within catchment area
Age	28 D. o. b. xx/xx/xx		
Date of referral	xx/xx/xx (Recent)		
Name of referrer	GP	Telephone	(xxx) xxx xxxx
Consultant	Dr xx	GP	Dr xx

Diagnosis   Schizophrenia   Ten year history

Current living situation

    Home alone

Reason for referral

    Lost confidence with going out and is not looking after themselves very well

Other services involved

    Counsellor

Any known history of violence?   No

Is the client aware of the referral?   Yes

Low priority   High priority

FIG. 2.2 Another referral example.

Go through the same process. Which referral is given higher priority?

To learn from those who have experience in the judgements and decisions of their domains we need to study experts in their specific specialities. How would occupational therapists with many years of experience in the field of community mental health make these types of judgements and decisions? Research was conducted in the United Kingdom with 40 experienced occupational therapists on 120 referrals of this type. It was found that four different judgement policies were being used. Policies differed according to whether the practitioner aimed to work in a generic or occupationally orientated way (Harries & Gilhooly, 2003a). A website has been developed to train novices to follow the occupationally orientated expert judgement policies. The website allows novices to practice on a set of referrals to learn how to calibrate their decisions. Training information is then provided about the expert policies, and then a second set of referrals is given for prioritisation. Feedback on how the decision maker has done in relation to the expert group is then provided. The training package has been shown to be effective in developing novices' referral prioritisation skills (Weiss et al., 2006) and is now a freely available evidence-based educational tool to be found at www.priscillaharries.com (Harries et al., 2012).

A second resource for developing professional decision-making capacity in occupational therapy driver assessment is https://fitnesstodrive.wordpress.com/training-aid/; this is also a free evidence-based resource developed by Harries et al. (2018). It is well documented that, when experienced, people are better at judging what is important and what is not (Shanteau et al., 1991); they are better at balancing the client's perspective with the realities of the environment and have a vision of their capacity for change. When a practitioner is new to a clinical or social domain it is difficult to make wise judgements or decisions; it is easy to feel overwhelmed as all new information can seem important. Experience is the only way to move forward; each time practitioners move to a new domain, they must start from the beginning and learn what is important in the new field. This new knowledge facilitates the store of scripts in memory (Abernathy & Hamm, 1994); these scripts are based on knowledge of similar clients and the narratives that have been heard. Recognition can then be used to pattern match between what has been experienced and any familiar situation that later arises.

Memory and Recognition

Research on memory has been conducted to identify how experienced clinicians organise memory chunks and how recall mechanisms facilitate recognition of previously encountered scenarios (Norman & Schmidt, 1992). Groen and Patel (1985) identified that novice problem solvers reasoned backwards from hypotheses generation to data, whereas experts reason forward using if-then rules (propositional reasoning). It is apparent that to use these propositional rules experts have to draw on their well-structured knowledge bases (Johnson-Laird & Shafir, 1993). However, when confronted with an unfamiliar problem, the expert will revert back to methods of hypothesis testing (Elstein et al., 1990). The use of scripts should not limit how a practitioner works with people but be used to develop an awareness of what is important to pay attention to and what change is possible.

Values

How people decide what is important when assigning weights or selecting an option is linked to their personal and professional values and the values of the setting in which the judgements and decisions must be made. In discussing how judgements have been made, values individuals hold can be brought to light. Some of these are from personal experience, some from professional experience. Where practitioners vary in their values, judgements will be made differently. In a health system that promotes parity and adherence to protocol, it is important to get to the core of an individual's thinking to identify thinking methods that result in best practice. Is it more important to help someone with managing self-care needs or to gain a work role? Do clients need to socialise? These issues are not black and white, and the clients themselves or carers are often able to help to focus priorities.

Values Inherent in Frames of Reference and Theoretical Frameworks

The differing theoretical frameworks that occupational therapists draw on are key to the process of judgement and decision making. These influence how phenomena are viewed and therefore where importance is placed both in terms of what is viewed as an issue that needs addressing

and how best that issue might be addressed. They view people from different perspectives and require attention to be given to different aspects of that person. Each frame of reference or theoretical framework has a different value system.

Psychoanalytic, client-centred, cognitive-behavioural, biomechanical, developmental, social, and occupational frames of reference (see Duncan, 2020) each hold links to what is viewed as important. The client-centred frame of reference, for example, requires the client to be heavily involved in the decision-making process, whereas the biomechanical frame of reference may be more practitioner led. Psychoanalytic theories require attention to past experiences, whereas cognitive-behavioural theories focus on the here and now. The value systems also vary between the conceptual models of occupational therapy practice. Research from the major conceptual models support their use as being relevant to a multiplicity of needs whether it be a person's social withdrawal or muscle weakness. And the use of conceptual models of practice does not restrict practitioners from also using a variety of frames of reference (such as the biomechanical, or client-centred frame of reference) depending on the presenting problem. However, not all occupational therapists practice in this way and many select their theoretical basis of practice from a range of frames of reference without necessarily using a conceptual model of practice as an occupational filter (Mallinson & Forsyth, 2000). In these cases practitioners aim to select a frame of reference that best fits the client's need and the context for the intervention, taking into account the strength of the theory's evidence base and the cost effectiveness of its use.

In the Vignette 2.1, Jean is not eating because she may have anorexia nervosa. An occupational therapist may view her needs from a psychoanalytic perspective. Her unresolved emotional conflict could be thought the result of prior life experiences. Her withdrawn, childlike state could be seen as a sign of emotional underdevelopment. A practitioner could involve the client in projective art, drama therapy, and creative group work to facilitate the psychosocial

---

VIGNETTE 2.1

Jean was seen at home by the occupational therapist from the community mental health team. The GP had referred the client due to her high anxiety levels, limited IQ, and a recent bereavement. Due to her anxiety Jean had also lost her job. During the interview the practitioner noticed how anxious and underweight Jean is. She also observed that there was a lack of food in the house. One aspect that the occupational therapist now wants to assess, through observation and interview, is why Jean is not eating enough to sustain her weight. Depending on the issues that present, the practitioner will choose interventions that are informed by differing theoretical frameworks. Each theory holds differing values that alter the focus of the intervention.

development of her emotional maturity. The ability to express herself, to develop a sense of self-efficacy and self-esteem, would be necessary before Jean will develop the wish to eat. Once partial psychosocial capacity is achieved, the practitioner would add an educational perspective (e.g., teaching skills in cooking, budgeting, and giving advice) as Jean resumes social and work activities.

If, however, Jean was not eating because she had severe rheumatoid arthritis, her needs would be viewed from a very different perspective. Her difficulties may be due to the physical weakness, pain, and limited range of movement that can cause problems with cutting up food, opening cans, and turning on taps. In this case a biomechanical and compensatory perspective may be taken (McMillan 2020). Joint-protection advice would be provided to try to reduce the risks of further hand function deterioration. Altering kitchen work surfaces may be suggested to allow heavy pans to be slid rather than lifted, so that ulna deviation is not exacerbated. Splints may be made by the practitioner to stabilise the radiocarpal and metacarpal phalangeal joints in a functional position. Fatigue management advice may be given to ensure periods of rest are balanced with periods of activity. Equipment such as tap turners, stair rails, and elastic shoelaces may be provided to maximise independence and thereby provide some privacy for dressing and bathing occupations. Advice and support to engage in valued leisure or work occupations would also be essential to ensure that Jean has a good quality of life.

If, however, a client with a physical disability has developed depression as a result of the capacity to cope with the disability, psychological theories may also be needed. Cognitive-behaviour theories would be used to promote positive thinking and to change/challenge cognitive distortions. However, an occupational therapist would not conduct cognitive-behaviour therapy in isolation but would use it alongside occupational engagement (Duncan, 2020). The benefits of engaging in a valued occupation that assists the client to recognise one's own skills and potential can help to reinforce positive thinking. The key is to find occupations that are matched to the individual's capacity and value system, thereby ensuring a sense of self-efficacy and achievement.

Some practitioners and theorists advocate selecting an occupational therapy conceptual model of practice before seeing a client to ensure the occupation focus of the intervention (Forsyth & Kielhofner, 2020); others do not. Regardless, the reasons for clients' needs have to be determined before it is known which specific frame of reference will be most valuable in guiding interventions. Some initial assessment is therefore needed before a theoretical frame of reference (such as the biomechanical or cognitive-behavioural frame) is chosen. This will then influence the

method of the full assessment and inform which issues need to be explored further. For example, if Jean has not been eating through:

- A lack of strength to open packets, turn on taps, hold cutlery (e.g., due to pain from rheumatoid arthritis) the practitioner may use a biomechanical frame of reference and compensatory approach, instructing in joint protection techniques and providing aids and adaptations.
- A lack of motivation (e.g., due to low mood from recent loss of her partner and work role) the practitioner may use a cognitive-behavioural frame of reference, advising on positive thinking strategies and planning graded, achievable goals.
- A lack of knowledge (e.g., budgeting difficulties, anxiety about abilities due to being recently bereaved) the practitioner may take an educational approach, practicing using transport, road safety, menu planning, shopping, cooking.
- A low IQ and limited skills (e.g., due to mild learning disability and recent loss of a partner/carer) the practitioner may take a developmental approach, educating Jean from her current level of ability up to her maximum level of capacity.
- A poor insight, denial, and bizarre eating behaviour (e.g., due to anorexia nervosa) the practitioner may take a psychodynamic approach, examining reasons for low self-esteem through therapeutic art sessions.

Therefore the way in which practitioners reason using conceptual models of practice and frames of reference can have a significant impact on the judgements and decisions in practice.

SUMMARY

This chapter has highlighted the importance of judgement and decision-making skills in practice. Occupational therapy clinical reasoning literature has been presented and discussed. Two judgement and decision-making models (the CCT and dual-process theory) drawn from cognitive psychology were described and discussed. These models highlight the difference between intuitive reasoning, which characterises artful practice, and rational reasoning, which is a more logical, deliberate, and conscious form of reasoning and characterises evidence-based ways of working. Historically the types of knowledge generated through artful practice and more evidence-based methods have been looked upon with equal worth within occupational therapy. However, both the CCT and dual-process theory highlight the superiority of the judgement and decision making that come from the logical, deliberate method (S2/N2), although most people tend to be naturally intuitive decision makers in practice (S1/N1). The chapter presented conceptual models of practice as one possibility that could increase the amount of S2 type judgement and decision making in practice. Practical examples were also given to illustrate the complexity of judgement and decision making in practice.

REFLECTIVE LEARNING

- What are the clinical judgements and decisions that I make in practice or have seen on placement?
- What examples of analytical and intuitive thinking do I practice or have I seen?
- What could I do to address my personal biases and heuristics as an occupational therapist?
- What values influence my judgements and decisions in practice?

REFERENCES

Abernathy, C. M., & Hamm, R. M. (1994). *Surgical scripts: Master surgeons think aloud about 43 common surgical problems.* Hanley & Belfus.

Alnervik, A., & Sviden, G. (1996). On clinical reasoning: Patterns of reflection on practice. *The Occupational Therapy Journal of Research, 16*(2), 98–110.

Barker, P. (2000). Reflections on caring as a virtue ethic within an evidence-based culture. *International Journal of Nursing Studies, 37*, 329–336.

Benner, P. (1984). *From novice to expert: Excellence and power in clinical nursing practice.* Addison-Wesley.

Chapparo, C. (1999). Working out: Working with Angelica-interpreting practice. In S. E. Ryan, & E. A. McKay (Eds.), *Thinking and reasoning in therapy: Narratives from practice.* Stanley Thornes.

Crabtree, M., & Lyons, M. (1997). Focal points and relationships: A study of clinical reasoning. *British Journal of Occupational Therapy, 60*(2), 57–64.

Creighton, C., Dijkers, M., Bennett, N., Brown, K., (1995). Reasoning and the art of therapy for spinal cord injury. *American Journal of Occupational Therapy, 49*, 311–317.

Crennan, M., & MacRae, A. (2010). Occupational therapy discharge assessment of elderly patients from acute care hospitals. *Physical & Occupational Therapy in Geriatrics, 28*(1), 33–34.

Degani, J. A. S., Shafto, M., & Kirlik, A. (2006). What makes vicarious functioning work? Exploring the geometry of human-technology interaction. In A. Kirlik (Ed.), *Adaptive perspectives on human–technology interaction* (pp. 179–196). Oxford University Press.

Doyle, S., Bennett, S., & Gustafsson, L. (2013). Occupational therapy for upper limb post-stroke sensory impairments: A survey. *British Journal of Occupational Therapy, 76*(10), 434–442.

Duncan, E. A. S. (Ed.). (2020). *Foundations for practice in occupational therapy* (6th ed.). Elsevier.

Elstein, A. S., Shulman, L. S., & Sprafka, S. A. (1978). *Medical problem solving: An analysis of clinical reasoning.* Harvard University Press.

Elstein, A. S., Shulman, L. S., & Sprafka, S. A. (1990). Medical problem solving: A ten year retrospective. *Evaluation and the Health Professions, 13*(1), 5–36.

Ericsson, K. A., & Simon, H. A. (1980). Verbal reports as data. *Psychological Review, 87*(3), 215–251.

Evans, J. (2003). In two minds: Dual-process accounts of reasoning. *Trends in Cognitive Science, 7*(10), 454–459.

Evans, J., & Over, D. (2004). *If.* Oxford University Press.

Eysenck, M. (1993). *Principles of cognitive psychology.* Lawrence.

Fawcett, J., Watson, J., Neuman, B., et al. (2001). On nursing theories and evidence. *Journal of Nursing Scholarship, 33*(2), 115–119.

Fleming, M. H. (1991a). Clinical reasoning in medicine compared with clinical reasoning in occupational therapy. *American Journal of Occupational Therapy, 45*(11), 988–996.

Fleming, M. H. (1991b). The therapist with the three-track mind. *American Journal of Occupational Therapy, 45*(11), 1007–1014.

Fondiller, E. D., Rosage, L. J., & Neuhaus, B. E. (1990). Values influencing clinical reasoning in occupational therapy: An exploratory study. *Occupational Therapy Journal of Research, 10*, 41–55.

Forsyth, K., & Kielhofner, G. (2020). The model of human occupation: Integrating theory into practice and practice into theory. In E. A. S. Duncan (Ed.), *Foundations for practice in occupational therapy* (6th ed., pp. 69–108). Elsevier/Churchill Livingstone.

Fortune, T., & Ryan, S. (1996). Applying clinical reasoning: A case-load management system for community occupational therapists. *British Journal of Occupational Therapy, 59*, 207–211.

Fossey, E. (1996). Using the occupational performance history interview: Therapist reflections. *British Journal of Occupational Therapy, 59*, 223–228.

Fugelsang, J. A., & Thompson, V. A. (2000). Strategy selection in causal reasoning: When beliefs and covariation collide. *Canadian Journal of Experimental Psychology, 54*, 13–32.

Fugelsang, J. A., Stein, C., Green, A., et al. (2004). Theory and data interactions of the scientific mind: Evidence from the molecular and the cognitive laboratory. *Canadian Journal of Experimental Psychology, 58*, 86–95.

Gale, J., & Marsden, P. (1985). Diagnosis: Process not product. In M. Sheldon, J. Brooke, & A. Recotr (Eds.), *Decision-making in general practice.* Macmillan.

Gathercole, S. (Ed.). (2003). *Short-term and working memory.* Taylor and Francis.

Gilovich, T., Griffin, D., & Kahneman, D. (Eds.). (2002). *Heuristics and biases: The psychology of intuitive judgement.* Cambridge University Press.

Goel, V., Buchel, C., Frith, C., et al. (2000). Dissociation of mechanisms underlying syllogistic reasoning. *Neuroimage, 12*(5), 504–514.

Groen, G. J., & Patel, V. L. (1985). Medical problem-solving: Some questionable assumptions. *Medical Education, 19*, 95–100.

Hagedorn, R. (1996). Clinical decision making in familiar cases: A model of the process and implications of practice. *The British Journal of Occupational Therapy, 59*, 217–222.

Hammond, K. R., & Brehmer, B. (Eds.). (1973). *Quasi-rational and distrust: Implications for international conflict. Human judgement and social interactions.* Rineholt & Winston.

Harries, P., & Gilhooly, K. (2003a). Generic and specialist occupational therapy casework in community mental health. *British Journal of Occupational Therapy, 66*(3), 101–109.

Harries, P., & Gilhooly, K. (2003b). Identifying occupational therapists referral priorities in community health. *Occupational Therapy International, 10*(2), 150–164.

Harries, P., Tomlinson, C., Notley, E., Davies, M., & Gilhooly, K. (2012). Effectiveness of a decision-training aid on referral prioritization capacity: A randomized controlled trial. *Medical Decision Making, 32*(6), 779–791.

Harries, P., Unsworth, C., Gokalp, H., Davies, M., Tomlinson, C., & Harries, L. (2018). A randomised controlled trial to test the effectiveness of decision training on assessors' ability to determine optimal fitness-to-drive recommendations for older or disabled drivers. *BMC Medical Education, 18*(27), 1–10.

Harries, P. A., & Harries, C. (2001a). Studying clinical reasoning, part 1: Have we been taking the wrong 'track'? *British Journal of Occupational Therapy, 64*(4), 164–168.

Harries, P. A., & Harries, C. (2001b). Studying clinical reasoning, part 2: Applying social judgement theory. *British Journal of Occupational Therapy, 64*(6), 285–292.

Hoffman, R. R. (1987). The problem of extracting the knowledge of experts from the perspective of experimental psychology. *AI Magazine*, 53–67.

Hooper, B. (1997). The relationship between pre-theoretical assumptions and clinical reasoning. *American Journal of Occupational Therapy, 51*, 328–338.

Johnson-Laird, P. N., & Shafir, E. (1993). The Interaction between reasoning and decision-making: An introduction. *Cognition, 49*, 1–9.

Kahneman, D., & Frederick, S. (2002). Representativeness revisited: Attribute substitution in intuitive judgment. In T. Gilovich, D. Griffin, & D. Kahneman (Eds.), *Heuristics and biases: The psychology of intuitive judgment* (pp. 46–71). Cambridge University Press.

Kahneman, D., Slovic, P., & Tversky, A. (Eds.). (1982). *Judgment under uncertainty: Heuristics and biases.* Cambridge University Press.

Kaptchuk, T. J. (2003). Effect of interpretive bias on research evidence. *British Medical Journal, 326*, 1453–1455.

Kielhofner, G. (2007). Model of human occupation. In *Theory and practice* (4th ed.). Lippincott Williams & Wilkins.

Koehler, J. J. (1993). The influence of prior belief on scientific judgments of evidence quality. *Organizational Behavior and Human Decision Processes, 56*, 25–28.

Kuipers, K., & Grice, J. W. (2009). The structure of novice and expert occupational therapists' clinical reasoning before and after exposure to a domain-specific protocol. *Australian Occupational Therapy Journal, 56*(6), 418–427.

Larkin, J. H. (Eds.). (1979). Information processing and science instruction. *Cognitive process instruction.* Franklin Institute.

Mallinson, T., & Forsyth, K. (2000). Components of the occupation filter. In E. A. S. Duncan (Ed.), *Foundations for practice in occupational therapy* (4th ed., p. 86). Elsevier/Churchill Livingstone.

Mattingly, C. (1991). What is clinical reasoning? *American Journal of Occupational Therapy, 45*(11), 979–986.

Mattingly, C., & Fleming, M. H. (1994). *Clinical reasoning: Forms of inquiry in a therapeutic practice.* Davis.

McKay, E. A. (1999). Lilian and Paula: A treatment narrative in acute mental health. In S. E. Ryan, & E. A. McKay (Eds.), *Thinking and reasoning in therapy: Narratives from practice* (pp. 53–64). Stanley Thornes.

McMillan, I. (2020). Assumptions underpinning a biomechanical frame of reference in occupational therapy. In E. A. S. Duncan (Ed.), *Foundations for practice in occupational therapy* (6th ed., pp. 152–164). Elsevier/Churchill Livingstone.

Mitchell, R., & Unsworth, C. A. (2005). Clinical reasoning during community health home visits: Expert and novice differences. *British Journal of Occupational Therapy, 68*(5), 215–223.

Munroe, H. (1996). Clinical reasoning in community occupational therapy. *British Journal of Occupational Therapy, 59*(5), 196–202.

Murphy, L. F., & Stav, W. B. (2018). The impact of online video cases on clinical reasoning in occupational therapy education: A quantitative analysis. *The Open Journal of Occupational Therapy, 6*(3), 1–11.

Nisbett, R., & Wilson, T. (1977). Telling more than we can know: Verbal reports on mental processes. *Psychological Review, 84*, 231–259.

Norman, G. R., & Schmidt, H. G. (1992). The psychological basis of problem-based learning: A review of the evidence. *Academic Medicine, 67*(9), 557–565.

Norman, G. R., Trott, A. L., Brooks, L. R., et al. (1994). Cognitive differences in clinical reasoning related to postgraduate training. *Teaching and Learning in Medicine, 6*, 114–120.

Paley, J., Cheyne, H., Dalgleish, L., et al. (2007). Nursing's ways of knowing and dual process theories of cognition. *Journal of Advanced Nursing, 60*(6), 692–701.

Paterson, M., Higgs, J., Wilcox, S., et al. (2002). Clinical reasoning and self-directed learning: Key dimensions in professional education and professional socialisation. *Focus on Health Professional Education: A Multi-Disciplinary Journal, 4*(2), 5–21.

Paterson, M. L. (2003). Professional practice judgement artistry in occupational therapy practice. Australia PhD thesis (unpublished). The University of Sydney.

Rassafiani, M., Ziviani, J., Rodger, S., & Dalgleish, L. (2008). Occupational therapists' decision-making in the management of clients with upper limb hypertonicity. *Scandinavian Journal of Occupational Therapy, 15*(2), 105–115.

Resch, K. I., Ernst, E., & Garrow, J. (2000). A randomized controlled study of reviewer bias against an unconventional therapy. *Journal of the Royal Society of Medicine, 93*, 164–167.

Roberts, A. E. (1996). Approaches to reasoning in occupational therapy: A critical exploration. *British Journal of Occupational Therapy, 59*(5), 233–236.

Roberts, M. J., & Sykes, E. D. A. (2003). Belief bias and relational reasoning. *The Quarterly Journal of Experimental Psychology, 56A*(1), 131–154.

Robertson, L. (1996). Clinical reasoning, part 2: Novice/expert differences. *British Journal of Occupational Therapy, 59*(5), 212–216.

Rogers, J. (1983). Clinical reasoning: The ethics, science, and art. *American Journal of Occupational Therapy, 37,* 601–616.

Rycroft-Malone, J., Seers, K., Titchen, A., et al. (2004). What counts as evidence in evidence-based practice? *Journal of Advanced Nursing, 47*(1), 81–90.

Sefton, A. J. (2001). Integrating knowledge and practice in medicine. In J. Higgs, & A. Titchen (Eds.), *Practice knowledge and expertise* (pp. 29–34). Butterworth Heinemann.

Shanteau, J. (1992). Competence in experts: The role of task characteristics. *Organizational Behavior and Human Decision Processes, 53,* 252–266.

Shanteau, J., Grier, M., & Berner, E. (1991). Teaching decision making skills to student nurses. In J. Baron, & R. V. Brown (Eds.), *Teaching decision making to adolescents* (pp. 185–206). Lawrence Erlbaum.

Smith, G. (2006). Telling tales—how stories and narratives co-create change. *The British Journal of Occupational Therapy, 69*(7), 304–311.

Stanovich, K. (2003). The fundamental computational biases of human cognition: Heuristics that (sometimes) impair decision making and problem solving. In J. E. Davidson, & R. J. Sternberg (Eds.), *The psychology of problem solving* (pp. 291–342). Cambridge University Press.

Stanovich, K., & West, R. F. (2003). Evolutionary versus instrumental goals: How evolutionary psychology misconceives human rationality. In D. Over (Ed.), *Evolution and the psychology of thinking* (pp. 171–230). The Debate Psychology Press.

Stark, S. L., Somerville, E., Keglovits, M., Smason, A., & Bigham, K. (2015). Clinical reasoning guideline for home modification interventions. *American Journal of Occupational Therapy, 69*(2), 1–8.

Stephens, M., Bartley, C., Betteridge, R., & Samuriwo, R. (2018). Developing the tissue viability seating guidelines. *Journal of Tissue Viability, 27*(1), 74–79.

Taylor, B., Robertson, D., Wiratunga, N., Craw, S., Mitchell, D., & Stewart, E. (2007). Using computer aided case based reasoning to support clinical reasoning in community occupational therapy. *Computer Methods Programs Biomed, 87*(2), 170–179.

Tempest, S., & McIntyre, A. (2006). Using the ICF to clarify team roles and demonstrate clinical reasoning in stroke rehabilitation. *Disability and Rehabilitation, 28*(10), 663–667.

Townsend, E., & Polatajko, H. J. (2007). *Enabling occupation II: Advancing an occupational therapy vision for health, well-being, & justice through occupation.* Canadian Association of Occupational Therapists.

Unsworth, C. A. (1996). Team decision making in rehabilitation. *American Journal of Physical Medicine and Rehabilitation, 75,* 483–484.

Unsworth, C. A. (2001). Studying clinical reasoning. *British Journal of Occupational Therapists, 64*(6), 316–317.

Unsworth, C. A. (2004). Clinical reasoning: How do pragmatic reasoning, worldview and client-centredness fit? *The British Journal of Occupational Therapy, 67*(1), 10–19.

Unsworth, C. A. (2005). Using a head-mounted video camera to explore current conceptualizations of clinical reasoning in occupational therapy. *American Journal of Occupational Therapy, 59*(1), 31–40.

Unsworth, C. A. (2011). Gaining insights to the clinical reasoning that supports an on-road driver assessment. *Canadian Journal of Occupational Therapy, 78*(2), 97–102.

Unsworth, C., Harries, P., & Davies, M. (2015). Using social judgment theory method to examine how experienced occupational therapy driver assessors use information to make fitness-to-drive recommendations. *The British Journal of Occupational Therapy, 78,* 109–120.

Unsworth, C. A., Thomas, S. A., & Greenwood, K. M. (1995). Rehabilitation team decisions on discharge housing for stroke patients. *Archives of Physical Medicine and Rehabilitation, 76,* 331–340.

Unsworth, C. A., Thomas, S. A., & Greenwood, K. M. (1997). Decision polarization among rehabilitation team recommendations concerning discharge housing for stroke patients. *International Journal of Rehabilitation Research, 20,* 51–69.

Upshur, R. E. G., VanDenKerkhof, E., & Goel, V. (2001). Meaning and measurement: An inclusive model of evidence in health care. *Journal of Evaluation in Clinical Practice, 7*(2), 91–96.

Wainwright, S. F., & McGinnis, P. Q. (2008). Factors that influence the clinical decision-making of rehabilitation professionals in long-term care settings. *Journal of Allied Health, 38*(3), 143–151.

Weiss, D., Shanteau, J., & Harries, P. (2006). People who judge people. *Journal of Behavioral Decision Making, 19,* 441–454.

3

Shared Decision-Making Skills in Practice

Edward A.S. Duncan

HIGHLIGHTS

- Person-centred practice is easy to discuss but challenging to deliver.
- Practitioners, consciously or unconsciously, use a variety of decision-making models in practice.
- Shared decision making is a valuable decision-making model for occupational therapists.
- Shared decision making requires at least two participants, the sharing of information and the making of a decision that is agreed by all parties.

- There are a variety of strategies that can be used to increase the likelihood of shared decision making taking place.
- It is important to measure your decision-making skills in practice, as many think they deliver shared decision making, but few actually do.

BACKGROUND

Whilst person-centred therapy was first developed by Carl Rogers (Rogers, 1939), it was not perhaps until the development of health promotion in the 1980s when the role of people in controlling and developing their own care became more prominent in international health care (World Health Organization, 1984). Within occupational therapy, client-centred practice (later known to and referred to in this chapter wherever possible as person-centred practice) was initially driven by Canadian occupational therapists (Canadian Association of Occupational Therapy/Department of National Health and Welfare, 1983), but has since become internationally recognised and embedded in ethical codes of conduct (Royal College of Occupational Therapists [RCOT], 2021). Parker (2006) described practitioners' views of person-centred practice as ranging from "quite simple" to "daunting." But what is person-centred occupational therapy?

Relationship Between Person-Centred Occupational Therapy and the Shared Decision-Making Model

Various definitions of person-centred occupational therapy exist. Law et al. (1995) provided the first definition,

describing it as "an approach to providing occupational therapy which embraces a philosophy of respect for and partnership with people receiving services. It recognises the autonomy of individuals, the need for person choice in making decisions about occupational needs, the strengths people bring to an occupational encounter and the benefits of the person-practitioner partnership and the need to ensure that services are accessible and fit the context in which a client lives" (p. 250). Key features of person-centred occupational therapy that emerged from the work of Law et al. (1995) include:

- Autonomy and choice
- Partnership (author's emphasis)/responsibility
- Enablement
- Contextual congruence
- Accessibility
- Respect for diversity

Later, Sumsion (2000) conducted research with British occupational therapists and developed the following definition of person-centred (or as she refers to it, client) occupational therapy.

Client-centred occupational therapy is a partnership [author's emphasis] between the client and the therapist that empowers the client to engage in functional performance and fulfils his/her roles in a variety of environments. The client participates actively in negotiating goals which are given priority and are at the centre of assessment, intervention, and evaluation. Throughout the process, the therapist listens to and respects the clients' values, adapts the interventions to meet the clients' needs and enables the client to make informed decisions [author's emphasis] (p. 308).

Building on this definition, Parker (2006) drew out the following key features of person-centred occupational therapy:
• The individual
• Partnership (author's emphasis)
• Respect and listening
• Empowerment
• Goal negotiation
• Language
• Informed decision making (author's emphasis)

Clear similarities can be seen between the key features highlighted by Law et al. (1995) and Parker (2006). Of particular relevance to the subject of this chapter, however, is the concept of *Partnership*, which is clearly highlighted in both definitions and summary features, and "informed decision making," which appears in Sumsion's (2000) definition and in Parker's (2006) summary, which, though now several years old, remain valid for practice today.

Delivering person-centred practice is easier said than done. Maitra and Erway (2006) conducted a study of person and occupational therapist perceptions of person-centred practice. They aimed to "conduct a comparative study of the perceptual involvement of clients and occupational therapists in the *shared decision* making [author's emphasis] process in health care facilities in the United States" and secondly, "to investigate whether there is a difference in the *shared decision making* [author's emphasis]" (p. 300). Despite the relatively small study (11 occupational therapists and 30 people were interviewed), interesting findings arose. The study indicated that whilst practitioners did involve people in the process of goal setting and treatment planning, a perceptual gap existed between the samples in relation to practitioners' use of person-centred practice and shared decision making: People did not always feel as if they participated in shared decision making, whilst practitioners believed they delivered it. Maitra and Erway's (2006) work is of interest as it nicely highlights the daily challenges of undertaking person-centred practice and clearly links the concept of person-centred practice to the centrality of partnership working and shared decision making by practitioners and the people with whom they work.

DECISION-MAKING MODELS

Whilst occupational therapy literature is now replete with literature about person-centred practice, very little has been written about shared decision making. Yet a great deal has been written about shared decision making in the broader health care literature (e.g., Bekker et al., 1999; Bugge et al., 2006; Charles et al., 1997) and is of relevance to occupational therapy practice today.

Shared decision making is one of many decision-making models in the health care literature. Before describing shared decision making in more detail, it is worth considering some of the other major models of decision making in practice. Principle amongst these are the paternalistic model, the physician (or in this context, practitioner) as agent model, and the informed decision-making model (Charles et al., 1997).

Paternalistic Model

The paternalistic model of decision making assumes that patients (as the word itself suggests) are passive recipients of care. This model is clearly outlined in the work of Talcott Parsons (1902–1979), an American sociologist, who conceptualised the sick role (Parsons, 1952), which clearly positions professionals as experts and patients (as the word itself suggests) as passive receivers of care. However, this definition is, as the vast literature of informed and shared decision-making literature within medicine illustrates, no longer an accurate blanket description of medical decision making in practice. Occupational therapists too followed this model for some time (Wilcock, 2002), until professional philosophical tensions moved the profession largely away from this model of decision making. However, whilst the profession's overarching philosophy of care has changed, paternalistic practice can still be found—even in practitioners who express the desire to be person centred (Danëls et al., 2002).

The following models of decision making have emerged, to a certain extent, as a reaction to the paternalistic model (Deber, 1994; Levine et al., 1992).

Practitioner as Agent Model

In the practitioner as agent model (a phrase adapted from the more commonly referred to physician as agent model; Charles et al., 1997) the professional retains overall control of the decisions that are made. However, in this model there is a clear expectation that practitioners will work to gain a comprehensive understanding of peoples' preferences, desires, and values and form their action plan on the basis of what they consider individuals would desire. Despite the good intentions of a practitioner to deliver the care that a person desires, this model of decision making remains incongruous

VIGNETTE 3.1

Mark is a 9-year-old boy with severe learning difficulties. He lives at home with his parents, his 13-year-old sister, and 11-year-old brother. Mark attends a local special needs school, and his teacher has reported that he wanders around, has difficulty concentrating, and frequently interrupts other children from their tasks. On the playground he often appears isolated from others. The school has requested an occupational therapy assessment to see how best to help Mark.

The occupational therapist visited Mark at school. As Mark has significant communication difficulties it was not possible to meaningfully interview him to understand his perspective and views. Instead, the occupational therapist observed him in the classroom and playground over several sessions and interviewed his teacher. The occupational therapist also visited Mark at home, observed his behaviour over two sessions, and interviewed his family. Mark's family reported that he is able to participate in a range of activities at home, and when the occupational therapist watches Mark at home being given support by his siblings he is observed to maintain his concentration for longer periods in play-type activities. The occupational therapist discusses options with Mark's family and teacher and with their agreement develops an intervention plan that engages Mark in small-group work within the classroom and supported play with peers on the playground. After 2 weeks of implementation of this plan, Mark is observed by the occupational therapist to be concentrating for longer periods in the classroom and socialising more on the playground. Mark's teacher reports that he appears more settled and disturbs the other children less.

with the philosophy of current occupational therapy practice. However, there may be times when this model is the closest one towards making partnership work (Vignette 3.1).

The Informed Decision-Making Model

"An informed decision is one where a reasoned choice is made by a reasonable individual using relevant information about the advantages and disadvantages of all possible course of action and in accord with the individual's beliefs" (Bekker et al., 1999, p. 1). Within an informed decision-making model, a practitioner's role is primarily about information sharing from the practitioner to the individual, but it is argued that whilst people wish to gain as much information about their condition or interventions as possible (Bekker et al., 1999), they do not consistently wish to be solely responsible for the decisions they make (Charles et al., 1997). Informed decision making has potential and has been provided in occupational therapy practice (Vignette 3.2), but it is not ideal for everyone: Some people will lack capacity to make informed decisions (Sumsion, 2000), whilst others lack the desire and will not wish to take on such responsibility.

The Shared Decision-Making Model

The shared decision-making model is increasingly put forward as the ideal decision-making process (Charles et al., 1997). It is the middle ground between paternalism and practitioner as agent, both of which take control away from the person, and informed decision making, which, while empowering people through the provision of information, also transfers the responsibility of intervention

decisions—a responsibility many prefer not to have (Charles et al., 1997).

It is important that practitioners ask people what sort of involvement they wish to have in their care and intervention (i.e., whether they wish practitioners to make [and communicate] decisions for them), whether they as individuals wish to make informed decisions based on information from practitioners, or whether to participate in a shared decision-making model of care.

Certain features of a decision-making process are required for it to be classified as a shared decision. A shared decision must involve the following:

- At least two participants
- The sharing of information, and the making of a decision (which should include an option to do nothing) that must be agreed upon by everyone (Charles et al., 1997).

SHARED DECISION-MAKING INTERVENTIONS

But how do you practice shared decision making? There are a wide variety of interventions that, when used appropriately, assist in making shared decisions. Three key interventions that are typically considered to support shared decision making are described in depth elsewhere in this book: Goal Setting in Occupational Therapy (see Chapter 7), and the Therapeutic Use of Self (see Chapter 8). However, there are various features of all therapeutic relationships that can either build or diminish the potential for shared decision making in practice (Braddock et al., 1997; Elwyn et al., 2000, 2005a).

VIGNETTE 3.2

Barry is an 86-year-old man. He has lived alone since the death of his wife 6 years ago. His main interests are his garden, his cat, and meeting his friends once a week for a pub lunch. Barry was admitted to his local hospital after falling at home. He fell in the kitchen after tidying up his dinner and had lain all night on the floor until being discovered by his daughter when she arrived the following morning to take him shopping. On arrival at hospital, it was noted that Barry's blood sugar levels were poor (he has diabetes), he had fractured his left hip, and was badly shaken by the experience.

Barry has made a better physical recovery than expected, and both he and the physiotherapists are happy with the progress he is making. His daughter and some of the clinical team, however, remain concerned that he will not be able to cope with living at home independently and fear he will fall again.

The occupational therapist carries out an assessment with Barry using the Canadian Occupational Performance Measure (Law et al., 1994). This assessment highlights that getting out of bed, walking distances, and bending down are some of the main occupational performance difficulties he is currently experiencing. Barry rates these activities highly (8–9) because it is necessary for him to continue to carry out the activities he is used to. Barry rates his current performance of these activities as 3, 2, 2, respectively, and his satisfaction as a consistent 2. The occupational therapist also presents Barry with some key figures and facts about the known dangers of returning home, for a man of his age, after having a fractured hip. Barry considers all this information but decides that despite his occupational performance difficulties and the potential dangers of returning home alone, he will return to his house. For Barry, the risk of future falls does not outweigh the risk of loss of identity, role, and routine that he feels giving up his home would entail. The occupational therapist designs an intervention plan to assist Barry to improve his areas of occupational performance difficulties and visit his house to carry out an environmental assessment.

Establishing a Partnership and Decision-Making Preference

The first stage in developing shared decision making is to establish a therapeutic partnership with the person (see Chapter 9 for further information). This is particularly important when working with people who have long-term conditions. As Montori et al. (2006) highlighted, a key characteristic of shared decision making in practice with people who have long-term conditions is "ongoing partnership between the clinical team (not just the clinician) and the patient" (p. 25). Once the relationship has been established, then practitioners should work to understand what type of role individuals wish to have within the relationship: Do they wish to see the professional as agent? Do they wish to be informed decision makers? Do they wish to partake in shared decision making? These issues must be communicated and understood very carefully: People are unlikely to immediately understand what you mean if you were to ask them a question such as, "What type of decision-making capacity do you wish to have in this relationship?" This information needs to be gained through careful discussion with each individual. It can often be more helpful to understand individuals' preferred format by presenting a series of options (Vignette 3.3). However, it should also be remembered that people may prefer different types of decision-making models depending on the nature of the decision being made, their current health status, and consequences of the decision in question. Individuals' decision-making preference is a dynamic concept that must be continually understood and responded to by practitioners.

Defining the Problem

Problem definition is, in effect, a process of assessment (see Chapter 6 for further information). It is through the assessment process that practitioners and people exchange information about a particular situation or problem. Assessment, and therefore problem definition, requires a two-way exchange of information. The practitioner must provide all the information about relevant intervention options, and people should share all their relevant history and their values relating to the potential intervention options presented by the practitioner. However, despite the relatively straightforward nature of the information exchange described earlier, research highlights that both practitioners and individuals with whom they work do not always share all the relevant knowledge with each other (Bugge et al., 2006). Whilst a study of the nonexchange of information has not been conducted within the context of occupational therapy, its occurrence across a broad range of clinical environments (Bugge et al., 2006) suggests that it will be no different in an occupational therapy context (Vignette 3.4).

VIGNETTE 3.3

Bethany is a 20-year-old woman. She is currently taking a year out of her psychology degree at University. She was diagnosed with chronic fatigue syndrome 8 months ago. Her symptoms commenced following a glandular fever–type illness, and her recovery has been hampered since by severe and disabling fatigue, lack of concentration, low mood, and poor concentration.

The occupational therapist visited Beth at home to carry out an assessment of her needs. Because of Bethany's condition, it was necessary to carry out the assessment over several sessions because Bethany was only able to concentrate for short periods of time and tired quickly. Initially Bethany was very hesitant of becoming involved with the occupational therapist as she was concerned that she would be made to do things she didn't want to or didn't have the energy to complete. The occupational therapist spent her initial meetings with Bethany listening to her talk about her life, condition, the difficulties she currently faced, and her hopes and desires for the future. As well as information gathering, a central task of these sessions was to build up Bethany's trust in the occupational therapist. Towards the end of the fourth session Bethany told the occupational therapist that whilst she did want to get better, she remained hesitant to engage in any active intervention as she feared she would lose control and become more sick. The occupational therapist reassured Bethany that her approach, and the approach of her team, was very much one of working together with people. Bethany was told that she had control of how she wished to involve her clinical team—if she wished them to tell her what to do, to give her advice, or to collaborate in making decisions together—as a core part of the whole team. Bethany appeared keen to work together with the team: she found the idea of them telling her what to do scary, but also did not want the responsibility of making all the choices herself. Bethany was reassured that she could be actively involved in all the decisions about her care and she would not be made to do anything she didn't want to.

Hesitantly at first, Bethany agreed to commence goal setting with her occupational therapist. Goals were set weekly and agreed upon together by both Bethany and her occupational therapist. It took several weeks of trial and error to set achievable goals that were, in Bethany's words, "challenging enough, but not too much." This was achieved through Bethany giving good feedback to the occupational therapist, in whom she had built increasing trust, and deciding together what the next appropriate goal should be.

VIGNETTE 3.4

Tim is a 54-year-old married businessman with two grown-up children. Two months ago he had a stroke that left him with muscle weakness (especially in his left arm), slightly slurred speech, and some loss of sight. Tim received stroke rehabilitation as an inpatient and was discharged 2 weeks ago. He has now been referred for continued community stroke rehabilitation at home. The occupational therapist visits Tim at home to see how he is doing. Tim's wife Sheena is present throughout the visit. During the interview they all discuss Tim's activities of daily living, leisure activities, and return to work.

What neither Tim nor his occupational therapist mention is Tim's sexual relationship with his wife.

The occupational therapist knows, from the discharge notes that she received, that Tim did mention worries about this at an early stage, to an occupational therapist during a kitchen session, but that this had not been taken forward by her or any member of the clinical team. The visiting occupational therapist does not mention it as she is uncertain of how to raise the subject (or indeed if she should raise the subject) in the presence of his wife; furthermore, she is not sure what she could recommend, or even if Tim still has concerns in this area of life.

Tim is indeed still concerned about his sexual relationship with his wife. In fact, it is his main concern; he has been able to discuss or began to address all the other issues. Tim does not mention it because he is unsure what his wife would think of him for discussing these issues with a younger lady (the occupational therapist), was unsure of how to raise the subject and maintain his composure, and was not even certain if the occupational therapist was the right person to talk to as the one in the hospital had not appeared that interested when he mentioned it during a kitchen session one day! The occupational therapy interview ends, and a continuing rehabilitation package is agreed upon by both the practitioner and Tim. His sexual dysfunction issues were not discussed and remain Tim's biggest source of anxiety and concern.

In Bugge et al.'s (2006) study, the following reasons were given by clients and practitioners for not exchanging relevant information during clinical encounters.

The environment was unconducive to sharing information (e.g., there were other people present during the meeting).
- The practitioner's behaviour put people off (e.g., practitioners appeared hurried, uninterested, or not listening to them).
- People wanted to present a particular self-image.
- People did not believe that certain pieces of information were important.

Practitioners' rationale for not exchanging information included the following:
- The environment was unconducive to sharing information; like people referred for services, practitioners were put off by the presence of others in the room (e.g., they would not ask people potentially embarrassing questions if others were present).
- Practitioners lacked knowledge about certain interventions.
- Practitioners decided not to share information about other interventions because they believed, without checking, that such interventions were not desired by the person.

None of these reasons seem beyond the realm of possibility within an occupational therapy encounter. It is therefore essential that all possible steps be taken to ensure that all the necessary information is exchanged between a person and the practitioner. A key step to ensure accurate problem definition is the active employment of the therapeutic use of self (see Chapter 9) as well as techniques such as active questioning of an individual to see if the individual wishes to ask anything that you have not already discussed.

Including the Individual in the Decision-Making Process

At first glance, including people in a shared decision-making process seems like an obvious statement to make; it wouldn't be shared if you didn't! Indeed, occupational therapy ethical guidelines state (except in exceptional circumstances, such as mental health legislation), "Clients have a right to make choices and decisions about their own health care" (p. 6). Yet how easy is it to truly achieve this in practice? Several studies illustrate the negative perceptions of peoples' involvement and participation in their own rehabilitation and illustrate the challenges of achieving true participation in practice (Becker & Kaufman, 1995; Danëls et al., 2002; Doolittle, 1992). Such is the discrepancy of philosophy and practice, that achieving true participation in the decision-making processes of

care has been claimed to be more "rhetoric than reality" (Lewis, 2003, p. 4). However, the challenges of involving people in meaningful participation must remain the goal of every practitioner. True participation and shared decision making are more likely to occur when practitioners ensure people understand their problems, explore their worries/fears/expectations, discuss options, and make collaborative decisions.

Ensuring People Understand Their Problems and the Decisions Required

It is vital that individuals, as well as practitioners, understand their problems and what, if any, decisions are required. To achieve this, practitioners must ensure that they communicate with everyone in a manner that builds confidence and rapport (see Chapter 9) and in language that is easy to follow and in the preferred media of the person with whom they are communicating (see Chapter 11). Building positive therapeutic engagement and educating individuals are both essential skills that are required if people are to understand their problems and the decisions that are required. However, the routine nature of building therapeutic relationships and educating people results in the complexity of truly achieving this is in practice being often overlooked (Vignette 3.5).

Exploring Peoples' Worries, Fears, and Expectations

Engaging in therapeutic assessment and interventions can be anxiety provoking. Anxiety negatively affects a person's ability to concentrate. This in turn can reduce individuals' abilities to exercise choice and engage in partnership working. Practitioners can help to reduce people's level of anxiety by explicitly eliciting and discussing individuals' worries, fears, and expectations about their health and care generally, and of occupational therapy in particular. Time and space should be given throughout sessions to enable people to ask questions. It can also be useful to explicitly ask people if they have any concerns (Vignette 3.6).

Discussing Different Intervention Options

Practitioners should discuss the differing therapeutic options that are available. Interventions have at least two options, as the option to do nothing is always available and ethically should be supported if that is the individual's desire (RCOT, 2021). Discussing options enables people to fully participate in the decision-making process and can reduce the fear of the unknown, as individuals who discuss available options will have a greater knowledge of what each intervention entails. A useful method of discussing potential interventions with people is to discuss the pros and cons (or advantages and disadvantages)

VIGNETTE 3.5

Carlo is a 10-month-old boy. He was born 4 weeks early and was noted to have low birthweight with asymmetric growth retardation on delivery. A diagnosis of mild cerebral palsy was made at a later date following a magnetic resonance imaging scan.

Carlo's development is being closely monitored by a paediatric community physiotherapist, paediatric community occupational therapist, and consultant paediatrician. Carlo had been seen by his physiotherapist for several weeks before the occupational therapy service receives a referral and arranges to visit him. The occupational therapist visits Carlo's home at the same time as the physiotherapist to carry out some joint working and to lessen the burden of health care professionals visiting the house each week. However, whilst Carlo's parents were informed why the physiotherapist was visiting,

they never received an explanation as to why the occupational therapy referral had been made, and this was not clearly explained by the occupational therapist when she visited.

During a series of joint visits, the occupational therapist assesses Carlo's motor, process, and communication skills and observes his response to a variety of stimuli. However, because of the nature of these visits, the occupational therapist never explained to Carlo's parents exactly why she was there, what she was looking for, and what she had to offer that was different from the physiotherapist. Because of this, Carlo's parents were puzzled about her role and what she was doing when she visited. To them, despite the complexity of analysis that the occupational therapist was undertaking, it just appeared as if she was there to hold toys for the physio!

VIGNETTE 3.6

Teresa is a 44-year-old woman who has suffered from depression for the last 12 years. She has been signed-off sick from her work for the last 3 months and has been referred to a return-to-work project by her job centre. Her initial appointment at the project is with an occupational therapist. When the occupational therapist commences his initial interview (a standard format of questions the project asks all new referrals) Teresa appears very anxious and responds to the practitioner's questions with minimal information. At a certain point the occupational therapist stops what he is doing and puts down his forms. He suggests to Teresa that it may be most helpful if she could start first of all by telling him all she thought he should know about her life and illness and how she felt about being referred to the project. Teresa responded well to this strategy and spoke openly about her life before she was diagnosed with depression as well as the impact the illness had had on her life and the life of her family. Teresa discussed how work had previously been

a very important part of her life—not only financially, but also socially. Teresa had worked as a seamstress in several clothing factories and had enjoyed the "buzz" and collegiality of working in these settings. Since being signed-off work, Teresa has missed these aspects and would love to regain these aspects of her life. Having engaged Teresa more fully within the interview, and having seen her relax as she spoke, the occupational therapist then asked Teresa if she had any particular views or concerns about attending the project. Teresa reported that she had lost a great deal of confidence since being signed-off and feared that if she returned to work (and in the process lost her government benefits) she may not manage to maintain her productivity at levels she used to, which could result in her dismissal and significant loss of income upon which she and her family depended. The occupational therapist was then able to discuss the work of the project in further detail and how they had managed similar situations in the past.

of each option (see Chapter 10 for further information) (Vignette 3.7).

Making Decisions

Having worked your way through each of the stages discussed, it is necessary to make choices and decisions about the direction of intervention. Fortunately, few of the decisions made by occupational therapists and the people with

whom they work have irreversible consequences, though some decisions (e.g., major environmental alterations to an individual's house or the decision to enter a nursing home) are less reversible than others (e.g., developing an activity schedule with a person who is depressed). Nevertheless, making decisions for and with people is a significant event. People should be asked if they wish further time to consider intervention options and (wherever possible) it should be

VIGNETTE 3.7

Lucy was referred to occupational therapy by her consultant psychiatrist following discussion at the weekly community mental health team meeting. She is 27 years old and lives with her parents and two younger brothers. She was recently discharged home after being admitted to an acute psychiatric ward for 2 months after being diagnosed with bipolar disorder and concern from her consultant psychiatrist and family that she may self-harm.

During the occupational therapy initial interview it became clear that Lucy was upset by her medical diagnosis and her recent experience of admission. Following her discharge Lucy felt that it was difficult to get back into her old routine and she had lost confidence in doing things she previously found simple. Until 6 months ago Lucy had attended college, where she had been studying business management. Lucy reported that she had previously been enjoying the course. When asked about her other interests she replied that she enjoys watching television, swimming, and using the Internet.

Lucy stated that in the future she hoped to run her own business.

The occupational therapist discussed the idea of Lucy returning to study as a goal they could work towards. Lucy was initially hesitant about working towards this as she was unsure if she would be able to manage—though at the same time she was unable to say what she did want to do. Lucy agreed with the occupational therapist that it would be a good idea to look at the pros and cons of working towards returning to college. Together Lucy and her occupational therapist sat down and drew up a list of the pros and cons of working towards returning to college. Having done this, Lucy felt that doing nothing would only lead her to increase her isolation, whilst she said she could see from the pros and cons sheet that working towards returning to college would not bind her to that choice, but would help her to take her first steps towards recovery and regaining the life she once had. She was still uncertain that she would make it back to college but agreed that it was worth working towards just now.

made clear that such decisions are open to review and can be altered if the people wish at a later date.

MEASURING SHARED DECISION MAKING IN PRACTICE

Given the centrality of the person in occupational therapy, and the policy imperatives to increasingly involve people in their care, shared decision making has now become increasingly relevant in health care; occupational therapy is no exception.

Occupational therapy is internationally recognised as having a person-centred philosophy, yet research into the practitioner–person partnership has shown that delivering person-centred practice is challenging, and there is a dissonance between the theory of person-centred practice and partnership working in practice (Danëls et al., 2002, Maitra & Erway, 2006). Research into shared decision-making practice in community rehabilitation has shown that delivery of shared decision making by occupational therapists in practice can be highly variable, from prescriptive and being practitioner driven to being collaborative, inquisitive, and empowering (Manhas et al., 2020).

The previous section described shared decision making as a method of ensuring person-centred practice and outlined ways in which practitioners can work to ensure that people are involved in their care to the level they wish to be and are facilitated to participate in shared decision making with

practitioners when so desired. As shared decision making is both a recognised good of practice and a challenging concept to deliver, practitioners should measure the degree of participation and shared decision making they deliver in practice as a routine core process measure. In this way they will truly be able to state whether they are being person centred.

Feedback

Individual's satisfaction with their involvement, participation, and shared decision making should be routinely included as part of practitioners' evaluations. Ideally this should occur while the practitioner and person are still working together so that changes can be made if the individual does not feel that there is an adequate partnership. It can feel awkward asking people for feedback on one's clinical performance. But questions such as, "Is there anything I am not doing that you would like me to do?" can provide opportunities for people to raise concerns about your style of partnership working. This can be achieved through interview, though people may not feel free to be honest in their evaluation, or by questionnaire, which provides some distance between the practitioner and the individuals and may enable some people to be more honest. Evaluations of practitioners are, however, fraught with difficulty as they may feel pressured to be overly positive or not report concerns they have for fear it would further affect their relationship. More objective measures of shared decision making are therefore highly desirable.

The OPTION Scale

The OPTION scale is an objective observational measure of shared decision making in practice (Elwyn et al., 2005b). It has been developed to evaluate the extent to which shared decision making occurs within a therapeutic encounter. While originally developed in primary care, the tool has been developed as a measure of any health care consultation (Elwyn et al., 2005b) and would be suitable to measure an occupational therapy contact when options are being considered and/or decisions made (e.g., during an intervention planning session).

The OPTION scale has been used to measure the shared decision-making ability of occupational therapists working in vocational rehabilitation (Coutu et al., 2015). In their cross-sectional study, Coutu and colleagues measured the shared decision-making ability of occupational therapists who had been trained in shared decision making. They found that basic shared decision-making practice occurred following 9 hours of coursework and 11 hours of prior reading. Despite this, some shared decision-making practices occurred less frequently; these include exploring people's concerns about how their problem should be managed, checking that individuals have understood the information, offering people opportunities to ask questions, and highlighting that they should review the decision (Coutu et al., 2015).

To score the OPTION scale, practitioners are required to record a session, with the people's permission, which is then listened to and rated using the OPTION scale.

Rating the OPTION Scale

The OPTION scale measures the extent to which a person is involved in the decision-making process within a session (Elwyn et al., 2005b). The scale itself consists of 12 items, which are each rated over a 5-point scale ranging from "The behaviour is not observed" to "The behaviour being exhibited to a very high standard" (Elwyn et al., 2005b, p. 93). The psychometric properties of the measure have been researched, and it has been shown to be a reliable and valid method of measuring the degree of shared decision making that occurs in a clinical encounter (Elwyn et al., 2005b). Further, research into the OPTION scale has highlighted that "practitioners with no previous training in shared decision making achieve very low levels of patient involvement in decision making" (Elwyn et al., 2005b, p. 58).

SUMMARY

Person-centredness has been the clarion call of occupational therapists since the early 1980s. Occupational therapy has built itself up to be focused on individual autonomy, based on choice, and centred on partnership working (Law et al., 1995; Parker, 2006; Sumsion, 2000, 2006). However, delivering person-centred occupational therapy has been acknowledged as daunting (Parker, 2006), and the perceptual gap that exists between the rhetoric and the reality of practice has been researched and reported (Danëls et al., 2002; Maitra & Erway, 2006).

Different models of decision making, and their contribution to person-centred practice, have been described within this chapter. While some models of decision making (such as the informed decision-making model) should rightly be recognised as being person centred, shared decision making (Charles et al., 1997) was presented as a model that is gaining wide endorsement and popularity as a usable method of working in partnership with people in a wide range of settings. A range of shared decision-making interventions, with practice scenarios to illuminate the concepts being discussed, were then presented.

Shared decision making, though increasingly researched within health care in general, has been surprisingly under-researched within the context of occupational therapy. As an approach to decision making, it has a great deal to offer practitioners who wish to narrow the gap between the rhetoric and reality of person-centred occupational therapy practice.

REFERENCES

Becker, G., & Kaufman, S. R. (1995). Managing an uncertain illness trajectory in old age: Patients' and physicians' views of stroke. *Medical Anthropology Quarterly, 9,* 165–187.

Bekker, H., Thornton, J. G., Airey, C. M., Connelly, J., Hewison, J., Robinson, M. B., Lilleyman J., MacIntosh M., Maule A. J., Michie S., Pearman A. D. (1999). Informed decision making: An annotated bibliography and systematic review. *Health Technology Assessment, 3*(1), 1–156.

Braddock III, C. H., Edwards, K. A., Hasenberg, N. M., Laidley, T. L., & Levinson, W. (1997). Informed decision making in outpatient setting: Time to get back to basics. *JAMA, 282,* 2313–2320.

Bugge, C., Entwhistle, V., & Watt, I. S. (2006). The significance for decision making of information that is not exchanged by patients and health professionals during consultations. *Social Science and Medicine, 63,* 2065–2078.

Canadian Association of Occupational Therapy/Department of National Health and Welfare. (1983). *Occupational therapy guidelines for client centred practice.* Author.

Charles, C., Gafni, A., & Whelan, T. (1997). Shared decision-making in the medical encounter: What does it mean? (or it takes at least two to tango). *Social Science and Medicine, 44*(5), 681–692.

Coutu, M. F., Légaré, F., Stacey, D., Durand, M. J., Corbière, M., Bainbridge, L., & Labrecque, M. E. (2015). Occupational therapists' shared decision-making behaviors with patients having persistent pain in a work rehabilitation context: A cross-sectional study. *Patient Education and Counseling, 98*(7), 864–870.

Danëls, R., Winding, K., & Borell, L. (2002). Experiences of occupational therapists in stroke rehabilitation: Dilemmas of some occupational therapists in inpatient stroke rehabilitation. *Scandinavian Journal of Occupational Therapy, 9,* 167–175.

Deber, R. (1994). Physicians in health care management: 7. The patient–physician partnership: Changing roles and the desire for information. *Canadian Medical Association, 151,* 171.

Doolittle, N. D. (1992). The experience of recovery following lacunar stroke. *Rehabilitation Nursing, 17,* 122–125.

Elwyn, G., Edwards, A., Kinnersley, P., & Grol, R. (2000). Shared decision making and the concept of equipoise: the competences of involving patients in healthcare choices. *British Journal of General Practice, 50*(460), 892–899.

Elwyn, G., Edwards, A., Wensing, M., Hood, K., Atwell, C., Grol, R. (2005a). Shared decision making. In *Measurement using the OPTION instrument.* Cardiff University.

Elwyn, G., Hutchings, H., Edwards, A., Rapport, F., Wensing, M., Cheung, W. Y., & Grol, R. 2005(b). The OPTION scale: Measuring the extent that clinicians involve patients in decision making tasks. *Health Expectations, 8*(1), 34–42.

Law, M. C., Baptiste, S., Carswell, A., McColl, M. A., Polatajko, H., & Pollock, N. (1994). *Canadian occupational performance measure.* Canadian Association of Occupational Therapists.

Law, M., Baptiste, S., & Mills, J. (1995). Client-centred practice: What does it mean and does it make a difference? *Canadian Journal of Occupational Therapy, 62*(5), 250–257.

Levine, M. N., Gafni, A., Markham, B., & MacFarlane, D. (1992). A bedside decision instrument to elicit a patient's preference concerning adjuvant chemotherapy for breast cancer. *Annals of Internal Medicine, 117*(1), 53–58.

Lewis, L. (2003). Is "participation" all just rhetoric? *Mental Health Nursing.* http://findarticles.com/p/articles/mi_qa3949/is_200311/ai_n9322083.

Maitra, K. K., & Erway, F. (2006). Perception of client-centred practice in occupational therapists and their clients. *The American Journal of Occupational Therapy, 60*(3), 298–310.

Manhas, K. P., Olson, K., Churchill, K., Vohra, S., & Wasylak, T. (2020). Experiences of shared decision-making in community rehabilitation: A focused ethnography. *BMC Health Services Research, 20*(1), 1–12.

Montori, V. M., Gafni, A., & Charles, C. (2006). A shared treatment decision making approach between patients with chronic conditions and their clinicians: The case of diabetes. *Health Expectations, 9*(1), 25–36.

Parker, D. M. (2006). The client-centred frame of reference. In E. A. S. Duncan (Ed.), *Foundations for practice in occupational therapy* (pp. 193–216). Elsevier/Churchill Livingstone.

Parsons, T. (1952). *The social system.* Free Press.

Rogers, C. R. (1939). *The clinical treatment of the problem child.* Houghton Mifflin.

Royal College of Occupational Therapists. (2021). Professional standards for occupational therapy practice, conduct and ethics. https://www.rcot.co.uk/publications/professional-standards-occupational-therapy-practice-conduct-and-ethics.

Sumsion, T. (2000). A revised definition of client-centred practice. *British Journal of Occupational Therapy, 63*(7), 15–21.

Sumsion, T. (2006). *Client-centred practice in occupational therapy.* Churchill Livingstone.

Wilcock, A. (2002). *Occupational for health. A journey from prescription to self health* (Vol. 2). College of Occupational Therapists.

World Health Organization. (1984). Discussion document on the concept and principles of health promotion. *Canadian Public Health Association Health Digest, 8L,* 101–102.

4

Doing Reflective Practice: Being a Reflective and Resilient Practitioner

Elizabeth Anne McKay

HIGHLIGHTS

- Engaging in thinking about your thinking is key to being a reflective practitioner.
- Participating with others in reflective processes should bring about changes in practice and service delivery.
- Reflection is a key skill for your own self-management and building your resilience.
- Reflective models/methods can facilitate your reflective ability—try them out to discover which you prefer.

- Sharing practice stories with peers and multidisciplinary team members enables understanding of each others' perspectives and offers new opportunities for working together.
- Reflection can occur before action, in the midst of action, or following action—it is important that action follows reflection

OVERVIEW

Reflection and reflective practice are terms that we all hear in our daily practice; we could assume that we all consider that they mean the same thing to all, but this may not be the case. This chapter returns to the basics regarding reflection and reflective practice, its historical development, and its importance and relevance to professional practice today. The concepts of doing reflection, being reflective, and becoming a reflective practitioner are integrated throughout the chapter. The terms will be defined and the key theorists discussed. The significance of reflection to individual and, importantly, teams of practitioners will be highlighted as a method for bringing about change in service delivery. Types of reflection, models, and methods to facilitate reflection are explored. Throughout the chapter, promoting-reflection activities are introduced; these can be done individually or with peers and offer strategies for enhancing doing reflection. The chapter concludes with highlighting signs and outcomes of reflection practice.

INTRODUCTION

In 2019, the Health and Care Professions Council (HCPC) and other UK regulators placed reflection as central to professional practice, an important element of our daily practice, and important to our own professional development through processes such as supervision (Point of Care Foundation, 2019). Significantly, reflection is a key process for practitioners' own self-management and for building their own resilience. Resilience is the concept that we can face problems or adversity and come back or bounce back with hope and meaning (Deveson, 2003).

Resilience has become extremely important in 2020 as the Covid-19 pandemic has changed much of our taken-for-granted personal and working lives. Resilience at the individual level is about maintaining self-awareness, self-monitoring, and importantly self-compassion. It is about being active in ensuring you are taking care of yourself and have strategies or a plan to help you, which of course may require you to seek support or guidance from your colleagues or friends (Mills et al., 2020). This is in no way a weakness or a limitation; it is a professional's duty to be the best, and sometimes this requires input from others. By self-reflecting you can monitor how you and others are doing and take action when necessary.

Reflection is something that can be used prior to events as well as most commonly postexperience. As you read through this text, whether you are a reader of books from beginning to end or a dipper into selected chapters, reflection should be part of that process so that you can make meaning of the chapter material in relation to your knowledge and experiences either as a student or practitioner. Consider the following: What does this mean for me? How did the service user experience that intervention? Could this be useful to my practice now or in the future? What could I bring into my practice or my team's practice now?

The concept of the reflective practitioner is something commonly discussed; the reflection process is something to build throughout your professional career. A recent review indicates that is should be embedded in all curricula and not dealt with in silo (Platt, 2014). For preregistration students, this means they are likely asked to reflect in class, during formative and summative assessment and when on placement, their learning with the practice educator. Given that, it is good to establish the reflective habit early on, whether you are a student, a novice therapist, or an expert practitioner. Throughout this chapter there are *Promoting Reflection* exercises for you to work on individually or with others; by completing these, you will be developing or enhancing your reflective abilities. Thus by the end of this chapter, you will be able to:

• Define reflection
• Discuss why it is imperative to professional practice
• Be aware of a range of models of reflection
• Be familiar with a range of strategies to promote your reflection, including storytelling and critical incidents
• Acknowledge the importance of self-management and developing your resilience

Box 4.1 asks you to undertake a reflective exercise.

This chapter will define reflection, its theoretical basis, and consider why reflection is important to individual occupational therapists and teams. It presents models to facilitate reflection and discusses activities for doing reflecting in and on practice to assist the development of becoming and being a reflective and resilient practitioner (Davies, 2019).

DEFINING REFLECTION

For clarity, it is useful to go back to dictionary definitions. Chambers 21st Century Dictionary (online) defines *reflect* as "to give an image of as in a mirror." The idea of holding a mirror up to gain a picture of practice is useful but limited as it only focuses on a specific frame in time. The term is also defined as "to consider meditatively." This develops the process of looking at or thinking more in depth and intentionally. The term *reflection* means careful and thoughtful consideration as the action of the mind by which it is conscious of its own operations; the individual is actively thinking about or examining one's thinking, a process called metacognition (Eraut, 1994).

Reflection is one of those words that is often used indiscriminately and that has many different meanings according to the user's perspective. Recently, practitioners and students were asked for their personal definitions of reflection (Table 4.1).

The therapists identified key aspects of reflection: reviewing their performance, examining it in detail, relating to their past knowledge and experiences and future

---

BOX 4.1   Promoting Reflection 1

Think back on some personal experience from the past 3 months; write it down. Take a few minutes to recall it: What happened, who was involved, when and where did it take place, why? Consider what you felt and thought about at the time.

Now consider how you think and feel about that event. What has changed, if anything? What did you learn from that event? Did it change how you thought or acted? How does it impact on your life today?

TABLE 4.1   Therapists' and Students' Definitions of Reflection

Therapists' Definitions of Reflection	Students' Definitions of Reflection
Looking back on thinking about something that has happened or something you have done, thinking how would I have done it differently or how would I deal with the same situation again.	Reflection is important to look back...what have you done right and what treatment you could improve in the future.
A systematic process to look at a situation in detail, to explore ideas for why the outcome occurred to learn new ways of dealing with this.	Reflection enables the person to return to the experience and analyse those experiences both good and bad.
To give thought to your actions/behaviour to improve/acknowledge what is going well.	To look back on your treatment and change it to adapt to different individuals—if it worked.
Reviewing your actions, appraising the efficacy of it, the theory behind it, your decision to do it.	
Looking at an event/issue and considering all aspects of it in terms of your past experience, knowledge base, and evidence.	

actions. Their definitions concentrate on retrospective reflection (i.e., reflection on action). Similarly, students' views of reflection were also retrospective.

The joint statement by Chief Executives of Statutory Regulators of UK Health and Care professionals (Point of Care Foundation, 2019) sets out the expectation that all staff should "be reflective practitioners, engaging meaningfully in reflection and the benefits it brings." This statement acknowledges the duty for practitioners to consider their own actions and their impact. The HCPC (2019) state:

> Our CPD guidance encourages registrants to learn and reflect on practice. In particular we reference developing evidence that suggests the most effective learning activities are often those that are interactive and which encourage self- reflection.

By reflecting, individuals consider their experiences to gain insights about their whole practice to improve the way they work and quality of care they provide to people. The importance of multidisciplinary reflection is highlighted for open discussion when they are going well, as when thing go wrong. Such discussions build resilience, improve well-being, and deepen professional commitment.

WHY IS REFLECTION IMPORTANT?

Reflection is an essential component for the competent and capable therapist practising in the 21st century. Developing reflective practitioners is now a requirement for pre-registration health programmes in the United Kingdom (HCPC, 2019). Practitioners are expected to self-reflect critically on personal performance and adopt a reflexive approach to problem solving. Reflecting on performance and acting on reflection is a professional imperative. Eraut (1994) highlighted that the failure not to engage in regular reflection is professionally irresponsible.

Today it is important that professionals are not only competent to practice but also educated for capability (Fraser & Greenhaugh, 2001). This means that given ever-changing practice contexts, against a backdrop of health and social care systems and processes that are constantly scrutinised for cost effectiveness, practitioners have to think and operate at the higher levels of the cognitive continuum—that is, they have to engage in self-evaluation and analysis of self. In short, practitioners require to manage themselves in their workplaces; self-monitoring and self-reflection are central to the development of ongoing self-management (Packer, 2013). Evidence indicates that self-management works. We require to look after ourselves, maintaining and improving our motivation for our work, ensuring that we monitor our mental and physical health (e.g., eat well and exercise), and acknowledging and seeking support if we are aware of issues arising (e.g., seek advice, use available services, or in some cases seek medical help).

Practitioners in working with others come into contact with stressful and traumatic situations that require them to review their practice against their own experience and knowledge of theory in their specialist area; thus reflection is about the process of therapy for all involved, not just about evaluating an intervention with a client (Kuit et al., 2001). Reflection is a bridge to linking the theory–practice gap; reflection on your own practice is an essential skill for lifelong learning.

Developing capability and capacity to adapt to meet changing needs is key to educating practitioners; therefore most professional educational programmes incorporate these factors. Cowan (2006) identifies essentials for developing capability into curricula. Curricula will include opportunities for learners to:

- Demonstrate competence through active learning methods.
- Develop capacity to cope through solving problems they have identified.
- Create their abilities through doing, making, and organising.
- Initiate and engage with others; not a stop-start activity.
- Reflect individually on doing practice.

At an individual level, therapists, whether novices or experts, still require to develop their critical thinking abilities through purposefully engaging in thinking about why and what it is they do in practice. What were they trying to achieve? How well was it done? How can their practice be different or improved in the future? Critical thinking is achieved through active learning methods, including the development of reflective processes; it is through reflection we integrate our thoughts and actions. The reflective process involves us in thinking about and critically analysing our actions with the goal of improving our professional performance and therefore our practice. Engaging in reflective practice requires individuals to assume the stance of observer of their own practice for them to be able to identify the assumptions and feelings underlying their practice and then to speculate about how these assumptions and feelings affect practice and how these can be modified for future practice (Osterman, 1990). Practitioners are the experts in what they learned from their varied professional experiences, whether these are through practice, reading, course attendance, or research. Being reflective involves you being an active agent, not a passive recipient.

MULTIPLE VOICES REFLECTING ON DOING PRACTICE

The reflective process is often regarded as an individual activity. However, there are compelling reasons for reflection to be done in collaboration with others. It is through working together as a team, or as a community of practitioners, that we can work to transform practice (Freire, 1972). As all our continued professional development occurs in cultural, social, and political contexts, the health and social care teams in which occupational therapists work are rich grounds for learning. Teams can share and discuss practice to make change to improve services for clients through collective reflection and subsequent collaborative action. Through working with others we are open to the possibility of change; our ways of understanding can be explored, challenged, and alternatives created. Winpenny et al. (2006) offer an illuminating account of group reflection. Through sharing our practice stories with others we become participants in our joint practice, gaining additional perspectives of a situation or an event and discovering new meanings or insights. Boud (2006) highlights the need for diverse methods of reflection that move the focus from the individual learner in the workplace to systems that support team and organisational reflection and action in the workplace—namely, productive reflection. Productive reflection should lead to action with and for others for the advantage of all involved, including the service users, the organisation, and wider society (Cressey & Boud, 2006).

To summarise, why is reflection important? Active reflection can enable individual therapists and teams to monitor, evaluate, and adapt their performance; as a result, their professional practice can be enhanced and the quality of service delivery to clients improved. Now the discussion moves into theory.

AN OVERVIEW OF REFLECTIVE PRACTICE

Reflective practice is embedded in educators' and practitioners' thinking, and it is found frequently in occupational therapy literature. There is an ever growing body of evidence; nonetheless, the research is dispersed across a range of disciplines, and it remains unclear regarding its impact on practice (Mann et al., 2009). A recent review from graduate medical education indicated that outcomes from reflection included increased learning of complex subjects, deepened professional values, improved attitudes, and comfort when dealing with difficult materials (Winkel et al., 2017). Nonetheless, there remains a need for patient level outcomes and professional capacities to be measured.

Dewey (1910) initially discussed reflection. Others have developed this concept over time, most notably, Schön (1983, 1987), Kolb (1984), Boud and Walker (1991), and Fish et al. (1989, 1991). Two models of reflection will be highlighted; these have been selected as occupational therapists and other health practitioners most often use them. The work of Brookfield (1990) will be presented, and the importance of storytelling as a reflective method will be examined (Mattingly, 1991).

Kolb's (1984) work on the learning cycle is considered first, as it is a useful starting point to examine experiential learning and how to develop understanding further. It provides a foundation from which reflective practice can be promoted (Fig. 4.1).

To illustrate the essentials of Kolb's work complete the task in Box 4.2.

Through completion of this task you have completed one full turn of Kolb's cycle. Stages 3 and 4 provide further input into concrete experience, and the learning cycle begins again.

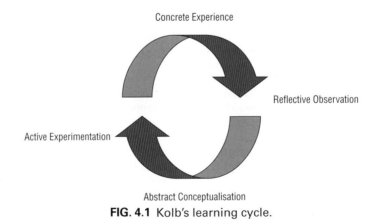

Concrete Experience

Reflective Observation

Active Experimentation

Abstract Conceptualisation

FIG. 4.1 Kolb's learning cycle.

BOX 4.2 Promoting Reflection 2

In pairs, think about a recent clinical event that occurred in your practice. Take turns and tell your story of that event.

Note: *at all stages partners may ask for clarification or ask questions; with stages 3 and 4 partners may offer alternative courses of action for consideration.*

1. Tell your story: describe your **experience.**
2. Share your **reflections** on that experience.
3. What **ideas/practical actions did you do/consider** to advance from that experience?
4. How did/will you **experiment** with your ideas/or practical actions?

BOX 4.3 Promoting Reflection 3

Can you recall the last time in your practice you were aware of thinking on your feet? Revisit that event; what prompted you to think on your feet, and why? What was the outcome? How did it feel?

New understanding or learning is dependent upon the integration of such experiences in relation to practice theory through reflection.

THE INFLUENCE OF SCHÖN

It is impossible to examine reflective practice without recognising the seminal work of Donald Schön (1983, 1987), who brought reflective practice and the reflective practitioner to the fore, as well as the concepts of reflection in action and reflection on action.

Schön examined the relationship between professional knowledge and professional competence; he proposed that practitioners should examine artistry in their own profession through observing and learning through reflection. Such so-called reflection on action or practice is core to professional development as recognised experts in a profession demonstrate artistry that cannot be taught through traditional methods (Fry et al., 2006). Furthermore, when working with noncomplex cases or situations, Schön proposed that experts demonstrate near automatic performance, or knowing in action. As experts in their specialist area, they know more than they can say or make verbally explicit; they are skilled and spontaneous in their performance but are often unable to articulate the dynamics of their practice fully. When questioned about their practice, they often describe the rules and procedures that underpin their practice—not what they did or what guided their thinking. Such rules and procedures remain static and unchanged and do not reveal how or why they performed in that manner.

This process of rethinking some part of our knowing in action leads to on-the-spot experimentation when the practitioner acts and thinks simultaneously (i.e., reflection in action). This process involves practitioners in reshaping their actions in the midst of the action. Schön considered that reflection in action was often a consequence of surprise when engaged in an experience that challenged our usual assumptions or knowledge. This process may be recognised as thinking on one's feet (Fish et al., 1991). The task in Box 4.3 asks you to recall a time from your own experience when you did just that.

Schön proposed a reflection in action coaching method for practitioners to use with learners, whether students or new staff, in their workplace to acquire new skills and insights. It involves three stages:

1. Follow Me: The coach explains and demonstrates a task, breaking it down at various points and then giving time for questions/clarifications. This facilitates learners to see the whole task completed and to understand the process and their relationship to it.
2. Joint Experimentation: This stage helps learners formulate what they want to achieve, and by working together through demonstration/questioning the coach and learners explore different ways of producing and completing the task.
3. Hall of Mirrors: Here learners and coach continually shift their perspectives with a task, taking turns to move the task to completion, with each giving their input/view of the task, giving a two-tier view of their interaction, which encompasses acting/questioning/reflecting/acting through this process to enable learners to complete the task.

Some aspects described in these three stages may be familiar strategies to you, although the language may differ. Nonetheless, using this method allows learners and coach to work collaboratively in developing reflection in action.

TYPES OF REFLECTION

It becomes clear when discussing reflection that there are some debates in the literature that often centre on this idea and its relationship to metacognition (Eraut, 1995). This involves some self-reflection to monitor one's own thinking. What is important is that reflection needs time, space, structure, and support to be developed. Three distinct types of reflection in relation to continuing professional development can be identified in the literature (Fade, 2007; Kinsella, 2000):

1. Looking forward (prospective or anticipatory reflection; reflection *for* action [Cowan, 2006])
2. Looking at present (spective; reflection *in* action)
3. Looking back (retrospective; reflection *on* action)

To illustrate these three concepts, consider the following: You are contemplating a change of job. You browse the professional journals and websites, which gives you an idea about what is out there, the jobs available, the location and type of clients, and the range of staff you might be working with (anticipatory). You go on a visit to a particular job location; while there, you stop to think about how you would complement or fit into this team. What could you offer here, and in what ways would this post help your career? What would it be like to work here? (reflection in action). Once the visit is completed, you review the experience: Who did you meet? What might you contribute? What was it like? (reflection on action). Now you must decide to apply or not to apply.

Let's Introduce Our Therapists

First, Alison: a therapist in her first year of practice; second, Donald: a senior therapist of 8 years. Both are having issues in their workplaces (Box 4.4).

Conscious forward thinking as described can help you prepare for a particular event or help you to decide on possible courses of action. This process allows you to reflect, evaluate, and propose solutions to manage yourself in the workplace.

> *Authors Reflection: I know that I often use anticipatory reflection prior to going to meetings, especially if I know that the meetings may be difficult or contentious. I plan what topics I would like discussed and if I'm presenting have a clear outline of what I wish to cover.*

MODELS OF REFLECTION

This section explores two models that can aid your ability to reflect on your own or with peers or team members. They offer you strategies and structures to guide and develop your skill as a reflective practitioner. These models offer a logical framework to make sense of complex information. Alternatively, there are other methods that are also useful to explore to enhance your reflective abilities such as the use of metaphors, literature (medical humanities), drawing, and photography (Denshire, 2005; Mattingly, 1998; McIntosh & Webb, 2006; Murray et al., 2000).

The well-known model developed by Boud et al. (1985) and Boud and Walker (1991) states that reflection is grounded in the personal foundation of experience of

---

BOX 4.4   Reflection for Action: Alison and Donald

1. Alison has been working on a community mental health team for the past 4 months. She has begun to notice that one of the service users is making increased demands on her time and often hanging back at end of sessions to chat over things with her. Alison is concerned that there may be an underlying issue. She has spoken with the service user in the first instance; however, nothing has changed. Other colleagues have commented on what they are seeing. Alison is becoming uneasy with this service user's attention. She is becoming worried and has decided to seek help from her supervisor to help her manage this situation. What could be Alison's reflections? These may include thoughts regarding anxiety, worry about her safety, concern that she is not able to manage the situation herself, and poor performance in others' view. **What else can you think of? How should Alison approach and discuss this situation with her supervisor?**

2. Donald is a senior therapist working in stroke rehabilitation. Lately, he feels he is less motivated, finding his post not so challenging and becoming less engaged in the wider service. He works on a busy stroke rehabilitation unit in a large general hospital. He manages two staff members and a health care assistant. He reports to the stroke unit manager. How might Donald discuss this in supervision? What would be feasible for him? What opportunities and professional development are open to him? **What else can you think of?**

---

the learner (Boud & Knights, 1996)—that is, the belief that all experiences to date have contributed to shaping who that person is now. Furthermore, it includes the notion of intent (i.e., the learner's intent in relation to an experience) as this gives a particular focus for use in learning contexts.

PREPARATION

The emphasis in Boud's model is on preparation prior to a learning event, which mirrors anticipatory reflection, as discussed previously. However, here there is a more in-depth approach to consideration of the learner, the milieu or the environment where the event will take place, and importantly the learner's skill set and strategies. Giving time to consider strategies, which one may use in that event, can help preparation and flexibility when in the situation. Box 4.5 describes Donald's experience.

BOX 4.5 Donald's Preparation

Let's return to Donald's situation

Donald is reviewing his expertise, skills, and strategies for his current post. He recognises that he has had little opportunity to research his current work and indeed has not taken up opportunities to develop his research development or capacity. He has reviewed his undergraduate studies, and has decided he would like to consider applying for further study in the future but requires a stepped approach to meeting this need.

EXPERIENCE

The middle section of the model deals with the learning experience. Learning occurs in context, which encompasses both the human and physical environment. We learn through our interactions within the environment. When in a specific context it is important to *notice* what is happening to ourselves in relation to the external factors. Learners can be assisted to this by others highlighting aspects that may be important. For example, a therapist may draw the learner's attention to how a client is positioned in a group task or to how the client sits in a chair. You may intervene in an *external* way (do something); for example, you talk with someone. Or it may be that you assist someone to complete a task as you become aware of the person having difficulties. Or you may intervene *internally* (think something); for example, noting some follow-up activity, such as reading more about a condition or a treatment. Self-vigilance for the person involved is key: Being aware of how one is acting and modifying actions in the midst of experience is reflection in action. See Box 4.6 for Donald's reflection in action.

The final aspect of the model is the reflective process (i.e., reflection on action). Following the event, the learner returns to the experience to review and describe what happened in as much detail as possible. The learner needs to attend to one's feelings: How did it feel? The learner must

---

BOX 4.6 Reflection in Action

At his monthly supervision session, Donald has come prepared to discuss his future as a stroke specialist. He indicates he has been looking for options to build his research capability. He has decided that he would like to consider applying for a PhD in the future. His supervisor suggests looking at a range of resources, including the people he works with regarding his future studies. Donald realises he could speak to his work colleagues and others who have completed studies to understand what might be involved in further study.

---

reevaluate the experience: What does it mean now? What may it mean for future actions or behaviour?

THE STRANDS OF REFLECTION MODEL

The strands of reflection model was developed by Fish et al. (1991); it differs from Boud's model in that it concentrates on providing a structured and systematic method to review an event or experience. There is no anticipatory reflection component. Practitioners like this model as it offers a structured method that they can see using, which assists them in being detailed and contextualised in reflection on action.

To aid the use of the model it is helpful to think of your experiences like a rope that is made up of several strings or strands; these strands are woven together and build a stronger or richer perspective to the reflective process. Within the model, four key strands come together to help reflection in an organised manner: factual strand, retrospective strand, substratum strand, and connective strand. Together they provide a means of reflecting upon your practice. They are not intended to be used independently; they seek to facilitate therapists to interpret their practice experiences. By separating the four strands, each can be looked at closely and then all four can be reformed as a whole from which the therapist can move forward. Box 4.7 unpacks Alison's reflections.

Factual strand: This strand acts to set the scene; briefly, it describes the context of the practice situation. Events are recalled in time order: What happened? How did you feel, think? Why? Therapists are asked to pinpoint any critical incidents that arose during the situation.

Retrospective strand: This strand considers what patterns are visible in the practice as a whole. It asks what aims were set, and if they were achieved. It asks practitioners to see themselves in relation to the practice event.

Substratum strand: This strand requires therapists to review what customs, traditions, and beliefs were brought into a situation or were already there. Furthermore, therapists consider what assumptions, beliefs, or values underpinned the actions they took and the decisions they made.

Connective strand: This strand brings it all together: What has been learnt from this practice experience and how will it relate to future practice? How can thoughts and actions specific to this situation be modified in light of experiences or further thought or reading? Finally, it considers the implications for future practice.

BOX 4.7 Illustrating Strands of Reflection—Alison's Meeting With Her Supervisor

Factual strand: Alison tells her supervisor about her situation; she gives specific examples of interactions she has had with the service user, dates, exchanges, and her feelings over this time. **Retrospective strand**: Alison recalls when she first became aware of the service user's attention and behaviour, thinking about how she responded and whether there are any patterns appearing. **Substratum strand:** Alison considered what beliefs and customs she brought to this situation or were already there. As she thought through the exchange, she considered that although she had worked in her normal manner with this service user, the service user was seeking her out. Her supervisor asked her to reflect on any similarities she may have with this person, which allowed her to recognise that she was a similar age and cultural background; although she came from a different town, it was very similar. She began to consider that the service user was looking perhaps for a friend or ally in the centre. **Connective strand:** Alison and her supervisor came up with a number of strategies for her to try over the coming weeks and to see if these had any impact. Alison would report back at her next supervision session. She was also encouraged to speak to her team members to alert them to her situation.

Strands of reflection and the process undertaken by Alison is described as the DATA method (Peters, 1991). DATA outlines the four stages of the process:

1. **D**escribe: What you did and what occurred
2. **A**nalyse: Why you choose this approach
3. **T**heorise: What assumptions influenced your initial choices (did they give an accurate explanation to what occurred)
4. **A**ct: If not, act by revising the assumptions or the approach

It's a useful shorthand way to remember those reflective steps.

OTHER METHODS FOR PROMOTING REFLECTION

The models here are not meant to be taken as the only methods for reflecting. Many other models exist in the literature. Practitioners can choose the model that they find most useful, indeed. HCPC (2019) does not indicate any particular model, only a systematic process. We each tune into different elements, so diversity is required. Moving away from specific models of reflection it is worthwhile to consider two other distinct methods that can assist in developing reflection further: storytelling (Mattingly, 1991) and critical incidents (Brookfield, 1990); both of these methods encourage sharing practice with others.

TELLING STORIES

We all tell stories of our practice informally with our colleagues on a daily basis. Telling stories or narrative is proposed as the primary form by which human experience is made meaningful (Polkinghorne, 1988). As personal meaning is offered through the individual's story, Mattingly (1991) considers that the story is particularly useful for addressing experiences and is therefore a useful tool for reflection. Mattingly (1998) regards storytelling as being "event and experience-centred, which create experiences for the listener or audience" (p. 8). Therefore the sharing and discussion of stories can aid all participants' reflections. Stories hold our experiences together, allowing links to the past, present, and crucially to the future. Through our own practice stories we are trying to make sense or give coherence to our actions and experiences and importantly give coherence and meaning to our clients' stories (Mattingly, 1998). Thus using stories to promote reflection is vital for therapists to develop their practice. Stories can be written or verbal. They can be sketches/vignettes or portraits of practice in words (Fish, 1998) that capture the essence of the story or can be developed to give detailed accounts of our practice (e.g., writing in reflective journals). Recalling our stories may be part of an individual's supervision session or a feature of team meetings. Living (1999) offers perspectives of a specific client from a range of different team members; each offers a slightly different view. Sharing our practice stories illustrates our thinking and practice and promotes reflection.

EXPLORING CRITICAL INCIDENTS

Critical incidents are not exactly what they sound like. They are not dramatic events such as life and death situations or crises; indeed, they are often small or common events that are meaningful to an individual often because these incidents touch the individual at an emotional level. The critical incident's significance lies with the practitioner and what the practitioner does following the event (Brookfield, 1990). The incident is described verbally or written, shared with others and the question asked: Why was the incident critical? McAllister (2003) offers a guideline for the analysis of critical incidents to promote advance practice. These include:

- Identify the critical incident.
- Crystallise the event.

- Clarify the nature of the problem or the issue.
- What are the lessons to be learnt here?
- Identify what you might do to address the problem or issue.

Critical incidents by nature are unplanned, so it is important that they are explored because they can be powerful learning tools for those involved.

When and how to reflect are questions often asked by practitioners. Reflection should take place when you are involved in something that is new or surprising, when faced with complex or difficult situations, after continuing professional development activities. What is important is that you take the time to reflect on such activities and monitor your own well-being and build your own resilience. Table 4.2 summarises a range of strategies for developing reflection both as an individual practitioner and as a shared task for peers and teams.

SIGNS OF REFLECTIONS

This chapter has looked at various ways of doing and being reflective. A question often asked is, How do we know that we are reflecting? Reflective processes can be observed in several ways; for example, the intensity of a discussion may be evidence of reflection, alternatively it may be the quality of silence, or it may be the nature of questions asked.

Consider the following (in first person):
- What was I aiming for when I did that?
- What exactly did I do?
- Why did I choose that particular action?
- What was I trying to achieve?
- What criteria am I using to judge success?
- How did the client feel about it?
- How do I know the client felt like that?

You can of course think of others in relation to your own or your team's practice. Change in practice, reconstructing a different way forward may evidence a reflective process in action. Changes may of course be small and cumulative; as a result, they may not be noticed immediately by others. Therefore it is important that you note such changes and share them with your colleagues.

OUTCOMES OF REFLECTION

The abovementioned models, storytelling, critical incidents, and other strategies identified must lead to action by the individual or the team. It is imperative that action follows reflection, otherwise the reflective process becomes a closed activity for the self; it will not lead to deeper commitment to your practice or build your self-management. The actions that result from reflection may take a number of forms, but they all have implications for practitioners and their practice:
- Practitioners may maintain their well-being and resilience.
- Practitioners/teams may gain new perspectives on an experience.
- Practitioners/teams may seek further knowledge or related research.
- Practitioners/teams may change their future behaviour in light of their reflections.
- Practitioners/teams faced with a similar situation in the future may have a readiness to apply different strategies or have a commitment to a specific course of action.

Reflection takes active involvement, time, structure, and support from others. It is important that reflection leads to action. Those actions have implications for your practice and ongoing continued professional development. Doing reflection is, after all, a professional imperative to being a reflective and resilient practitioner. Through engagement in such activities throughout their career, therapists are able to begin to negotiate the reality of the practice world whilst being active in their own self-management as reflective and resilient practitioners. To conclude, we draw on the words

TABLE 4.2 Techniques for Doing and Being Reflective				
	Individual	**Peers**	**Mentors**	**Multidisciplinary Teams**
Prebriefing and debriefing	√	√	√	
Storytelling (written/oral)	√	√	√	√
Exploration of attitudes and beliefs		√	√	√
Reflective questions	√		√	
Continuing professional development portfolio*	√		√	√
Reflective journal	√			
Wait time or think time		√	√	
Critical incidents		√	√	√
Directing attention		√	√	

*Royal College of Occupational Therapists Career Development Framework.

of Drucker, an American educator, who offers a timely message: "Follow effective action with quiet reflection. From the quiet reflection will come even more effective action."

SUMMARY

This chapter has highlighted the importance of reflection and reflective practice; it has considered the significance of reflective practice for the practitioner, both at an individual and at a team level. Being a reflective practitioner is a key skill in today's health and social care environment. Reflection on practice and experience is necessary for continuing professional development, self-management, and building resilient practitioners able to face adversity and to continue to provide services at difficult times. Key theorists have been included to trace the historical and recent development of reflective practice. A number of models and a range of methods for developing reflection in practice have been introduced and illustrated. Readers are encouraged to use the Promoting Reflection boxes in their work setting.

REFERENCES

Boud, D. (2006). Relocating reflection in the context of practice: Rehabilitation or rejection? Paper presented at Professional Lifelong Learning: Beyond Reflective Practice. http://www.leeds.ac.uk/medicine/meu/lifelong06/.

Boud, D., & Knights, S. (1996). Course design for reflective practice. In N. G. Gould, & I. Taylor (Eds.), *Reflective learning for social work: Research, theory and practice* (pp. 23–34). Aldershot Hants.

Boud, D., & Walker, D. (1991). In the midst of experience: Developing a model to aid learners and facilitators. Paper presented at the National Conference on Experiential Learning Empowerment Through Experiential Learning: Explorations of Good Practice. University of Surrey.

Boud, D., Keogh, R., & Walker, D. (Eds.). (1985). Promoting reflection in learning: A model. In D. Boud, R. Keogh, & D. Walker (Eds.), *Reflection: Turning experience into learning.* Kogan Page.

Brookfield, S. (1990). Using critical incidents to explore learners' assumptions. In J. Mezirow, et al. (Eds.), *Fostering critical reflection in adulthood: A guide to transformative and emancipatory learning.* Jossey-Bass.

Chambers 21st Century Dictionary. (1999). https://chambers.co.uk/book/the-chambers-dictionary/#.

Cowan, J. (2006). *On becoming an innovative university teacher: Reflection in action.* Society for Research into Higher Education & Open University Press.

Cressey, P., & Boud, D. (2006). The emergence of productive reflection. In D. Boud, P. Cressey, & P. Docherty (Eds.), *Productive reflection at work: Learning for changing organisations.* Routledge.

Davies, N. (2019, May 8). *Cultivating resilience as a nurse.* Independent Nurse.

Denshire, S. (2005). "This is a hospital, not a circus": Reflecting on generative metaphors for a deeper understanding of professional practice. *International Journal of Critical Psychology, 13,* 158–178.

Deveson, A. (2003). *Resilience.* Allen and Unwin.

Dewey, J. (1910). *How we think.* University of Chicago.

Drucker, P. (n.d.). Brainy Quote. https://www.brainyquote.com/quotes/peter_drucker_120337.

Eraut, M. (1994). *Developing professional knowledge and competence.* The Falmer Press.

Eraut, M. (1995). Knowledge creation and knowledge use in professional contexts. *Studies in Higher Education, 10,* 117–133.

Fade, S. (2007). Learning and assessing through reflection: A practical guide. Making practice-based work. www.practice-basedlearning.org.

Fish, D. (1998). *Appreciating practice in the caring profession: Refocusing professional development and practitioner research.* Butterworth Heineman.

Fish, D., Twinn, S., & Purr, B. (1989). *How to enable learning through professional practice.* West London Press.

Fish, D., Twinn, S., & Purr, B. (1991). *Promoting reflection: Improving the supervision of practice in health visiting and initial teacher training.* West London Institute.

Fraser, S. W., & Greenhaugh, T. (2001). Coping with complexity: Educating for capability. *British Medical Journal, 323,* 799–803.

Freire, P. (1972). *Pedagogy of the oppressed.* Penquin.

Fry, H., Ketteridge, S., & Marshall, S. (2006). *A handbook for teaching and learning in higher education. Enhancing academic practice.* RoutledgeFalmer.

Health and Care Professions Council. (2019). Continuing professional development. http://www.hcpc-uk.org/registrants/cpd/.

Kinsella, E. A. (2000). *Professional development and reflective practice: Strategies for learning through professional experience— A workbook for practitioners.* CAOT Publications ACE.

Kolb, D. A. (1984). *Experiential learning; experience as the source of learning and development.* Prentice Hall.

Kuit, J. A., Reay, G., & Freeman, R. (2001). Experiences of reflective teaching. *Active Learning in Higher Education, 12(2),* 128–142.

Living, R. (1999). The team's story of a client's experience of anorexia nervosa. In S. E. Ryan, & E. A. McKay (Eds.), *Thinking and reasoning in therapy.* Stanley Thornes.

Mann, K., Gordon, J., & MacLeod, A. (2009). Reflection and reflective practice in health professions education: A systematic review. *Advances in Health Sciences Education, 14,* 595–621.

Mattingly, C. (1991). Narrative reflection on practical actions: Two learning experiments in reflective storytelling. In D. A. Schön (Ed.), *The reflective turn.* Jossey Bass.

Mattingly, C. (1998). *Healing dramas and clinical plots. The narrative structure of experience.* Cambridge University Press.

McAllister, L. (2003). Using adult education theories: Facilitating others' learning in professional practice settings. In G. Brown, S. A. Esdaile, & S. E. Ryan (Eds.), *Becoming an advance healthcare practitioner.* Butterworth Hieneman.

McIntosh, P. W. (2006). Creativity and reflection: An approach to reflexivity in practice. Paper presented at Professional Life-long Learning: Beyond Reflective Practice. http://www.leeds.ac.uk/medicine/meu/lifelong06/.

Mills, J., Ramachenderan, J., Chapman, M., Greenland, R., & Agar, M. (2020). Prioritising workforce wellbeing and resilience: What COVID-19 is reminding us about self-care and staff support. *Palliative Medicine*, 34(9). https://doi.org/10.1177%2F0269216320947966.

Murray, R., McKay, E., Thompson, S., & Donald, M. (2000). Practising reflection: A medical humanities approach to occupational therapist education. *Medical Teacher*, 22(3), 276–281.

Osterman, K. F. (1990). Reflective practice: A new agenda for education. *Education and Urban Society*, 22(2), 133–152.

Packer, T. L. (2013). Self-management interventions: Using an occupational lens to rethink and refocus. *Australian Occupational Therapy Journal*, 60(1), 1–2.

Peters, J. M. (1991). Strategies for Reflective Practice. *New Directions for Adult and Continuing Education. 51*, 89–96.

Platt, L. (2014). The wicked problem of refelctive practice: A critical literature review. *Innovations in Practice*, 9(1), 44–53.

Point of Care Foundation. (2019). Benefits of becoming a reflective practitioner. http//www.pointofcarefoundation.org.uk.

Polkinghorne, D. (1988). *Narrative knowing and the human sciences.* State University of New York Press.

Schön, D. (1983). *The reflective practitioner: How professionals think in action.* Basic Books.

Schön, D. (1987). *Educating the reflective practitioner.* Jossey Bass.

Winkel, A. F., Yingling, S., Jones, A. A., & Nicholson, J. (2017). Reflection as a learning tool in graduate medical education: A systematic review. *Journal of Graduate Medical Education*, 430–439.

Winpenny, K., Forsyth, K., Jones, C., Evans, E., & Colley, J. (2006). Group reflective supervision: Thinking with theory to develop practice. *British Journal of Occupational Therapy*, 69(9), 423–428.

Professional Skills for Practice

5

Assessment Skills for Practice

Susan Prior, Nichola Duffy, and Edward A.S. Duncan

HIGHLIGHTS

- Assessment is a term used to describe both a process and a tool.
- Assessments ensure that interventions meet the needs of individuals, can measure change, and reflect the unique contribution of occupational therapy to practice.
- Top-down approaches to assessment, whilst lacking in objective evidence, have a strong theoretical rationale that supports their use in practice.

- There are a variety of different forms that assessments can take.
- Standardised and nonstandardised assessments each have strengths and weaknesses in practice.

OVERVIEW

Accurate assessment is an essential component of occupational therapy. But what exactly is assessment and at what stage of therapy should it be carried out? How do practitioners choose which assessments to use? These questions, among others, are discussed in this chapter. The chapter commences by examining why occupational therapists carry out assessments and considers why other stakeholders (such as the service manager or regularity body) feel strongly that assessment should be a core part of practice.

The chapter tackles head-on the debate about whether conceptual models of practice should be selected prior to or following (or not at all) the initial assessment process. Other factors that influence the selection of an assessment in occupational therapy are then described and discussed.

Assessments can be undertaken in various formats, and these are each described in turn with key points highlighted for when they are appropriate to use. The chapter concludes with discussion about the appropriateness of using standardised and nonstandardised assessments in practice. Case vignettes are used throughout the chapter to illuminate relevant issues.

WHAT IS ASSESSMENT AND WHY ASSESS?

Assessment is a term used to describe both a process and a tool. The process of assessment aims to develop practitioners' understanding of people as occupational beings,

recognising their strengths and challenges. Assessment is the initial stage of the occupational therapy process where information is gathered (Pentland et al., 2018), establishing if intervention is required (American Occupational Therapy Association [AOTA], 2020). Effective assessment supports practitioners to appropriately carry out the second stage of the process: developing individualised intervention strategies tailored to people's values and priorities (AOTA, 2020). Assessments are used at the evaluation stage of the occupational therapy process, identifying changes from the initial assessment and determining the effectiveness of the interventions (Pentland et al., 2018).

Assessments and the assessment process help to ensure that occupational therapy practice not only meets the needs of people but also reflects the unique contribution that occupational therapy practitioners can make to the health and well-being of people. AOTA (2020) suggests that assessments that reflect occupational therapy values should be the initial tools used by occupational therapists, providing an occupational profile at the beginning of the occupational therapy process. These include assessments drawn from two conceptual models of practice: the Model of Human Occupation (MOHO; Taylor, 2017) and the Canadian Model of Occupational Performance and Engagement (CMOP-E; Polatajko et al., 2007). This is known as a top-down approach to assessment (Kramer, 2020), where practitioners first consider individual's occupational roles, performance, and skills. Without this understanding it will

| | | | Profession (When |
Individual	Practitioner	Service	Outcomes Are Published)
To be listened to and understood by the practitioner	Better understanding of a person initially and throughout therapy	To ensure that resources are being used in the most effective way	Developing an evidence base upon which other practitioners may draw
Establishing a collaborative relationship			
Occupational therapy is tailored to individual need	Time is spent focusing on people's needs and priorities	To evidence need for new resources to develop new services	To allow others to build on previous work
Provides evidence of change and allows reassessment of goals	Professional development providing material for reflective learning	To identify areas where intervention is ineffective, and practice needs to be reviewed or redirected	
To identify when therapy is no longer required			

TABLE 5.1 The Value of Evaluation

be much harder to understand what the consequences of specific problems will be on people's lives. For example, the impact of limited grip strength will be different for a needlework artist and a manual labourer. Thereafter a practitioner may decide to further investigate specific performance components. It is at this stage that measurement of grip strength (in this example) may or may not be appropriate.

It is often the case that practitioners may not discover anything new by conducting an assessment; the same information may have been gathered through informal conversation and observation. However, by gathering information systematically through a standardised assessment a practitioner can be confident that a comprehensive review has been completed, and this can then be used for comparison at a later stage of therapy.

An occupational therapy assessment may have considerable consequences for an individual. It could indicate whether they are safe to be discharged from hospital or to continue living at home, or it may identify goals of getting back to work or entering education. These implications have considerable impact on their lives, so it is each practitioner's professional responsibility to ensure that all assessments are conducted sensitively, thoroughly, and reliably.

In addition to the direct clinical requirements of carrying out assessments, practitioners may be required to assess by service managers to demonstrate the service's clinical effectiveness. Professional or regulatory bodies also insist that practitioners use assessments in practice. For example, in the United Kingdom the Health Professions Council (2018) Standards of Proficiency for Occupational Therapists requires that registrants must be able to use assessment techniques and to gather, analyse, and evaluate

information. Assessment, therefore, as both a process and a tool, is an essential component of the occupational therapy process.

Who Benefits From Assessment?

At times external influences and the drive for evidence-based practice led practitioners to consider the assessment strategies that they are using. But, whilst evaluating outcomes of intervention is important for occupational therapy services and helps demonstrate their effectiveness, it is vital not to lose sight of the value that this evaluation will have for individuals and practitioners (Table 5.1).

Assessment may occur throughout therapy, but assessments should only be carried out when necessary. So why would an occupational therapist decide to conduct an assessment? There are various reasons.

At the beginning of occupational therapy involvement:
- To determine need for occupational therapy intervention
- To understand an individual's current strengths and needs in relation to their occupational performance
- To gain an accurate picture of an individual's lifestyle prior to illness or injury
- To determine current and predict future functional ability
- To provide a baseline assessment prior to intervention
- To assist in goal setting for intervention
  Throughout occupational therapy involvement:
- To evaluate the effectiveness of an intervention programme
- To review, adapt, or redesign an intervention
- To identify needs best met by other services leading to referral onto other agencies

VIGNETTE 5.1

Mrs. Jones attends the local day hospital; she has been experiencing depression since the death of her partner 6 months ago. She was first seen by a member of the local authority access team who conducted the locality's single shared assessment used by both health and local authority staff. The assessment identified needs in the area of diet and meal preparation as Mrs. Jones was no longer preparing meals, occasionally snacking instead. Following the assessment Mrs. Jones initially agreed to Meals on Wheels; however, 2 weeks later she asked for this service to be discontinued, expressing frustration and saying that she did not need meals delivered.

An occupational therapist was asked to assess Mrs. Jones to gain a greater understanding of her needs by carrying out an OCAIRS (Forsyth et al., 2005), which identified that her routine and habits around meal preparation tasks had changed. She had always enjoyed preparing meals with her partner but expressed that she wasn't "the cook in the relationship," leaving all the supermarket shopping and meal ideas to her partner. She expressed that these tasks now felt overwhelming, as the closest supermarket was quite far away and extremely busy.

An AMPS assessment (an observational measure of activities of daily living, which rates a person's effort, efficiency, safety, and independence in carrying out familiar tasks demonstrated that Mrs. Jones had the necessary skills to prepare her meals.

Following discussions with Mrs. Jones and the multi-professional team, Meals on Wheels was discontinued, and Mrs. Jones received support to create a list of meal ideas and ingredients needed that she could access regularly and add to. She also received support from a local community project to set up a reoccurring online supermarket order that she felt confident using and preferred to use the local shop to buy any other items needed, which also formed part of her new morning routine.

At the end of occupational therapy involvement:
- To identify appropriate time for discharge from services
- To determine ongoing needs for support
- To make recommendations for alternative or additional services

Shared (or Needs) Assessments

Occupational therapists may work within clinical settings where they contribute to assessments where there is a multiprofessional shared responsibility to gather information. This is likely to be an important aspect of their role with other team members relying on the occupational therapist to assess an indiviudal's independence in activities of daily living. However, a therapist should consider if this shared assessment should be informed by a profession-specific assessment. Shared assessment tools tend to be global measures and are therefore useful for screening strengths and difficulties; however, they are insufficient to gain the detail an occupational therapist would require to plan an appropriate intervention. Supplementing the shared assessment with an occupational therapy tool will be vital as illustrated in Vignette 5.1.

HOW TO SELECT AN ASSESSMENT?

There are numerous assessment tools that occupational therapists could use in practice, so how do practitioners know which to select? Practitioners use a wide variety of types of assessment, the selection of which depends on the information they wish to gather. Frequently more than one type of assessment may be required to gain a comprehensive understanding of a situation or a person's functioning, among others. Various factors should be considered when deciding which type of assessment to use.

A practical guideline to assessment selection is offered by the Allied Health Professions (AHP) Outcome Measures UK Working Group (2019) who recommend consideration of the following:
- Outcome of interest and how this will be measured
- Acceptability and utility of assessment tool
- Its measurement properties

Conceptual Models and Selecting Assessments

In considering the outcome of interest to occupational therapists and people receiving occupational therapy leads us to the argument of whether to use the top-down assessment approach previously discussed. Or stated another way, which comes first, the assessment or the choice of conceptual model? This occupational therapy alternative to the better-known chicken and egg scenario has taxed the profession for a number of years and continues to do so today.

The top-down approach suggests that an occupation-focused conceptual model of practice is selected as the first stage of the occupational therapy process (ensuring, amongst other issues, that the assessment and therefore the outcome of interest is occupationally focused) and from that point an initial or screening assessment can take place. Following this assessment, it may then be necessary to conduct further, more specific assessments depending on the initial assessment's findings. A good example of this way of practising and selecting assessments is outlined by Forsyth (2017). A process to select appropriate MOHO (Taylor, 2017) assessment tools is outlined very clearly in a flow chart. Similarly, the Canadian Occupational Performance Measure (COPM-E) (Polatajko et al., 2007) is intrinsically linked to the COPM-E (Law et al., 2019). Law et al.'s (2019) argument for using the COPM-E as an initial assessment is "the tone of the therapeutic relationship lets the person know you will be working as partners and helps to focus your further assessment and intervention on the issues that they feel are priorities."

Both the MOHO and the CMOP-E have been developed within a generally Western societal context. Interestingly, the Western perspective of occupational therapy practice has been criticised for being excessively reductionistic, linear, and scientific (Iwama, 2009). It is beyond the scope of the current chapter to consider whether the differences between Western and Eastern perspectives are truly significant in occupational therapy practice and if so what its effect on the assessment process would be.

It is important to highlight that using a top-down approach to practice does not restrict the practitioner to only using assessments that have been developed within the selected conceptual model; there may be times when an unstructured assessment is appropriate, and an impromptu assessment opportunity may also occur when the practitioner has not had time to prepare a more structured assessment process.

The alternative bottom-up approach provides a focus on discrete body impairments (Doucet & Gutman, 2013), which may also be used to complement the initial top-down approach. Indeed, a specific issue may be best understood from a specific frame of reference (e.g., mood and the cognitive-behavioural frame of reference). Therefore, following an initial assessment guided by an occupation-focused conceptual model, a more specific assessment may be selected. The use of a top-down approach to assessment therefore does not restrict practitioners to using assessments solely associated with that model.

Students and practitioners rightly question which of these two differing approaches is more effective. Does it matter if a top-down approach to assessment is used or not? To date, there does not appear to be any research that has rigorously studied this question. However, at a theoretical level, an argument can be made that a top-down approach is least likely to leave practitioners vulnerable to making errors through peoples' known limitations—specifically in working memory capacity and personal biases in information gathering. In other words, using a top-down approach may minimise the errors that practitioners make. Various issues leave practitioners vulnerable to making assessment errors.

Given that the maximum number of pieces of information a person can hold in working memory is 7 ± 2 (Miller, 1956), clearly it can be seen that listing an extensive range of factors that should be considered when assessing an individual (without placing them in the context of a well-developed structured assessment) is likely to lead to practitioners accidentally omitting some aspects of the assessment. Miller's research therefore lends weight to the idea that practitioners should consider using a top-down approach and intentionally use a conceptual model of practice when initially conducting an assessment.

It has also been clearly evidenced in a range of studies in differing contexts that individuals are not reliable information gatherers and are biased in the manner in which information gathered from assessments is analysed (Paley et al., 2007). Assuming that occupational therapists are no different (and there is no reason to assume they are), it can be seen that if practitioners do not impose an assessment structure that has been thoroughly tested they leave themselves open to bias, focusing in on areas of particular interest to themselves, potentially not giving due weight to certain issues raised by people who are referred, and emphasising some issues more than others when reporting the findings of their assessment. Each of these dangers is lessened when a practitioner uses a structured scoping or initial assessment founded in a conceptual model of practice. Practitioners are in effect forced to consider the range of aspects covered in the assessment, thus lessening the potential for bias or omission. For example, both the MOHO screening tool (MOHOST; Parkinson et al., 2006) and the COPM (Law et al., 2019) contain specific questions that cover each of the aspects that are included within their respective conceptual models. This assessment structure ensures that individual practitioners gather information about the whole range of occupational functioning (as conceived by each respective model) and are less likely to succumb to personal biases and shortcuts or accidentally omit certain aspect of the assessment.

As with so many areas of practice, research into the superiority of differing assessment approaches is needed before it can be said with confidence whether it is more beneficial to use a top-down assessment approach. However, the well-established literature surrounding heuristics and biases (Gilovich et al., 2002) and existing knowledge about human's limited working memory capacity (Miller, 1956) lends strength to the theoretical arguments that support using a top-down assessment approach.

Finally, this top-down occupation-focused approach to assessment is also coherent with the World Health Organization's (WHO; 2001) International Classification of Functioning, Disability and Health (ICF), which conceptualises a person's level of functioning as a dynamic interaction

VIGNETTE 5.2

The rapid response team has been asked to visit Mr. MacDonald by his general practitioner (GP). He was found, having fallen this morning, by a neighbour. The GP visited and has decided not to admit Mr. MacDonald as he has only sustained minor bruising. However, the GP would like occupational therapy and physiotherapy to assess him and refers Mr. MacDonald to the rapid response service.

The rapid response service is a busy service that responds to referrals within 24 hours. Their priority is to ensure peoples' safety at home. They use a quick checklist to assess the home environment and individuals' functional abilities. They visit Mr. MacDonald in the morning spending about 30 minutes with him. From the assessment, the occupational therapist identifies that a toilet frame, bed rail, and highback chair would improve his safety, and the physiotherapist recommends a walking frame. The team is able to deliver and fit these items the same day.

The occupational therapist is confident that the situation has improved but recognises there are longer-term issues her service is not able to deal with. They recommend that Mr. Macdonald be seen by the community rehabilitation service who can offer a longer-term input aiming to increase his independence and safety. This team conducts a more thorough assessment through interview and observation over two home visits.

---

between one's health conditions, environmental factors, and personal factors.

Work Context

The acceptability and utility of any assessment tool will be influenced by the area of practice an occupational therapist works in. The priorities of the service and time available each influence the selection of appropriate assessments (Vignette 5.2).

In a long-term setting there may be benefits in investing time in comprehensive assessments to ensure that an intervention programme is thorough, while there may not be the time available to conduct several assessments in acute settings where practitioners are required to make quick decisions based on rapid assessments. As in the case of Mr. MacDonald in the vignette, this may result in referral onto another service where longer term needs are suggested.

Decisions about assessments may also be influenced by the clinical specialism; some assessments are designed for particular areas of practice, while others can be applied across most areas. Assessment manuals often provide guidance about when using it would be inappropriate (e.g., using a self-report assessment with a person who has limited insight). Occupational therapists also work in a variety of settings, including hospitals, clinics, and in people's homes. There may be some practical limitations that restrict the available range of assessments for use (e.g., if the equipment is not easily portable).

Occasionally an occupational therapist may be asked to assess an individual only to provide a report (e.g., in a compensation claim). However, usually assessments are a means to an end—that is, to begin, review, or end a programme of intervention. It is therefore important that practitioners consider what to do with the information that they gather.

Standardised assessments provide a structure for organising information into a logical format and may provide information for interpreting the findings. Practitioners may also have gathered information from one or several assessments. Taking time to formulate all the information gathered through the assessment process into a conceptualisation of the individual is an important step in the assessment process and vital to enable appropriate planning of an intervention. The conceptualisation, drawn from the information gathered, will provide a portrait of a person's occupational life and needs. This information should be considered as a whole. In collaborative therapeutic relationships, practitioners should return to the person they are working with, share their understanding, and confirm whether the individual views the situation in a similar way (see Chapter 3 for further information as this issue is often much easier to suggest than to truly achieve). Sharing and confirming your understanding is an important step towards developing shared goals.

Report writing is a useful way of synthesising the findings of assessments, provides a document in the clinical records to demonstrate occupational therapy's intervention, and can be used to compare future assessment findings (see Chapter 11). Some assessments provide a quantitative summary of findings (e.g., the Assessment of Motor and Process Skills [AMPS]; Fisher & Bray Jones, 2012), but a narrative interpretation of findings is also useful to describe what this means for the person in question.

The Type of Information Required

The type of information required will also influence the type of assessment used. Practitioners wishing to gain a broad understanding of a person may decide to use a general screening tool. Alternatively, where more detailed information is desired about an individual's specific abilities, a structured observational measure may be more appropriate. Which assessment is ultimately selected depends on a variety of issues, including individual ability, timing, and the form of assessment the practitioner wishes to undertake.

The Ability of an Individual to Participate in the Assessment Process

People who are nonverbal or have very low levels of concentration will be unable to participate in interviews; people who are unable to read will not be able to complete self-assessment forms without assistance.

The Timing of the Assessment

An assessment at the start of therapy will initially be broad in nature: practitioners will frequently conduct a screening procedure or initial interview to ascertain whether an individual requires occupational therapy, and if so, broadly what the issues are. Towards the end of therapy, assessments are likely to be much more focused to measure (whether narratively or numerically) what difference (if any) occupational therapy intervention has made.

Forms of Assessment

Several different forms of assessment exist and have been mentioned within the chapter so far. Each method of assessment has its strengths and weaknesses.

Case Note Review

Frequently people have already seen several health care professionals before they meet an occupational therapist. Looking through multidisciplinary notes (where available) is an excellent way in which to gain some extra knowledge about people before a practitioner sees them for the first time. Frequently case notes are interdisciplinary, and there may not be separate case notes held by each professional discipline. Either way, there are often medical case notes that are held separately, and these can contain additional valuable background information.

Some practitioners prefer not to look at case notes before they meet someone and may suggest this to students. The rationale for this is that it is best to form your own initial impressions without having your assessment tainted by the clinical information and reasoning of others. There are several other reasons why reviewing people's notes before meeting them is very sensible:

- People may already have related their story, background, and key clinical features to several clinicians before you get involved. Having to repeat this information can be intensely frustrating and gives the impression that services do not communicate with each other.

- Individuals may have recently (or historically) undergone a traumatic life event, which practitioners may inadvertently touch upon during an assessment if they were not aware of them. Examples of this include death of a family member or close friend and experiences of sexual abuse.
- It may be necessary to conduct a risk assessment for meeting someone. Some people may have histories of violent or sexually inappropriate behaviour. It cannot be guaranteed that such information would always be included in a referral. Not knowing this information before a meeting could place the practitioner in danger.
- Case note reviewing can help a practitioner to understand an individual's case and context in much greater detail than most referral forms allow. Reading case notes can assist in developing further areas of assessment such as interviews or observational assessments.

Observation

Observation is an essential assessment skill for every practitioner. Observational assessments can be either structured or unstructured. An excellent example of an unstructured observational assessment process, and the richness of information that can be gained through this process, is recounted in the book *Dibs in Search of Self* (Axline, 1964). This section outlines various forms of observational assessments commonly used in practice.

Using the theoretical framework of the MOHO, observation can also be used to understand both the performance and participation levels of persons' occupational functioning. An observation of performance skills could include assessing their dressing ability poststroke, while an observation of occupational participation could include assessing persons with multiple sclerosis working in their office to see if any adaptations are required. In regard to unstructured observations of individuals' skill level, the practitioner may also wish to conduct a structured observation of their communication and interaction or motor and process skills. Two well-known assessments developed from the MOHO enable practitioners to do this and provide extremely detailed information about people's actual abilities (Fisher & Bray Jones, 2012; Forsyth et al., 1998) (Vignette 5.3).

The environmental location of both participation and performance skills are highly dependent on the environment in which they occur: How persons complete an activity can significantly differ between an occupational therapy department and their home, for example. This differentiation in skill level may be due to environmental differences (e.g., the kitchen in the occupational therapy department is at a more suitable height than the home kitchen), but it can also be due to volitional differences.

VIGNETTE 5.3

Mrs. Harris is a 78-year-old widow, who lives alone and has no local family. After a recent home visit, the district nurse has referred Mrs. Harris to the community rehabilitation team. The district nurse was concerned that Mrs. Harris is not looking after herself and her home environment is deteriorating. The occupational therapist on the team is asked to visit to carry out a functional assessment.

During the visit it quickly becomes apparent that Mrs. Harris is a poor historian and has limited insight into the difficulties she is experiencing; she does not know why the district nurse has asked for this assessment. When discussing her daily routine Mrs. Harris reports going to the shops every morning, and coming home to do some housework before cooking her own lunch. There is only out-of-date food in the fridge and no signs of recent cooking even though it is early afternoon. The occupational therapist decides that to get an objective assessment of Mrs. Harris's abilities she should carry out an AMPS assessment. This is suggested to Mrs. Harris, who agrees.

Volition is most easily understood as the thoughts and feelings people have about what they have done, are doing, and will be doing in the future (Lee & Kielhofner, 2017). Volitional deficits can have a significant effect on a person's functioning. Some people may be able to accurately articulate these issues, others (such as individuals with severe mental health needs or learning difficulties) will find this harder. In these cases, it is useful to carry out an observational assessment.

While it can therefore be very important to observe an individual in the environment in which the activity will normally take place, it can also be useful, depending on the reason for the assessment, to observe a person in a variety of settings. This variation in environment can be used to good effect to demonstrate an individual's occupational potential. The Volitional Questionnaire (de las Heras et al., 2007) (a structured assessment developed from the MOHO) provides an excellent method of measuring volition through observation. This assessment can be used to good effect when a practitioner wishes to understand in greater depth why an individual performs better in one environment than another, or to demonstrate the significance of this altered behaviour to other members of the clinical team.

Interviews

At their most basic level, interviews involve a practitioner asking questions from an individual to gain a better picture of the individual's occupational performance. Like observation, interviews can generally be categorised as unstructured or structured.

Unstructured Interviews

Unstructured interviews are those in which the practitioner is not following a standardised interview assessment or formal information-gathering schedule.

Unstructured interviews may vary in their formality and presentation. At their most informal, a practitioner may conduct an unstructured interview whilst participating in another task. An example of this is the interview that occurs when an individual and practitioner are jointly preparing a meal, doing the dishes, or driving somewhere in a car. Participating in such activities can make information sharing for some people much easier, and often a practitioner is able to gather more information from a person whilst participating in such tasks than when formally sitting down in a room together with the specific aim of talking!

Of course, it will often be appropriate and feasible to sit down together to interview a person. In these situations, even when the interview is unstructured, it is important to consider factors that will improve the interview process. These factors can be broadly categorised as expectations (of both practitioner and individual) and environment (where the interview will take place) and are equally relevant and worthy of consideration when carrying out structured assessments.

People should be informed in advance of the reason for an interview, the time and location that it will take place, and the length of time it will take. Having provided appropriate information practitioners should also have gained people's consent to be interviewed.

The physical and social environment where an interview is to take place should be closely considered. Interviews should be carried out in a peaceful setting, free from distractions and interruptions. Let other people know that an interview is taking place so that unnecessary interruptions are avoided. Consideration should be given to the seating arrangements of both parties: a 90-degree angle of seats that are comfortable and allow the feet of both practitioner and individual to be flat on the floor is ideal (Fig. 5.1). Seats should be the same height so neither party is looking up or down on the other. It is important that people are as relaxed as possible during interviews, so practitioners need to employ all their skills in the therapeutic use of self (see Chapter 9).

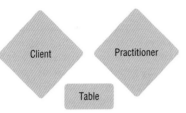

FIG. 5.1 Seating plan for one-to-one interviews.

Structured Interviews

Structured assessments have a relatively fixed format. They may form the basis of an initial assessment developed by a department or service, which contains a list of questions that are asked of everyone who enters the service. Alternatively, a practitioner may wish to gather particular information about occupational functioning and may use a structured assessment from a conceptual model of practice. One such example is the Occupational Circumstances Assessment Interview and Rating Scale (OCAIRS) (Forsyth et al., 2005), which is developed from the MOHO and now has specific formats and guiding questions for physical, general mental health, and forensic settings (Vignette 5.4). It is important to read the instructions for all structured assessments carefully because some require the use of precise words in questions, whilst others (including the majority of those associated with the MOHO) provide examples of questions to use but have specific guidelines for scoring the assessment. Familiarity with structured interview assessments is essential to enable the interview to flow smoothly. They can feel awkward to use at first, due to a lack of experience, but frequent use helps practitioners to feel more comfortable with them, which in turn helps the interview to flow more like a good conversation.

Self-Report Questionnaires and Checklists

Self-report questionnaires and checklists are commonly used in practice. They can be generic, such as measures of disability and functional impairment (e.g., WHO Disability Assessment Schedule 2.0 [Üstün et al., 2010]), of depression (e.g., Patient Health Questionnaire–9 [Kroenke & Spitzer, 2002]), or occupation specific such as measures of individuals' self-assessment of their occupational roles (Role Checklist [Scott, 2019]) or occupational competence (Occupational Self-Assessment [Baron et al., 2003]). Whilst questionnaires and checklists do not provide a depth of information about a person, they can be very useful methods of gathering specific information.

When deciding whether to use a self-report method of assessment consideration should be given to the individual's eyesight quality, as well as reading, comprehension, and concentration levels.

Assessments That Combine Information-Gathering Methods

Some assessment measures do not fit nicely into either observation, interview or self-report categories, as they use a combination of methods to gather information. Two examples of such measures are the MOHOST (Parkinson, 2006) and COPM (Law et al., 2019).

The MOHOST was developed by a group of practitioners in the United Kingdom who worked with people who were very low functioning. The practitioners wished to use a broad screening assessment to gather information about the general occupational functioning difficulties of the people they worked with, but they found the interview structure of assessments such as the OCAIRS (Forsyth et al., 2005) too intense and challenging for this population. Over time and in collaboration with academic

---

VIGNETTE 5.4

James is a long-term user of mental health services, who lives independently in the community supported by his keyworker (a community psychiatric nurse). The keyworker is concerned that he is isolated and has no social network. She has discussed her concerns with the occupational therapist (Beth); they plan a joint visit for James's next appointment.

However, on introducing James to Beth he immediately refuses to work with her. James explains that he has seen occupational therapists in the past and they always wanted him to join sports and art groups. He tells her he has no interest in these activities. Beth asks him about what he does enjoy, and he tells her about his interest in computers. Beth explains that if he were to agree to work with her, she would initially interview him using the OCAIRS (Forsyth et al., 2005). Beth explained that this would help her to fully understand what is important to him and what, if any, difficulties he was having. Beth told James she would then share her assessment with him and then they would be able to discuss what they could work on together. She guaranteed that as James was not interested in sports or art group, she would not ask him to attend these. Beth recognised that by using this interview as an initial assessment her intervention could be tailored to James's specific needs and they could work in collaboration to set meaningful goals.

VIGNETTE 5.5

Potter House is a new residential rehabilitation unit built in the community as an intermediary step between hospital and independent tenancy as part of the neurorehabilitation service. The multiprofessional team has been asked to consider appropriate assessments to be used at monthly intervals during a person's stay in the unit. It is planned that residents will be in the unit for between 3 and 12 months.

The practitioner considers that it will be important to gain a comprehensive picture of a person's occupations in self-care, work, and leisure pursuits; they want to be able to identify areas of need and the individual's priorities.

They are particularly aware that while in hospital people tend to follow the routine of the busy ward and priorities tend to be set by the clinical team. This has led to people finding it difficult on discharge as they feel overwhelmed with the responsibility of planning for the future. The occupational therapist decides to use the COPM. The therapist recognises that this assessment gathers information about people's self-perception of their occupational performance and facilitates individuals setting their own priorities for rehabilitation. The therapist anticipates that through supporting people in setting their own goals the transition to independence may be assisted.

---

colleagues they developed the MOHOST. Whilst primarily an observational measure, information can also be gathered through case note review, interview, and even third-party information gathering from relatives or other care staff to inform the scoring of the MOHOST.

The COPM (Law et al., 2019) combines an interview format with a self-report rating of satisfaction and importance. This assessment is closely linked with the COPM-E and addresses the three occupational performance areas covered by the model: self-care, productivity, and leisure (Vignette 5.5).

STANDARDISED AND NONSTANDARDISED ASSESSMENTS

Standardised Assessments

The final area of concern with regard to choosing assessments raised by the AHP Outcome Measures UK Working Group (2019) is the measurement properties of assessments. Measurement properties of assessments are improved through standardisation procedures. Assessments can be standardised in two main ways: in terms of their process, materials, and scoring instructions; and by normative standardisation (i.e., by providing statistics that outline what healthy so-called normal individuals could expect to score on the assessment) (Simon & Kramer, 2020). Grampurohit (2020) outlines the importance of standardised assessments for occupational therapists. Standardised assessments can provide objective information about the health status or occupational functioning of a person. Such objectivity is important as it provides a very useful outcome measurement of a person's progress and can form the basis of decision making that is more defensible than a practitioner's judgement alone. Further, and as previously discussed, human memory is very fallible (Schacter, 2011),

and self-reporting is recognised to be a very subjective process, with tenuous reliability and open to numerous biases. All of these reasons provide a sound rationale for using standardised assessments. Taking these factors into account Laver Fawcett (2014) rightly concludes that it is an ethical responsibility to select, use, and report standardised outcome measures and to contribute valid and reliable outcome measures to service evaluation and research. Given this, why do nonstandardised assessments continue to be used in practice?

Nonstandardised Assessments

Nonstandardised assessments continue to form a part of practitioners' assessment toolkit for a variety of reasons, some of which are more defensible than others! These include:

- Lack of an existing structured (standardised) assessment (Forsyth, 2017)
- Individual resistance to completing a standardised assessment (Forsyth, 2017)
- Augment information collected by standardised assessments (Forsyth, 2017)
- An opportunity presents itself to gather information and the practitioner is unable to use a standardised measure (Forsyth, 2017)
- Lack of training or confidence in using standardised assessments
- Standardisation of assessment process being perceived as a lack of flexibility
- Unhelpful culture of the therapeutic environment (e.g., "Standardised assessments! We don't use those here!")
- Lack of accountability (practitioners are still too rarely called to account for the differences they do/or do not make in peoples' lives)

Nonstandardised assessments lend themselves to those serendipitous moments in therapy when a person shares some information during the course of intervention that helps the practitioner to understand their occupational performance in a new or more profound manner. Further, there is no standardised measure that can help a practitioner to understand what it means to an individual to be affected by the illness or disability they themselves are experiencing. However, this does not mean that due care and attention should not be made to the process of gathering this sort of information. Forsyth (2017) outlines three strategies that support the dependability of the information gathered by unstructured means: evaluating context, triangulation, and validity checks.

Evaluating Context

The circumstances in which a person shares information often influences the degree of confidence a practitioner has in the information received: Information shared by a child who is refusing to go to school may be interpreted quite differently if given in the presence of their schoolteacher than in a one-to-one interview scenario.

Triangulation

Information that is yielded in a nonstructured assessment should be checked, using an alternative source, for accuracy: This can be achieved by observing the person do the activity they discussed or by asking another person who knows them well (e.g., nurse or spouse) for their perspective of the situation.

Validity Checks

It is important that practitioners ensure that their understanding of information shared is accurate. This can be done by:
- Reflecting on the information and asking if it fits with what is already known about the person
- Continuing to collect information through a variety of assessment methods to either confirm or refute the information already gathered
- Checking with the person to see if there is agreement with the practitioner's interpretation

Thus, although Laver Fawcett's (2014) argument that lack of use of standardised assessments, where they are already developed, could place practitioners and people at risk is true, sound reasons to use nonstandardised assessments also exist (Forsyth, 2017). The challenge for the discerning practitioner is to have the skill to know when to use each to their best effect.

SUMMARY

This chapter has described what, why, where, and when practitioners should consider undertaking assessments in practice. Basic information about the various types of

assessments and the appropriate stages at which assessments could be carried out were presented. More contemporary issues, such as whether a top-down approach to conducting assessments is appropriate, were also discussed. It was suggested that, while objective evidence of the superiority of a top-down assessment approach over a more traditional assessment strategy is still lacking, there are well-grounded theoretical arguments that support the use of an assessment strategy that commences with the selection of an occupation-focused conceptual model of practice and initially uses assessments drawn from the model.

REFERENCES

Allied Health Professions (AHP) Outcome Measures UK Working Group. (2019). *Key questions to ask when selecting outcome measures: A checklist for allied health professionals.* Royal College of Speech and Language.

American Occupational Therapy Association (AOTA). (2020). Occupational therapy practice framework: Domain and process (4th ed.). *American Journal of Occupational Therapy, 74*(S2).

Axline, V. M. (1964). *Dibs in search of self.* Mansion.

Baron, K., Kielhofner, G., Iyenger, A., Goldhammer, V., & Wolenski, J. (2003). *The occupational self-assessment, version 2.1.* University of Illinois, Model of Human Occupation Clearinghouse.

de las Heras, C. G., Geist, R., Kielhofner, G., & Li, Y. (2007). *The volitional questionnaire (version 4.1).* University of Illinois, Model of Human Occupation Clearinghouse.

Doucet, B. M., & Gutman, S. A. (2013). Quantifying function: The rest of the measurement story. *American Journal of Occupational Therapy, 67*(1), 7–9.

Fisher, A. G., & Bray Jones, K. (2012). In *Assessment of motor and process skills. Development, standardization, and administration manual* (vol. 1). (7th rev. ed.). Three Star Press.

Forsyth, K. (2017). Assessment: Choosing and using standardized and nonstandardized means of gathering information. In R. R. Taylor (Ed.), *Kielhofner's model of human occupation: Theory and application* (pp. 173–186). Wolters Kluwer.

Forsyth, K., Deshpande, S., Kielhofner, G., Henriksson, C., Haglund, L., Olson, L., Skinner, S. and Kulkarni, S. (2005). *Occupational circumstances assessment and interview rating scale (v. 4).* University of Illinois, Model of Human Occupation Clearinghouse.

Forsyth, K., Salamy, M., Simon, S., & Kielhofner, G. (1998). *Assessment of communication and interactional skills (v. 4).* University of Illinois, Model of Human Occupation Clearinghouse.

Gilovich, T., Griffin, D., & Kahneman, D. (Eds.). (2002). *Heuristics and biases: The psychology of intuitive judgment.* Cambridge University Press.

Grampurohit, N. (2020). Psychometric properties related to standardized assessments: Understanding the evidence for reliability, validity and responsiveness. In J. Hinojosa, & P. Kramer (Eds.), *Evaluation in occupational therapy: Obtaining and interpreting data* (pp. 109–122). American Occupational Therapy Association.

Health Professions Council. (2018). Standards of proficiency for occupational therapists. Accessed at https://www.hcpc-uk.org/standards/standards-of-proficiency/occupational-therapists.

Iwama, M. K., Thomson, N. A., & Macdonald, R. M. (2009). The Kawa model: The power of culturally responsive occupational therapy. *Disability and Rehabilitation, 31*(14), 1125–1135.

Kramer, P. (2020). Philosophical and theoretical influences on evaluation. In J. Hinojosa, & P. Kramer (Eds.), *Evaluation in occupational therapy: Obtaining and interpreting data* (pp. 13–24). American Occupational Therapy Association.

Kroenke, K., & Spitzer, R. L. (2002). The PHQ-9: A new depression diagnostic and severity measure. *Psychiatric Annals, 32*(9), 509–515.

Laver Fawcett, A. (2014). Routine standardised outcome measurement to evaluate the effectiveness of occupational therapy interventions: Essential or optional? *Ergoterapeuten, 4,* 28–37.

Law, M., Baptiste, S., Carswell, A., McColl, M. A., Polatajko, H., & Pollock, N. (2019). In *Canadian occupational performance measure* (5th rev. ed.). COPM Inc.

Lee, S. W., & Kielhofner, G. (2017). Volition. In R. R. Taylor (Ed.), *Kielhofner's model of human occupation: Theory and application* (pp. 38–56). Wolters Kluwer.

Miller, G. A. (1956). The magical number seven, plus or minus two: Some limits on our capacity for processing information. *Psychological Review, 63*(2), 81.

Paley, J., Cheyne, H., Dalgleish, L., Duncan, E. A., & Niven, C. A. (2007). Nursing's ways of knowing and dual process theories of cognition. *Journal of Advanced Nursing, 60*(6), 692–701.

Parkinson, S., Forsyth, K., & Kielhofner, G. (2006). *The model of human occupation screening tool (MOHOST) (version 2.0).*

University of Illinois, Model of Human Occupation Clearinghouse.

Pentland, D., Kantartzis, S., Clausen, M. G., & Witemyre, K. (2018). *Occupational therapy and complexity: Defining and describing practice.* Royal College of Occupational Therapists.

Polatajko, H. J., Townsend, E. A., & Craik, J. (2007). Canadian model of occupational performance and engagement (CMOP-E). In *Enabling occupation II: Advancing an occupational therapy vision of health, well-being & justice through occupation* (p. 23). Canadian Association of Occupational Therapists.

Schacter, D. L. (2011). *How the mind forgets and remembers: The seven sins of memory.* Souvenir Press.

Scott, P. J. (2019). *Role checklist (V3) participation and satisfaction.* University of Illinois, Model of Human Occupation Clearinghouse.

Simon, R. L., & Kramer, P. (2020). Administration of evaluation and assessments. In J. Hinojosa, & P. Kramer (Eds.), *Evaluation in occupational therapy: Obtaining and interpreting data* (pp. 63–76). American Occupational Therapy Association.

Taylor, R. R. (Ed.). (2017). *Kielhofner's model of human occupation: Theory and application.* Wolters Kluwer.

Üstün, T. B., Kostanjsek, N., Chatterji, S., & Rehm, J. (Eds.). (2010). Measuring health and disability: Manual for WHO disability assessment schedule (WHODAS 2.0). World Health Organization.

World Health Organization. (2001). The international classification of functioning, disability and health (ICF). http://www.who.int/classifications/icf/en/.

6

Activity Analysis

Kirsty Forsyth

HIGHLIGHTS

- Activity analysis is the process for finding and/or adjusting an occupation to achieve some therapeutic benefit or allow a person to engage in a former or new occupational role.
- The demands of an occupation can only be identified in relation to the client or client group who is receiving occupational therapy.

- Analysis that is based on theory provides the additional benefits of the explanatory power of theory to identify the activity characteristics and how they influence a client.
- This chapter presents a theory-driven approach to activity analysis consisting of four steps.

OVERVIEW

Activity analysis is a process for finding and/or adjusting an occupation to achieve some therapeutic benefit or allow a person to engage in a former or new occupational role. Its aim is to find a fit between the characteristics and needs of a client or client group and an occupation. While there are a number of approaches to activity analysis, basing it on theory both provides a structure for the analysis and brings the explanatory power of theory to help identify activity characteristics and how they influence a client or group.

This chapter presents a theory-driven approach to activity analysis. It begins by identifying key principles underlying activity analysis. Then the chapter presents and discusses four key steps in theory-driven activity analysis. The application of these steps is illustrated through the following case examples.

Selma is an occupational therapist providing service to Elsie, a 72-year-old who has osteoarthritis as well as a fracture in her right dominant hand, and is having challenges bathing. Elsie has been referred to occupational therapy. The therapist needs to complete an analysis of the bathing challenges for Elsie, to support her reengaging with this activity.

Vincent is an occupational therapist providing services to children with special needs in a primary school classroom. He typically works with pupils (students) who have cerebral palsy and are integrated into regular classrooms. A common task Vincent must address is how to enable these pupils to engage in typical classroom activities such as taking notes and completing exams.

Gwen works as an occupational therapist in a residential home. The director of the residential home has approached her and asked if she could initiate some group activities designed to reduce the social isolation observed among many residents with limited cognitive function. Gwen is concerned to identify group activities she can implement that provide opportunities for engaging in meaningful activities but that will not be too difficult for the residents. Additionally, she recognises that since all groups are voluntary she will need to find activities that will be motivating to entice residents to participate.

Philip is an occupational therapist working in an industrial setting. His responsibilities typically include making recommendations for how clients with a variety of impairments can complete work tasks efficiently and without sustaining further injury.

While each of the practitioners described here face quite different tasks, each will have to engage in a process that is ordinarily referred to in occupational therapy as activity analysis. The aim of this chapter is to provide a practical approach to activity analysis in the context of contemporary practice, which emphasises the importance of theory and evidence.

OVERVIEW OF ACTIVITY ANALYSIS

Activity analysis is one of the oldest occupational therapy processes. It emerged out of occupational therapists' need to find and/or adjust an occupation to achieve some therapeutic benefit or allow a person to engage in a former or new occupational role. Basically, the core of all activity analysis is to find a fit between the characteristics and needs of a client or client group and an occupation. The analysis of occupations and their use within therapy is one of the unique skills of the occupational therapist (Duncan, 2021). Despite being an essential skill for any occupational therapist, there is not a single definition or set of agreed-upon procedures for activity analysis in the field. In fact, a variety of different discussions can be found on the topic over the decades (Bryant et al., 2014; Crepeau, 2003; Fidler & Fidler, 1963; Lamport et al., 2001; Mosey, 1986; Schell et al., 2019).

Discussions of activity analysis do agree that the core of the analysis involves asking questions about the occupation. These questions are designed to help the practitioner understand what doing the occupation involves and what therapeutic potential the activity might have. The following are examples of the types of questions one might ask about an occupation. Is it a simple or complex occupation? Where does the occupation take place? What are the stages or sequences of the occupation? Does the occupation require more than one performer? Sometimes the questions that are asked are based on the type of client or client group that the therapist has in mind when doing the activity analysis. So, for instance, if the client has an impairment that affects movement, the practitioner may focus on asking questions about the kinds of movements required for doing the occupation.

Some authors offer a structure for doing activity analysis. In some instances, these structures try to include all things that need to be considered to determine what capacities are needed for doing an occupation. This approach to activity analysis will seek to describe physical, sensory, cognitive, social, emotional, and cultural demands of the occupation. Box 6.1 shows an example of such a structured approach to activity analysis.

Occupational theories have long been advocated as an appropriate framework for activity analysis (Crepeau, 2003; Katz and Toglia 2018). Crepeau (2003) outlined theory-focused activity analysis. This approach to activity analysis examines the properties of an activity from the perspective of a particular practice theory. She notes that this approach is most appropriate when analysing an occupation in terms of its appropriateness for a particular client or a particular group of clients who share a common impairment or challenge.

This chapter takes the position that activity analysis should always be theory driven. An analysis that is based on theory provides the additional benefits of the explanatory power of theory. Using an occupational therapy theory as the structure for activity analysis serves not only to provide a structure or a framework for the analysis but also an explanation of how the elements identified operate together to support or prevent a person engaging with occupation. Traditional structured approaches to activity analysis that provides lists of issues to consider (or lists of questions) offer the first part of what a theory offers (i.e., a structure), but they cannot provide the explanation that enriches the activity analysis making it more comprehensive.

TOWARDS A DEFINITION OF THEORY-DRIVEN ACTIVITY ANALYSIS

Before discussing the process of theory-driven activity analysis, some key principles that should guide the process are outlined.

Principle 1: Theory-Driven Activity Analysis Should Reflect the Occupation-Centred Approach That Characterises the Field's Contemporary Perspective

From the early 1990s onwards, occupational therapy has emphasised that practice should be occupation focused (Christiansen, 1999; Clark, 1993; Fisher, 1998, 2014; Gillen & Greber, 2014; Polatajko, 1994; Trombly, 1993, 1995; Wong & Fisher, 2015; Wood, 1998). Along with this is the theme that, while underlying performance components are recognised as necessary to occupational performance, they must always be viewed in the larger context of the client's occupational life. This top-down approach (Trombly, 1993) means that thinking in occupational therapy always begins with asking what clients want and need to do in their occupational lives and then proceeds to consideration of personal and environmental barriers and supports to performance.

Principle 2: Theory-Driven Activity Analysis Should Be Part of the Therapeutic Reasoning Process Whereby Practitioners Plan a Course of Action for a Particular Client or a Group of Clients

Analysis is most useful when it is employed as a step in the therapeutic reasoning that guides practice with a given client or client group. As noted at the beginning of this chapter, analysis is undertaken to make specific decisions about selecting and adapting an occupation to meet the needs of a specific client or group. Thus the analysis occurs and relational questions arise about how the characteristics of an occupation compare with the characteristics of a client or group. Analysis therefore should always be done

BOX 6.1

Having identified the purpose, sequence, and duration of the performance of the activity and the spaces, tools, and materials required, it may be necessary to ask any of the following questions and to identify how, when, and where within the activity or tasks any particular skills or changes in demands and requirements are needed.

Physical Skills
Position
What is the starting position when carrying out the activity—sitting, standing, lying?
Any changes that occur during the sequence of performance of the activity?

Movements
Which joints are involved and what movements are required?
Which muscle groups are involved at specific stages?
What ranges of specific movements are required at each joint?
Is the action unilateral or bilateral?
Is the movement required: active, static, or passive?
Repetitive assisted or resisted? Fast, slow, smooth, or irregular?

Strength
Does the activity require a high, moderate, or low level of muscle strength?
Is the effort continuous or intermittent?
Does the activity require high, medium, or low levels of stamina and endurance?

Coordination
Does the activity require gross or fine motor coordination?
Is the coordination unilateral or bilateral?
Where does the coordination take place: hand/hand, hand/eye, lower limbs?

Hand Function
Does the activity require grip: cylinder, ball, hook, plate, pincer, tripod grip?
What levels of manipulative or dexterous movements are needed?
Are any precise actions needed?
Are both hands required equally?

Sensory and Perceptual Skills
Does the activity require vision: short and/or long distance, colour recognition?
Auditory: Is hearing necessary to identify particular sounds, tones, or volume?

Gustatory: Does the activity involve the ability to identify or discriminate between tastes?
Olfactory: Is the ability to identify or discriminate between smells necessary?
Touch: Does the activity require gross or fine sensation? Is the ability to distinguish shapes, textures, or temperatures necessary?
Are stereognosis, proprioceptive, or vestibular skills required?

Cognitive Skills
Is the level of thinking concrete or abstract?
What level of concentration does the activity require? Is it constant or changing?
Is short-term, long-term, or procedural memory required?
Are organisational skills needed: logical thinking, planning, decision making, problem solving?
Is specific level of numeracy or literacy required?
Does the activity involve time recognition and time management skills?
What levels of responsibility and control does the activity involve?
Are there any opportunities for use of imagination, creativity, or improvisation?

Social Interaction Skills
Is the activity carried out with others?
Is the interaction formal or informal, cooperative, competitive, in parallel or compliant?
What forms of communication are involved: receptive (listening and interpreting), expressive (verbal, written, technological), nonverbal, touch?
Does the activity involve attention to others through debate or negotiation?

Emotional Skills
Does the activity require insight or ability for expression?
Are attitudes and values inherent in the activity?
Is the activity likely to demand conflict, handling feelings, testing reality, or role identity?
Does the activity require patience managing impulses or self-control?

Cultural Demands
Is the activity specific to certain cultural groups in terms of gender, ethnicity, class, or age?
What is the sociocultural symbolic meaning of the activity?
Does the activity require particular cultural values, approaches, or techniques?

to determine how the occupation can be used as part of therapy or modified to allow the clients to engage in occupation as part of their overall occupational participation. Analysis is always undertaken with reference to a particular individual or group. To illustrate this point, it is helpful to return to the examples from the beginning of this chapter. In these instances, analysis would be undertaken to:

- Determine how to change the environment to support Elsie engage in bathing
- Determine how typical classroom occupations can be adapted to allow pupils with cerebral palsy to do them
- Identify occupations appropriate for implementation with a group of adults with cognitive impairments
- Recommend strategies for clients with impairments to complete work occupations efficiently and safely

Principle 3: Theory Driven–Activity Analysis Should Be Both Theoretical and Empirical

The most efficient way to do analysis that is theoretical and empirical is to base it on conceptual practice models. Conceptual practice models are bodies of knowledge in occupational therapy that provide explanations of some phenomena of practical concern in the field, while providing a rationale and methods for therapy (Kielhofner, 2009). Since conceptual practice models include both theoretical concepts and empirical testing of those concepts and their application in therapy, using them allows a practitioner to be both theoretically and empirically based when doing analysis. Practice-based theories have the added advantage of providing an understanding of how different elements of analysis relate to each other and provides an insight into the change process (Creek, 2002).

Each model of practice addresses different phenomena. Most of the traditional models (biomechanical, sensory integration, cognitive disabilities, cognitive-perceptual, motor control) address some aspect of the underlying capacity for performing occupation. In contrast, the model of human occupation (MOHO) (Taylor, 2017) addresses the motivation for occupation, the lifestyle or pattern of occupation in a person's life, and the environmental context. This model also offers a unique view of skills (Taylor, 2017) that have been recommended as an important dimension of task/activity analysis (Crepeau, 2003; Watson & Wilson, 2003).

Let us briefly consider how these principles would frame analysis by returning to one of the examples at the start of this chapter. Consider Vincent who typically works with children who have cerebral palsy in a mainstream school. Vincent will routinely use analysis to determine what gaps exist between the physical, interpersonal, cognitive, and sociocultural demands of the various activities required for being a student and the characteristics of the students

he serves. His use of analysis will help him recommend ways that the student can be better integrated into the daily activity stream of a classroom. His analysis will lead him to a series of solutions that enable children to engage in the occupational role of student. To undertake analysis Vincent can use the MOHO as a broad framework for considering the interpersonal, social, and cultural aspects of the analysis as well as the skills involved in classroom activities. He can also employ the motor control model that addresses issues of movement that these children face. To the extent that his clients may have cognitive or sensory problems he might also employ other models that address these concerns as well. Because his analysis is guided by these conceptual practice models, he would go beyond a simple taxonomy of elements to consider and instead be able to create a more in-depth explanation of the gaps between necessary activities and his pupils' characteristics, which will guide him in seeking ways to close those gaps. Vincent would also have the reassurance that the conceptual practice models that he uses have an identifiable evidence base.

THE PROCESS OF THEORY-DRIVEN ACTIVITY ANALYSIS

This section presents a process of theory-driven activity analysis consisting of four steps. These steps are as follows:

- Identify the appropriate practice model(s) to guide the analysis
- Select the occupation to be analysed
- Generate questions to guide the analysis
- Identify ways the occupation(s) can be adapted and/or graded

The following section discusses the four steps of analysis in detail. The process of activity analysis will be illustrated with one of the cases presented at the start of this chapter: Selma is a practitioner who is supporting Elsie with bathing challenges.

Step 1. Identify the Appropriate Practice Model(s) to Guide the Analysis

Before selecting the models one should reflect on the person or group for which the analysis is being done. It is the characteristics of the person or group for which the analysis is being done that should influence the choice of conceptual practice models to be used for the activity analysis.

The conceptual practice model(s) chosen to guide the analysis should reflect the following:

- The occupational and client-centred focus of contemporary practice
- The unique impairment status of the client

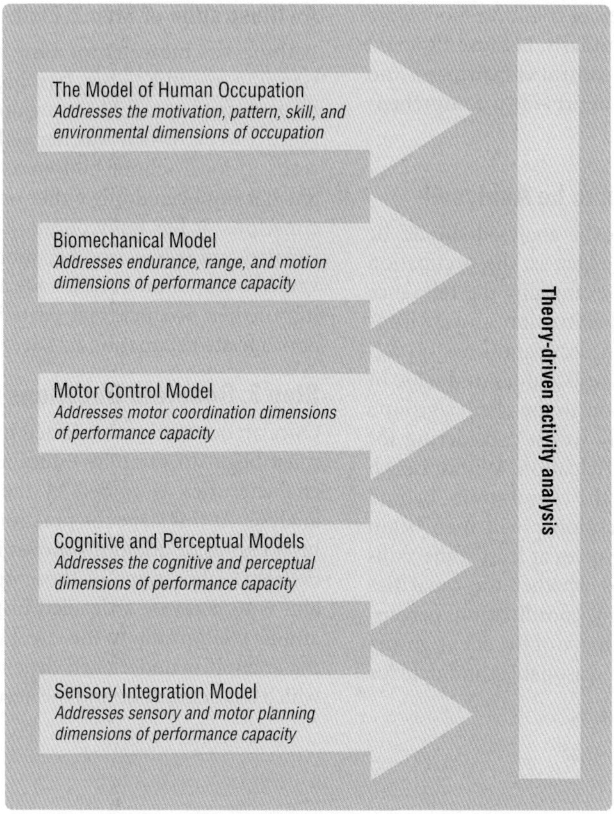

FIG. 6.1 Theory-driven activity analysis.

The MOHO provides a comprehensive view of key aspects of occupation and client centredness (Taylor, 2017). MOHO is one of the most frequently used modes in occupational therapy practice (Lee et al., 2008). Moreover, it is designed to be used in combination with models that address performance components and therefore easily dovetails with such models.

In addition to MOHO, one should select additional models that address the impairment(s) experienced by the client or client group. If the client has a cognitive impairment, one should choose an appropriate cognitive model; if the client has muscle weakness, one should choose the biomechanical model. If the client has problems controlling motion, one should choose the motor control model. Moreover, if the client has problems with all these, one should include all the relevant models (Fig. 6.1).

Illustration of Step 1: Selecting Models for an Analysis of Bathing for Elsie

Elsie is a 72-year-old Scottish woman who has osteoarthritis and is having difficulty bathing. As described, MOHO would be appropriate to understand the broader occupational issues Elsie faces in relation to bathing. MOHO provides an analysis structure for considering such factors as the value of bathing for Elsie, the usual routine within which the bathing occupation happens, the responsibilities Elsie holds that are reliant on bathing, and the sense of efficacy Elsie feels towards bathing. MOHO will also call attention to the physical and social environment and how it may impact on Elsie's bathing. In short, MOHO provides an analysis framework that views bathing in the context of Elsie's occupational participation. Additionally, MOHO will provide a detailed framework for examining what skills Elsie will need to employ to complete bathing.

Other models of practice will also be important for this analysis. Because Elsie has osteoarthritis, has fractured her right dominant hand, and has orthopaedic limitations, the biomechanical model would provide a structure for considering whether Elsie has the strength and range of motion to get in and out of the bath and whether she has enough endurance to complete bathing safely.

On review of medical notes and feedback from the multidisciplinary team it would be noted that Elsie did not have any cognitive challenges and therefore cognitive models are not necessary for this analysis. Similarly, because Elsie did not have any sensory or motor control impairments, no additional models were required to provide a comprehensive analysis of her bathing.

Step 2: Select the Occupation to be Analysed

Selection of the occupation(s) to be analysed should be guided by a top-down approach. That is, the occupation selection should always begin by examining the relevance of the occupation to the volition, habituation, and environment of the client or group. If an occupation has no relevance to the person's/group's interests, values, and sense of competence and if it is not relevant to the client's/group's roles or lifestyle, then it is hardly worth considering for occupational engagement or participation. Without such relevance, it has no meaning for the client/group. Behind these first considerations, a practitioner will then begin to ask whether the occupation involves at least some skills that the client/group possess and whether the capacities required (e.g., strength, movement, coordination, perception, and cognition) overlap with those of the client/group. If not, then the occupation is not a reasonable candidate for the client/group.

An Illustration of Step 2: Elsie

Bathing has meaning for Elsie and is a part of her long-standing routine. Elsie has high standards of personal hygiene for herself. She previously attended a social club twice a week, which was her only leisure activity. She also reads to local schoolchildren as a volunteer once a week. She has not been doing either occupation because she feels conscious of her body odour. This is causing Elsie to feel isolated and is lowering her mood. Bathing, therefore, is a valued occupation in Elsie's life and is significantly impacting on her occupational participation. It is therefore an appropriate occupation to select for analysis.

Step 3: Generate Questions to Guide the Analysis

Once an occupation is selected for analysis, the practitioner must begin to carefully examine it in light of the client's characteristics as guided by the model(s) being used for analysis. At this stage the practitioner moves from the more broad kinds of questions shown in Table 6.1 to much more detailed elaborations of those questions in Table 6.2. The aim is to generate a detailed inspection of the occupation and its relationship to the client's characteristics. Thus how the analysis is undertaken depends on the client/group for which it is being done and the needs that are being addressed.

TABLE 6.1 Examples of Broad Questions to Guide Analysis

MOHO-Based Questions

What is Elsie's sense of efficacy with bathing?
Does Elsie value bathing? If so, why?
Does Elsie find bathing enjoyable?
What is Elsie's routine of bathing?
When in the day does Elsie bathe?
Does Elsie have full responsibility of bathing?
What of Elsie's responsibilities are dependent on bathing?
What physical and/or mental capacities are affecting her bathing?
What physical environment does Elsie bathe in?
What social supports does Elsie have to support bathing?

Biomechanical-Based Questions

What range of motion does Elsie have at her knee joints?
What muscle strength does Elsie have in her limbs?
Do Elsie's physical capacities allow Elsie to transfer in and out of the bath?
Does Elsie have reduced strength in her right dominant hand following her fracture?
Does Elsie have enough physical endurance to complete the full bathing occupation?
Does Elsie have pain anywhere that restricts movement?
Does Elsie have enough physical flexibility to be able to reach her toes and her back while bathing?
Does Elsie have contractures that may be restricting range of motion or strength?

MOHO, Model of human occupation.

TABLE 6.2 Examples of Detailed MOHO Questions to Guide Analysis

MOTOR SKILLS

Posture: Can Elsie stabilise and align her body while moving and in relation to bathing objects?

Can Elsie steady her body and maintain trunk control and balance while sitting, standing, walking, reaching, or while moving, lifting, or pulling objects while bathing?

Can Elsie maintain the vertical alignment of the body over the base of support while bathing?

Can Elsie place her arms and body in relation to bathing objects in a manner that promotes efficient arm movements?

Mobility: Can Elsie Move Her Entire Body or a Body Part in Space When Bathing?

Can Elsie ambulate on level surfaces, including turning around and changing direction while bathing?

Can Elsie stretch or extend her arm and, when appropriate, her trunk to grasp or place bathing objects that are out of reach?

Can Elsie actively flex, rotate, or twist her body in a manner and direction appropriate to bathing?

Coordination: Can Elsie move body parts in relationship to each other and to the bathing environment?

Can Elsie use different parts of her body together to support or stabilise bathing objects during bilateral motor tasks?

Can Elsie use dexterous grasp and release, as well as coordinated in-hand manipulation patterns while bathing?

Can Elsie use smooth, fluid, continuous, uninterrupted arm and hand movements while bathing?

Strength and Effort: Can Elsie generate muscle force appropriate to actions needed in bathing?

Can Elsie push, shove, pull, or drag bathing objects along a supporting surface or about a weight bearing axis?

Can Elsie carry bathing objects while ambulating or moving from one place to another?

Can Elsie raise or hoist bathing objects off a supporting surface?

Can Elsie regulate or grade the force, speed, and extent of movements?

Can Elsie pinch or grasp to securely hold handles or other bathing objects?

Energy: Can Elsie have enough physical exertion and sustained effort over time while bathing?

Can Elsie persist and complete an activity without evidence of fatigue, pausing to rest, or stopping to catch her breath?

Can Elsie maintain a rate or tempo of performance across an entire bathing occupation?

PROCESS DOMAINS AND SKILLS

Energy: Can Elsie sustain and appropriately allocate mental energy while bathing?

Can Elsie maintain a rate or tempo of performance across an entire bathing experience?

Can Elsie maintain attention focused on bathing?

Using Knowledge: Can Elsie seek and use knowledge while bathing?

Can Elsie select appropriate tools and materials for bathing?

Can Elsie employ tools and materials according to their intended purposes while bathing?

Can Elsie support, stabilise, and hold tools and materials in an appropriate manner while bathing?

Can Elsie use goal-directed task performance that is focused towards the completion of bathing?

Can Elsie seek appropriate verbal/written information by asking questions or reading directions?

Temporal Organisation: Can Elsie initiate, logically order, continue, and complete the steps and action sequences required when bathing?

Can Elsie start or begin doing an action or step without hesitation while bathing?

Can Elsie perform an action sequence of a step without unnecessary interruption and as an unbroken, smooth progression?

Can Elsie perform steps in an effective or logical order for efficient use of time and energy while bathing?

Can Elsie finish or bring to completion single actions or steps without perseveration, inappropriate persistence, or premature cessation while bathing?

Organising Space and Objects: Can Elsie organise bathing space and objects?

Can Elsie look for and locate tools and materials through the process of logical searching while bathing?

Can Elsie collect needed or misplaced bathing tools and materials?

Can Elsie logically position or spatially arrange bathing tools and materials in an orderly fashion while bathing?

Can Elsie return/put away bathing tools and materials, and restore her immediate space to original condition?

Can Elsie modify the movement of the arm, body, or wheelchair to avoid or manoeuvre around existing obstacles that are encountered in the course of moving the arm, body, or wheelchair through space while bathing?

(Continued)

TABLE 6.2	**Examples of Detailed MOHO Questions to Guide Analysis** (*cont.*)

Adaptation: Can Elsie relate to the ability to anticipate, correct for, and benefit by learning from the consequences of errors that arise in bathing?

Can Elsie respond appropriately to nonverbal environmental/perceptual cues that provide feedback regarding bathing progression?

Can Elsie modify her action or locate objects within the bathing area in anticipation of or in response to circumstances/problems that might arise in the course of bathing or to avoid undesirable outcomes?

Can Elsie change environmental conditions in anticipation of or in response to circumstances/problems that arise in the course of bathing or to avoid undesirable outcomes?

Can Elsie anticipate and prevent undesirable circumstances/problems from recurring or persisting while bathing?

MOHO, Model of human occupation.

Since activity analysis is done with reference to a particular individual, not all concepts from each model will be necessary to generate necessary questions. Communication and interaction skills questions were not generated since bathing was a solitary activity and process skills questions were not generated because she did not have any cognitive challenges that may impact her processing skills.

Step 4: Identify and Test Ways Occupation(s) Can Be Adapted and/or Graded Based on Identified Gaps Between the Activity and the Person

Occupations can be adapted and/or graded, for example:
- Providing adaptive equipment
- Modifying how the occupation is done
- Providing assistance/encouragement
- Making environmental alterations

Since step 4 involves coming up with possible strategies to address identified gaps between the activity and the person/group, it is important that these strategies be tested to see whether they work.

An Illustration of Step 4: Adapting Elsie's Bathing

Links between the theory base and Elsie's case example are highlighted in parentheses. Elsie had previously been provided with a bath board and tap spray (MOHO—physical object) in 2003 and had been using this equipment independently until about 4 weeks ago. She reported she is no longer bathing for a variety of reasons, including:
- She was physically having more difficulty due to osteoarthritis stiffening in her knees (biomechanical—range of motion)
- She has decreased confidence (MOHO—personal causation) due to lack of power in her dominant hand following a fracture (biomechanical—strength), which she feels reduces her ability to grip (MOHO—skill) the side of the bath
- Water goes on the floor and she is anxious (MOHO—personal causation) she will slip on the lino floor

(MOHO—physical environment) when she gets out. She has fallen in the house recently and so has a legitimate fear.

Not bathing is affecting other occupations. Her only leisure activity is going to the social club twice a week (MOHO—role) and she reads to local schoolchildren as a volunteer once a week (MOHO—role). She has not been doing either activity in the last 2 weeks because she feels conscious of her body odour. This is causing Elsie to feel isolated (MOHO—disengaged from roles).

The practitioner originally decided on the strategy of using a bath hoist since this was the least costly and involved a kind of adaptation that could be made. To assess the suitability of a bath hoist (MOHO—physical object) it was tried out with Elsie. During the assessment Elsie physically struggled to get her legs over the side of the bathtub due to restricted range of motion at her knee joints (biomechanical—range of motion) and required physical assistance (MOHO—social environment). This kind of physical effort against resistance is contraindicated by her high blood pressure and irregular heartbeat. Moreover, when she was trying to transfer off the bath hoist her foot caught on the leg of the wash hand basin and she required physical assistance (MOHO—social environment) to move it. Elsie was visibly fearful during the assessment (MOHO—personal causation), which exacerbated her chronic obstructive airways disease (MOHO—performance capacity). To manage a bath hoist Elsie would need physical help (MOHO—social environment) due to physical restrictions (biomechanical), anxiety (MOHO—personal causation), and medial conditions (MOHO—performance capacity). Elsie, however, lives alone and does not have physical support available (MOHO—social environment). Thus it was determined that a bath hoist was not an adequate solution for closing the gap between the demands of bathing and Elsie's characteristics. As a result, the practitioner determined that the only option for bathing would be to have a walk-in shower with nonslip flooring (MOHO—physical environment), which she could manage independently and would allow her to feel she can return to her volunteer responsibility and her social club (MOHO—roles).

SUMMARY

This chapter presented an approach to theory-driven activity analysis. We argue that the demands of an occupation can only be identified in relation to the client/client group who is receiving occupational therapy. We also argue that an analysis that is based on theory provides the additional benefits of the explanatory power of theory to identify the activity characteristics and how they influence a client. That is, theory-driven occupational analysis provides a framework that not only identifies areas of analysis but also provides a theory that supports an explanation of how the identified elements operate together to support or prevent a person engaging in an occupation.

REFERENCES

Bryant, W., Fieldhouse, J., & Bannigan, K. (2014). *Creek's occupational therapy and mental health* (5th ed.). Elsevier.

Christiansen, C. (1999). Defining lives: Occupation as identity: An essay on competence, coherence, and the creation of meaning: Eleanor Clark Slagle lecture. *American Journal of Occupational Therapy, 53,* 547–558.

Clark, F. A. (1993). Occupational embedded in a real life: Interweaving occupation science and occupational therapy. *American Journal of Occupational Therapy, 47,* 1067–1077.

Creek, J., III. (2002). The knowledge base of occupational therapy. In J. Creek (Ed.), *Occupational therapy and mental health* (pp. 29–49). Churchill Livingstone.

Crepeau, E. B. (2003). Analyzing occupation and activity: A way of thinking about occupational performance. In E. B. Crepeau, E. S. Cohn, & B. A. Boyt Schell (Eds.), *Willard and Spackman's occupational therapy* (10th ed.). Lippincott, Williams & Wilkins.

Duncan, E. A. S. (Ed.). (2021). *Foundations for practice in occupational therapy* (6th ed.). Elsevier Health Sciences.

Fidler, G., & Fidler, J. (1963). *Occupational therapy: A communication process in psychiatry.* Macmillian.

Fisher, A. G. (1998). Uniting practice and theory in an occupational framework. *American Journal of Occupational Therapy, 54*(7), 509–521.

Fisher, A. G. (2014). Occupation-centred, occupation-based, occupation-focused: Same, same or different? *Scandinavian Journal of Occupational Therapy, 21*(1), S96–S107.

Gillen, A., & Greber, C. (2014). Occupation-focused practice: Challenges and choices. *British Journal of Occupational Therapy, 77*(1), 39–41.

Katz, N., & Toglia, J. (Eds.) (2018). Cognition, occupation, and participation across the life span: Neuroscience, neurorehabilitation, and models of intervention in occupational therapy. AOTA press. Maryland.

Kielhofner, G. (2009). *Conceptual foundations of occupational therapy* (4th ed.). FA Davis.

Lamport, N., Coffey, M., & Hersch, G. (2001). *Activity analysis and application building blocks of treatment.* SLACK Incorporated.

Lee, S. W., Taylor, R., Kielhofner, G., & Fisher, G. (2008). Theory use in practice: A national survey of therapists who use the model of human occupation. *American Journal of Occupational Therapy, 62*(1), 106–117.

Mosey, A. (1986). *Psychosocial components of occupational therapy.* Raven Press.

Polatajko, H. J. (1994). Dreams, dilemmas, and decisions for occupational therapy practice in a new millennium: A Canadian perspective. *American Journal of Occupational Therapy, 48*(7), 590–594.

Schell, B. A. B., Gillen, G., Crepeau, E., & Scaffa, M. (2019). Analyzing occupations and activity. In *Willard and Spackman's occupational therapy* (pp. 320–333). Lippincott, Williams & Wilkins.

Taylor, R. (2017). *Kielhofner's model of human occupation: Theory and application* (5th ed.). Lippincott, Williams and Wilkins.

Trombly, C. (1993). The issue is—anticipating the future: Assessment of occupational functioning. *American Journal of Occupational Therapy, 47*(3), 253–257.

Trombly, C. (1995). Occupation: Purposefulness and meaningfulness as therapeutic mechanisms: Eleanor Clark Slagle Lecture. *American Journal of Occupational Therapy, 49*(10), 960–972.

Watson, D. E., & Wilson, S. A. (2003). *Task analysis: An individual and population approach* (2nd ed.). American Occupational Therapy Association.

Wong, S. R., & Fisher, G. (2015). Comparing and using occupation-focused models. *Occupational Therapy in Health Care, 29*(3), 297–315.

Wood, W. (1998). It is jump time for occupational therapy. *American Journal of Occupational Therapy, 52*(6), 403–411.

7

Goal Setting in Occupational Therapy: A Client-Centred Perspective

Lesley Scobbie and Sally Boa

HIGHLIGHTS

- Client-centred goal setting is fundamental to occupational therapy practice.
- Goal setting is only one part of the process; goal pursuit requires other goal-related activities.
- There are many formal and informal approaches to goal setting; there is currently no universally accepted gold standard evidence-based approach.

- Relevant theory and principles of client-centred care can guide practice.
- People with communication difficulties should be supported to participate in the goal-setting process in a way that suits them.
- Occupational therapy interventions should be guided by client-centred goals.

INTRODUCTION

The aim of this chapter is to provide an overview of client-centred goal setting relevant to occupational therapy practice. We begin by defining key terms used within this chapter, introduce the World Health Organization (WHO) International Classification of Functioning, Disability and Health (ICF), and describe key features of a client-centred approach. We view these as important foundations to interdisciplinary goal-setting practice. Different approaches to goal-setting practice are then presented. In particular, we focus on (1) those that incorporate outcome measurement (SMART goals, goal attainment scaling [GAS], and the Canadian Occupational Performance Measure [COPM]) and (2) those that are theory based (the goal-setting and action planning [G-AP] framework, and goal-setting and action planning palliative care [G-AP PC]). Case studies are used to illustrate the use of goal-setting approaches in practice. We discuss methods to support involvement of people with communication difficulties in the goal-setting process and conclude the chapter by considering implications for occupational therapy practice.

Defining Rehabilitation, Rehabilitation Goal, Goal Setting and Goal Pursuit

Rehabilitation is a person-centred, goal-orientated process that helps people to play an active role in managing their own health (Wade, 2020). Goal setting is viewed as an integral part of the rehabilitation process (Wade, 2005, 2009; Wade & de Jong, 2000). Levack and Siegert (2014) define a rehabilitation goal as: "A desired future state to be achieved by the person with a disability as a result of rehabilitation activities" (p. 11). They go on to differentiate between goal setting and goal pursuit. The former is defined as "the establishment or negotiation of rehabilitation goals" and the latter as "activities beyond the selection of rehabilitation goals that are implemented in order to enhance the level of goal attainment." This differentiation is important as it highlights that goal setting is only one part of the process, and that further goal-related activities are required to support clients in the pursuit of rehabilitation goals.

International Classification of Functioning, Disability and Health

The WHO-ICF (WHO, 2001) is a framework that aims to provide an international, standard language for describing and measuring health and disability. This framework aims to provide an international, standard language for describing and measuring health and disability. It supports multidisciplinary rehabilitation professionals to think holistically, incorporating environmental and personal factors. Using the ICF, clients can be supported to identify and work toward goals that are important to them at the levels of impairment (body function/ structure), activity

65

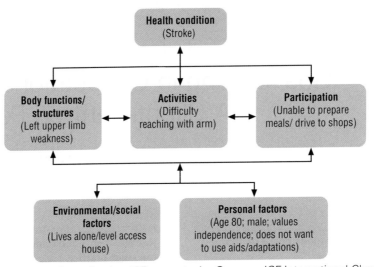

FIG. 7.1 World Health Organization ICF case study: George. *ICF,* International Classification of Functioning, Disability and Health.

(execution of a task or action), and participation (involvement in a life situation). Goals can also be considered in relation to the environment (physical, social, and attitudinal environment) or personal factors (such as coping styles or habits).

The following case study illustrates how the ICF can help the rehabilitation professional think holistically about a client (Fig. 7.1). George is 80 years old (personal factor) and has had a stroke (health condition) resulting in moderate weakness in his left arm (impairment). He is unable to reach for objects with his left arm (activity) and consequently has difficulty preparing meals and driving his car (participation). George lives on his own in a level access house (environmental factor). He has always taken great pride in his ability to be independent (personal factor). He is very motivated to improve and wants to be independent, without relying on aids and adaptations (personal factor).

A Client-Centred Approach

Maintaining a client-centred approach to goal-setting practice ensures that rehabilitation goals reflect clients' individual needs and preferences and priorities (Rosewilliam et al., 2011). Occupational therapists aspire to be client centred (Hammell, 2013; McAndrew et al., 1999). However, there is evidence to suggest that it is challenging for health and social care rehabilitation staff (from now on referred to as "staff") to deliver client-centred goal-setting practice for a variety of reasons. These can include organisational barriers (e.g., lack of time); client-related issues (e.g., communication and cognitive difficulties), and discrepancies between staff and client perspectives (e.g., what constitutes an important goal) (Barnard et al., 2010;

Hunt et al., 2015; Lloyd et al., 2018; Plant et al., 2016; Rosewilliam et al., 2011). There is also evidence to suggest that clients may not always share their personal goals with staff (Boa et al., 2019). However, strategies and techniques have been identified to support a client-centred approach (e.g., taking time to listen to the client, building trust, sharing expertise, working collaboratively, talking about goals explicitly, and promoting autonomy) (Boa et al., 2019; Cott, 2004; Fleming et al., 2013; Hunt et al., 2015; Lawler et al., 1999; Leach et al., 2010).

APPROACHES TO GOAL-SETTING PRACTICE

There are many different approaches to the setting and pursuit of rehabilitation goals. For a comprehensive overview of the main approaches, see *Rehabilitation Goal Setting: Theory, Practice and Evidence* (Siegert & Levack, 2015). In this section, we will summarise some of those relevant to occupational therapy practice. Approaches may be formal or informal. Formal goal-setting approaches have been defined as "an approach that is able to be replicated in practice due to the availability of written standardised guidelines regarding the procedure of administration" (Prescott et al., 2015). However, there are many informal approaches that have been developed within rehabilitation teams or by individual staff (Scobbie et al., 2015). It is therefore not surprising that goal-setting practice can be highly variable both within and between rehabilitation settings. In the following section, we discuss two groupings of formal goal-setting approaches: those that incorporate outcome measurement and those that are theory based. Practice considerations are highlighted for each approach.

BOX 7.1   SMART GEM Criteria

Specific: 1. Desired performance; 2. Conditions for performance; 3. Context for performance

Measurable: 4. Method of measurement; 5. Criteria for performance outcome

Activity-related: 6. Activities or interventions used

Review: 7. Review date specified

Time frame: 8. Time frame for achievement of goal

BOX 7.2   Goal Setting Using GAS

+2: To independently make lunch in 15 min three times/ wk within 4 wk

+1: To independently make lunch in 15 min seated on a perching stool three times/wk within 4 wk

Zero: To make lunch seated on a perching stool with daughter supervising in 15 min three times/wk within 4 wk

-1: To make lunch with minimal assistance from daughter in 15 min whilst seated on a perching stool three times/wk within 4 wk (current status)

-2: To make lunch with moderate assistance from daughter in 15 min whilst seated on a perching stool within 4 wk

---

GAS, Goal attainment scaling.

Goal-Setting Approaches Incorporating Outcome Measurement

SMART goals, GAS, and the COPM are examples of formal goal-setting approaches that incorporate outcome measurement.

SMART Goals

The concept of SMART goals has become an enduring feature of goal-setting practice (McPherson et al., 2015). The acronym SMART has been used in different ways over time (Wade, 2009), but typically stands for **s**pecific, **m**easurable, **a**ttainable, **r**elevant, and **t**imely (McPherson et al., 2015). The features of a SMART goal allow clinicians to determine whether goals are achieved. Bowman et al. (2015) developed the SMART Goal Evaluation Method (SMART-GEM). The SMART-GEM's scoring and grading scale provides a structure to support occupational therapists and other health professionals to write SMART rehabilitation goals. It also provides an objective outcome measurement tool that can be used to audit the content of rehabilitation goals (Box 7.1).

The eight criteria listed under SMART-GEM domains are reviewed and the written goal is assigned a lettered grade depending on how many of the criteria have been met (A = 8 criteria met; B = 7 criteria met, C = 6 criteria met, D = 5 or less criteria met). The grade provides a measure of the degree to which the goal meets the criteria set out in the SMART-GEM approach.

Practice considerations: Developing SMART goals allows staff to judge whether goals have been achieved. Although setting SMART goals has gained considerable traction in clinical practice, there is growing consensus that a focus on setting SMART goals may foster a professionally led, rather than client-centred, approach to goal-setting practice (Hersh et al., 2012; McPherson et al., 2015; Scobbie et al., 2020). As well as disempowering active engagement in the rehabilitation process, this risks reducing the client's motivation as set goals may not reflect their individual needs, preferences, and priorities.

Goal Attainment Scaling

Setting SMART goals is an important first step in the process of GAS (Bovend'eerdt et al., 2009; Turner-Stokes, 2009; Turner-Stokes et al., 2009). Prior to starting the rehabilitation intervention, goals are set on a 5-point scale. **Zero** indicates the expected level of goal attainment; **+1** and **+2** indicate higher, and much higher, than expected levels of goal attainment; and **-1** and **-2** indicate lower, and much lower, than expected levels of goal attainment. At a predetermined review date, the outcome score for each goal is rated (by the team and the client/carers) by judging actual client performance against the predefined levels. Box 7.2 provides an illustrated example of how a rehabilitation goal can be set using the 5-point GAS scale.

Practice considerations: GAS has been recommended as a sound measure of outcome in physical rehabilitation settings (Hurn et al., 2006); however, the methodologic limitations of using goal attainment as an outcome measure have been highlighted (Tennant, 2007). Turner-Stokes (2009) acknowledges that GAS depends on "the clinician's ability to predict outcome, which requires knowledge and experience" (p. 368). This can limit its usefulness in routine clinical practice as (1) it is not always possible to accurately predict clinical outcomes, and (2) staff may not have the prerequisite knowledge and experience to set SMART goals with confidence. Finally, GAS does not include a planning stage to support clients in the pursuit of their goals (Stevens et al., 2013); nor has it been designed to support (or positively score) adaptive goal adjustment (Scobbie et al., 2020).

The Canadian Occupational Performance Measure

The COPM (Carswell et al., 2004) is an occupational therapy client-reported outcome measure. A semistructured

---

BOX 7.3   Use of the COPM in Practice—A Case Study Example

Sheila has rheumatoid arthritis. She suffers from joint pain and deformity in her hands. This affects her ability to engage in valued occupations.

Using the Canadian Occupational Performance Measure (COPM), the occupational therapist and Sheila engage in a structured and supportive discussion about the problems she is experiencing in the domains of self-care, productivity, and leisure. Sheila identifies cooking the family meal as one of her biggest problems within the productivity domain. Using the visual analogue scale, Sheila rates the importance of this problem as 9; her current performance as 3, and her satisfaction with her performance as 4. Sheila's goal is to cook the family meal independently.

The occupational therapist delivers interventions to help Sheila reach her goal. This includes provision of adaptive equipment, education about joint protection techniques, and use of wrist splints. Sheila's goal was reviewed at the end of the intervention period and rescored in relation to performance and satisfaction with performance. Sheila's performance score improved to 6, and her satisfaction with performance score to 9. This indicates a clinically significant improvement. Both the occupational therapist and Sheila were happy with this outcome and moved on to consider another goal.

---

interview is used to identify client problems within the domains of self-care, productivity, and leisure. Identified problems provide the basis for setting rehabilitation goals. A 10-point visual analogue scale is used to obtain client-reported measures of importance, performance, and satisfaction with performance for each identified problem. Performance and satisfaction scores are summed and averaged before and after the intervention period to produce a score out of 10. A difference of two or more between the initial and follow-up scores indicates a clinically significant improvement. Box 7.3 illustrates the use of COPM in practice.

Practice considerations: As well as supporting client-centred goal-setting practice (Larsen et al., 2018), the COPM has been shown to be a valid, reliable, and sensitive measure of change in occupational performance over time (Carswell et al., 2004; Cup et al., 2003; Yang et al., 2017). The COPM is also supported by a web-based resource with access to training and published evidence (http://www.thecopm.ca/about/). Thus the COPM can be used to both inform and evaluate occupational therapy interventions. A potential limitation of the COPM is that it was developed for use by occupational therapists using the Canadian

Model of Occupational Performance as its conceptual basis. Consequently, it may be less useful in settings where goal setting is an interdisciplinary process. Like GAS, the COPM does not include a planning stage to support clients in the pursuit of their goals (Stevens et al., 2013); nor has it been designed to support adaptive goal adjustment (Scobbie et al., 2020).

Theory-Based Goal-Setting Approaches

Theory is important as it helps occupational therapists to understand and articulate what they do, why they do it, and what they think the outcome will be (Melton et al., 2009; Scobbie & Dixon, 2014). Theory can inform what the key components of interventions are and inform predictions about how they are likely to impact on outcomes (Medical Research Council, 2008; MRC Population Health Science Research Network, 2014). This allows for replication and testing of interventions, which are important prerequisites for theory development, knowledge generation, and development of the evidence base.

The G-AP Framework and G-AP Palliative Care

The G-AP framework, and the adapted version of this, G-AP PC, are examples of theory-based approaches to goal-setting practice. The former was developed for use with stroke survivors in community rehabilitation settings (Scobbie & Dixon, 2014; Scobbie et al., 2009, 2011, 2013, 2020); the latter for use with people who have life-limiting conditions in palliative care settings (Boa, 2013; Boa et al., 2014, 2019). Both frameworks are designed to inform collaborative, client-centred goal-setting practice with clients being supported to attain and (if necessary) adjust their rehabilitation goals. The knowledge, expertise, and perspectives of staff, clients, and carers is valued equally and considered throughout the process of goal setting and pursuit. G-AP and G-AP PC include four theoretically informed key stages, each of which include specific goal-related activities (Fig. 7.2).

Theories underpinning the development of G-AP and G-AP PC include self-efficacy theory (Bandura, 1997), goal-setting theory (Locke & Latham, 2002), heath action process approach (Schwarzer, 1992), hope theory (Gum & Snyder, 2002; Snyder et al., 2006), Bye's (1998) framework for affirming life whilst preparing for death, and self-regulation theory (Carver & Scheier, 2001). Each stage of G-AP and G-AP PC will now be described, with reference to underpinning theory.

Stage 1: Negotiating and Setting Rehabilitation Goals
Goal negotiation: An important first step in the G-AP process is to listen to and understand clients' perspectives about their current status and what their hopes are for the future. This creates the foundation for client-centred goal-setting

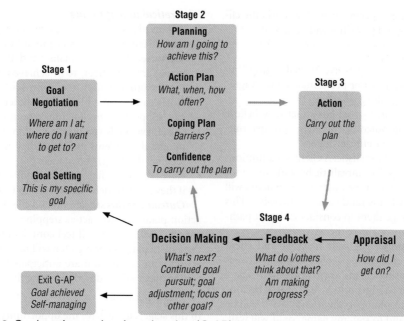

FIG. 7.2 Goal setting and action planning (G-AP) and palliative care (G-AP PC) framework.

conversations to develop. Clients should be supported during this conversation in a way that suits them. Useful open questions to start the conversation might include, "How do you think you are doing just now?" "What's going well and not so well?" "What would you like to focus on in the next month or so?" A helpful question to start the conversation in palliative care settings is, "What's important to you in the next wee [short] while?" This question allows clients to consider what they might like to achieve, whilst acknowledging in a sensitive manner the limited time they may have available. Clients with communication or cognitive difficulties may require additional support at this stage (see the section Using Accessible Methods to Support People With Communication Difficulties in the Goal-Setting Process, later).

Theoretical underpinning

- Developing goal intentions (supporting clients to think about what they would like to achieve) builds motivation (health action process approach).
- Goals direct behaviour, and clients need to have a sense of personal agency; that is, clients benefit from having a sense of personal agency and control therefore thy should be supported to identify goals that are personal and important to them (hope theory).
- Clients can simultaneously work toward goals about living whilst preparing for death, thus enabling them to consider what is important to them beyond the limits

of their illness (Bye's affirming life: preparing for death framework).

Outcome of this stage: Staff will have a clear understanding of what the client's needs, preferences, and priorities are. This will support the identification of valued goals that clients will be motivated to pursue.

Goal setting: Having understood the client's perspective, staff can then support clients to identify specific goals they would like to pursue. Goals can be suggested by staff and/or the client (or carer) and collaboratively discussed. It does not matter who comes up with the goal, as long as it is agreed. General goals, such as "I want to get back to normal" or "I want to do the things I used to do" can be discussed and refined into a specific, challenging goal(s). Useful questions to prompt client-centred goal-setting conversations might include, "Think about something specific you'd like achieve around... getting out more... feeling less anxious... moving your arm better... etc." or "What about (staff member suggests a goal based on knowledge of the client's needs, preferences, and priorities), would that be something you would like to focus on?" or "So, you would like to be more independent in the house, can you think of something in particular you would like to do independently?" Thinking about goals can be challenging for clients, particularly in palliative care settings. It can be helpful if staff listen and pick up on cues (e.g., "You've said you would like to improve your walking. Is there somewhere particular you would like to be able to walk to?").

Outcome of this stage: Specific goals that reflect the client's needs preferences and priorities will be agreed.

Theoretical underpinning
- Specific goals that clients perceive as challenging (but not overly so) result in better performance than vague, "do your best" type goals (goal-setting theory).
- Clients will be motivated to set goals that they believe will result in a good outcome for them (positive outcome expectancies) (self-efficacy theory).
- Goals may not always be realistic. A client-set ambitious goal (perhaps perceived as unrealistic by staff) may motivate the client. If they prove unattainable, clients will better understand what is (and is not) achievable. This in turn will encourage them to consider different pathways to goal attainment (hope theory).

Outcome of this stage: The staff member and client will agree on specific, challenging goal(s) to pursue. Goals should be described using clients' own words and reflect their needs, preferences, and priorities (e.g., "I will be confident talking on the telephone to my friends" or "I will be able to use my right hand to sign my name" or "I will walk with my dogs in the field at the back of my house").

Stage 2: Action planning and Coping Planning
Action planning: Action plans act as incremental stepping stones to goal attainment. An action plan details what clients must do, where they must do it, and when (e.g., "I will do my arm exercises, sitting at the kitchen table, twice a day for the next week" or "I will use my mindfulness app, before bedtime, every day for the next week" or "I will practice walking to the gate and back every day this week using my stick"). Action plans meet the SMART rule; they are specific (detail exactly what the client must do), measurable (success of completion easily assessed), achievable (represents the next incremental step, therefore should be highly achievable), relevant (the link between the action plan and the goal should be clear), with a time frame (the date for action plan completion should be agreed).

Coping planning: Clients are supported to consider barriers that may get in the way of action plan completion, and to develop a coping plan to overcome them. For example, a client may identify fatigue as being a barrier to completing a daily exercise programme. A coping plan that prompts them to complete their exercises in the morning when they have the most energy may support them to overcome this barrier.

Measuring confidence: Clients are then supported to think about how confident they feel about completing the plan. This can be done using a visual analogue scale or by just asking them. A lack of confidence (score <7 on a 10-point visual analogue scale) would suggest the plan should be modified or discussed further to optimise the chances of successful completion.

Theoretical underpinning
- Action plans and coping plans motivate clients initiate and sustain behaviours in pursuit of their goals. Goals supported by action plans (and if necessary, coping plans) are more likely to be achieved than those that are not (health action process approach).
- Goals can become blocked or difficult to achieve; staff can support clients to think about different pathways to achieve goals (pathways thinking) and to anticipate potential problems and how they might be overcome (agency thinking) (hope theory).
- Clients are more likely to successfully complete their plan if they are confident they can do so (self-efficacy theory).

Outcome of this stage: Staff and clients agree on SMART action plans that will act as stepping stones to achieving a specific goal. Clients will feel confident they can complete the agreed plan. A coping plan will be in place if barriers to action plan completion are anticipated. Action plans and coping plans will be described using the client's own words.

Stage 3: Action
In this stage, clients have the opportunity to carry out their plan, either independently or with support for someone else (e.g., a family member or staff member).

Outcome of this stage: Clients will have direct experience of carrying out their plan. The experience of successes and/or setbacks at this stage will inform appraisal, feedback, and decision making at the next stage.

Stage 4: Appraisal, feedback, and decision making
Staff and clients collaboratively appraise the outcome of the action plan and progress toward the goal; staff can provide clients with specific feedback. Collaborative appraisal and feedback will inform decisions about what to do next. Successful action plan completion will encourage development of the next action plan and continued pursuit of the goal. The experience of a setback or failure to complete the action plan should encourage a supportive discussion around why it was unsuccessful. Understanding the reason(s) for the setback or failure will inform decisions about whether to (1) continue goal pursuit with a new or revised action plan or coping plan, (2) consider adjusting the goal to make it achievable, or (3) disengage from the goal and consider other achievable goals.

Theoretical underpinning
- Appraisal and feedback support reflection and learning from successes and setbacks. This can inform helpful adjustments to goal-related behaviour (goal setting theory).
- Reviewing goals is important because even when goals are no longer achievable, mourning the loss of unattainable goals is an important aspect of adapting to disability. Reminders of previous achievements and positive self-talk can motivate clients to seek alternative

pathways to achieve existing goals or set and work toward new ones (hope theory).

- Behaviour is goal directed and feedback controlled. Perceived progress will result in enhanced emotional well-being and motivate continued goal pursuit. A perceived discrepancy between current performance (what the client is able to do) and the goal (what the client needs to do to achieve the goal) will motivate increase in effort if the goal is still considered achievable. If the goal is considered unachievable, the goal will be adjusted or effort redirected to other achievable goals (self-regulation theory).

Outcome of this stage: Progress will be collaboratively reviewed, feedback provided, and informed decision made about how to progress. Goal decision options include continued goal pursuit if satisfactory progress is being made or goal adjustment or disengagement if goals are proving too difficult to achieve.

G-AP: Case Study Example—Jenny

The following anonymised case study illustrates use of G-AP in clinical practice. Jenny is a 50-year-old woman who had a stroke resulting in right-sided weakness and dysarthria. Jenny lives at home with her husband Jim and their 8-year-old son, Colin. Jenny was fully independent prior to her stroke. She enjoyed going to the gym, walking, and spending time with her family. Jenny lives in a small town; the shops and school are nearby.

Stage 1. Negotiating and setting rehabilitation goals: The occupational therapist talked to Jenny about how she felt she was currently doing and what she hoped to achieve in the future. Jenny talked about her difficulties walking, which meant that she could not walk Colin to school; she found this upsetting. One of the first goals she prioritised was to be able to walk Colin to and from school.

Stage 2. Planning: Jenny and her occupational therapists and physiotherapist discussed action plans or stepping stones to help her achieve her goal. A series of action plans were agreed to improve Jenny's strength in her right leg and her exercise tolerance (Box 7.4).

Stage 3. Action: Jenny completed her exercises programme three times a day, but she was not able to do all of the repetitions because she felt too tired. She was able to walk to the local park and back as planned with Jim walking beside her.

Stage 4. Appraisal, feedback, and decision making: Jenny was happy with her progress but remained apprehensive about tripping. She was disappointed she had not managed to complete all of her exercise programme. Jenny's occupational therapist and physiotherapist provided positive feedback and reassured her that she was making good progress. Her exercise programme was adjusted to optimise her chances of success. Jenny agreed the next action plan with her occupational therapist and physiotherapist

---

BOX 7.4   Action Planning Examples

Goal: Jenny will be able to walk Colin to and from school

Action plan 1. Complete home exercise programme 3x a day for the next week

Any barriers? *Yes, I might be too tired to do the exercises.*

Coping plan: *Do exercises after breakfast, lunch, and dinner because that's when I have the most energy.*

Confidence to carry out the plan: 0————————
7——**9**——10

Action plan 2. Jenny will walk to the local park and back 3x this week using her stick.

Any barriers? *Yes, I'm frightened of tripping and falling.*

Coping plan: *Jim will walk with Jenny (on her right side) until she is confident she can do it by herself.*

Confidence to carry out the plan: 0————————
7——**9**——10

(to walk to the local park and back every day for the next week using her stick).

Outcome: By working through a series of action plans, Jenny met her goal of being able to walk Colin to and from school. This was an important step forward in her recovery as she felt she was fulfilling her role as Colin's mum.

G-AP PC: Case Study Example—Mary

The following anonymised case study illustrates the use of G-AP PC in a palliative care setting.

Mary was admitted to the hospice for end-of-life care. She was asked to think about what was important to her in the next wee [short] while. Initially, she found it difficult to think about goals beyond her illness, but on reflection, thought she would like to go out with her daughter, preferably away from the hospice. Conversations, guided by staff using the theory-based questions (Box 7.5), resulted in the following goal, action, and coping plan, which in turn led to a positive client-centred outcome (Box 7.6).

A few days after Mary had achieved her goal, her condition deteriorated and she died in the hospice. Staff and her daughter were very glad that they had been able to support Mary to achieve this important goal, right at the end of life, leaving her with a sense of elation and achievement and her daughter with a positive memory of her final days of life.

The case study demonstrates the importance of having an explicit, theory-based framework to underpin the goal-setting process. Without it, Mary may not have been

BOX 7.5   Questions to Guide Staff Through G-AP PC

Stage 1: Negotiate and set goal
- "What's important to you in the next wee while?"
- "What would you like to work toward at the moment?"

Stage 2: Agree an action plan and (if necessary) coping plan
- "What do you need help with and who do you need to ask?"
- "Can you think of anything that might get in the way of completing the plan?"
- "How confident do you feel about completing this plan?"

Stage 3: Carrying out the plan: provide support, as agreed

Stage 4: Appraise performance, provide feedback and decide what to do next
- "How did you get on—what went well, what didn't go so well?"
- "How do you feel?"
- "Is it still important to you?"
- "What's next?"

G-AP PC, Goal-setting and action planning palliative care.

supported to pursue her goal, and without a clear coping plan she may not have been able to address the potential barriers to goal achievement.

Practice considerations: G-AP and G-AP PC create a structured, theory-based process to inform a client-centred goal-setting practice in community-based stroke rehabilitation and palliative care settings. Both can be used (by all members of the care team) to support clients to attain and (if necessary) adjust their rehabilitation goals. Unlike GAS and COPM, G-AP and G-AP PC have not been designed for use as an outcome measure (neither include a scoring system).

SUPPORT PEOPLE WITH COMMUNICATION DIFFICULTIES IN THE GOAL SETTING PROCESS

Goal setting is based on a conversation where a client's priorities are firstly elicited and then the specific goal negotiated and agreed. Therefore it is critical that clients with communication difficulties are supported to understand and participate in the process (Brown et al., 2020). Including people with communication difficulties in the goal-setting process can be challenging due to a range of factors. For example, (1) people with communication difficulties may have difficulty understanding the concepts

BOX 7.6   Mary's G-AP PC Case Study

G-AP Stage	Theory-Informed Questions	Mary's Responses
Stage 1	"What's important to you in the next wee while?"	"To go out with my family."
	"What would you like to work towards at the moment?"	"I'd like to go out for lunch with my daughter, preferably away from the hospice."
Stage 2	"How confident do you feel?"	1 2 3 4 5 6 7 8 ⑨ 10 "Very!"
	"What do you need help with and who do you need to ask?"	"I need to arrange it with my daughter."
	"Can you think of anything that might get in the way?"	"I might get tired, so I need to arrange to have my wheelchair brought in from home. I might get sore, so I will need to take my pain relief with me."
Stage 3	Carrying out the plan	The next day at handover, the nurse noticed that Mary was due to go to an outpatient appointment at the hospital. She suggested that Mary's daughter take her and they could go out for lunch. She took her wheelchair and the pain medication as planned.
Stage 4	Appraisal and feedback	Mary went out for lunch and then did some shopping with her daughter. She felt "wonderful" but was glad she had taken her wheelchair and medication, as planned. She planned to do this again.

G-AP PC, Goal-setting and action planning palliative care.

and possibilities and expressing ideas and prioritising issues (Bornman & Murphy, 2006); (2) staff who are not speech-language therapists may have less confidence supporting people with communication difficulties through the goal-setting process (Cameron et al., 2018); and (3) the client's communication partner may take on the role of speaking for the person with the communication difficulty, providing a further barrier to the client's involvement (O'Halloran et al., 2008).

Accessible Information

The importance of creating a supportive environment (e.g., quiet room with minimal distraction) and use of supportive conversation strategies (e.g., giving the client extra time to process information and respond) has been highlighted (Brown et al., 2020). It is recognised that verbal and written information should be adapted so that it is accessible to people with communication difficulties (Brown et al., 2020; Rose et al., 2011). A range of strategies commonly used by multidisciplinary staff has been summarised (Dörfler & Kulnik, 2020) (Box 7.7). The strategies used should be adapted to each client according to the client's strengths, needs, and personal preferences, as well as the topic being discussed.

A SMARTER Approach

In their goals and aphasia project, Hersh et al. (2012) recognised the challenges of genuinely including people with aphasia in the goal-setting process. They identified an underlying set of principles that can support greater collaboration between people with aphasia, families, and staff. They have developed the familiar acronym SMART, into SMARTER. The SMARTER approach is summarised in Box 7.8.

> ### BOX 7.7 Strategies Used to Support People With Communication Difficulties
>
> - Use real objects to point to/use
> - Make use of the immediate surroundings to demonstrate/point to/interact with
> - Point to body parts
> - Use gestures
> - Read the client's body language
> - Observe the client's behaviour
> - Use a calendar to get an overview of activities/achieved goals/to mark dates
> - Show or view pictures/photos
> - Use a communication book/board
> - Use drawings to convey a point
> - Write things down

> ### BOX 7.8 SMARTER Approach to Goal-Setting Practice
>
> **S**hared: Emphasises that goal setting should be an interpersonal collaboration between the client, the member of staff and the family.
> **M**onitored: Goals and progress toward them should be continuously evaluated, not only by professionals but by clients and families, too.
> **A**ccessible: Communication should be adapted and tailored to the needs of the person with aphasia and goals should be written down in a way that the person with aphasia can understand.
> **R**elevant: Goals should be relevant to the person's life.
> **T**ransparent: There should be a clear link between therapy tasks/activities and the person's goals.
> **E**volving: Goals should change with time, so the process of goal setting should be flexible and iterative.
> **R**elationship centred: The process of goal setting should be based on the therapist-client relationship.

The SMARTER approach to goal setting emphasises the need for a relationship-based approach, with flexibility at all levels, and emphasises the need for skilled staff to approach the goal-setting process with adaptability and sensitivity. Although developed for people with aphasia, the principles of SMARTER are relevant to all client groups.

Talking Mats

A talking mat is an evidence-based communication tool explicitly designed for use by all members of the care team to support a client's communication. Talking mats is used internationally, in both clinical practice and in research settings (Murphy, 2009; Murphy & Boa, 2012; Murphy et al., 2010). Talking Mats supports interaction using three sets of picture communication symbols - topics, options and a visual scale - and a space on which to display them (see https://www.talkingmats.com/about-talking-mats/#howitworks).

Talking mats can be used to support clients with communication difficulties to identify and work toward their personal goals. As an example, Gill had a brain tumour that affected her ability to communicate. She had severe word-finding difficulties, and her response to yes/no questions was unreliable. Staff found it very difficult talk with Gill about the goals she wanted to work on during her rehabilitation. Talking mats were used to get to know Gill and to begin to find out what was important to her (Fig. 7.3). Gill used a symbol set relating to interests. Supported by talking mats, she was able to have a conversation about her interests and hobbies. When she picked up the arts and crafts

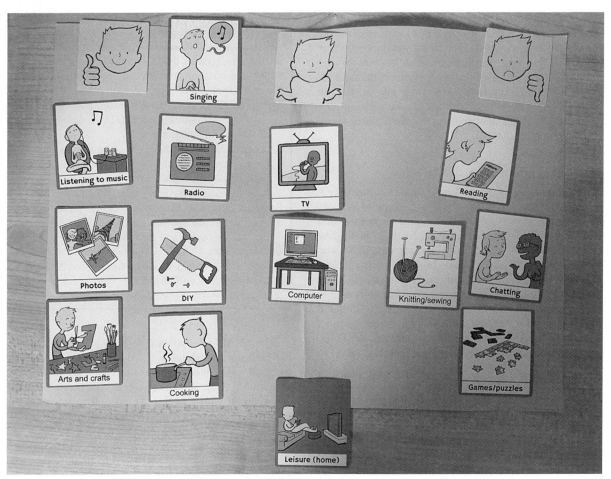

FIG. 7.3 Gill's talking mat.

symbol and photos symbol, she became animated and was able to tell staff that she wanted to finish creating a memory book of photos that she had been making for her family.

By using talking mats to support Gill's communication, rehabilitation staff were able to find out about what was important to her and agree a client-centred goal: to finish her memory book. Staff and family members supported Gill to work toward and achieve her goal.

IMPLICATIONS FOR OCCUPATIONAL THERAPY PRACTICE

There is currently no available gold standard evidence-based approach to guide goal-setting practice in rehabilitation settings (Levack et al., 2015). In this chapter we

have presented an overview of approaches to goal-setting practice relevant to occupational therapy practice, highlighting practice considerations for each. Occupational therapists (and other rehabilitation staff) need to decide which approach, or combination of approaches, can be delivered within their setting to best meet the needs of their client group. We suggest a useful starting point is to review current goal-setting practice in your setting (Scobbie & Dixon, 2014). In practical terms, this would mean taking a reflective approach to critiquing current goal-setting practice. Box 7.9 provides questions (informed by the aforementioned theories and features of client-centred practice) to guide you, which you could use collectively as a service or individually as an occupational therapist, to reflect on and develop your goal-setting practice.

BOX 7.9 Questions to Inform Critique of Current Goal-Setting Practice

1. Are clients provided with information about the goal-setting process and how they can participate?
2. Are clients supported to tell staff about their individual needs, preferences, and priorities?
3. Are client-centred goals collaboratively agreed to direct rehabilitation efforts?
4. Are clients supported to develop action plans to act as stepping stones to achieving their goals?
5. Are clients supported to think about barriers to successful action plan completion and how they can be overcome?
6. Is client confidence to successfully complete the action plans assessed?
7. Is progress collaboratively reviewed and feedback provided by staff on an action plan–by–action plan basis?
8. Are clients supported to adjust or disengage from goals proving too difficult to achieve?
9. Are clients provided with an accessible copy of their goals, action plans, and progress?
10. Are clients with communication difficulties supported to participate in the goal-setting process in a way that suits them?

SUMMARY

The process of setting and pursing goals presents occupational therapists with an ideal opportunity to engage in client-centred rehabilitation practice. Agreeing and working toward client-centred goals will optimise client motivation and ensure that occupational therapy interventions are tailored to meet individual client's needs, preferences, and priorities. However, in the absence of an evidence-based goal standard, there are many formal and informal goal-setting approaches and methods to choose from. We suggest that a good place to start is to review your practice in relation to how client centred it is and whether it is theory driven. By doing this, occupational therapists, together with other rehabilitation staff, can decide which aspects of current practice to retain, which to review and update, and to identify any missing components. This reflection can inform decisions about whether use of any of the formal goal-setting approaches might enhance client-centred goal-setting practice. Regardless of the approach chosen, goal-setting practice should be client centred, delivered using effective interpersonal skills and subject to ongoing reflective practice. Whilst challenges will inevitably be encountered, client-centred goal-setting practice will reap many rewards for occupational therapists as they are able to focus on the unique occupations that really matter to each individual client in their care.

REFLECTIVE LEARNING

- How might the WHO ICF model help you think about person-centred goals?
- Reflect on some goals you have documented recently. To what extent have you used the client's own words? How much do they reflect the person's story, values, and valued occupations?
- To what extent do you empower clients to set and purse their personal goals? Is there anything you could do differently?
- Are there any benefits and challenges to involving family members in the goal-setting process?
- To what extent do you work with other members of the multidisciplinary team to help clients set and pursue their personal goals? Could this teamwork be improved?
- Do clients' personal goals directly inform the occupational therapy interventions you deliver? If not, why not?

REFERENCES

Bandura, A. (1997). *Self efficacy—the exercise of control.* W.H. Freeman.

Barnard, R. A., Cruice, N., & Playford, E. D. (2010). Strategies used in the pursuit of achievability during goal setting in rehabilitation. *Qualitative Health Research, 20,* 239.

Boa, S. (2013). The development and evaluation of a goal setting and action planning framework for use in palliative care (G-AP PC). PhD thesis, University of Stirling.

Boa, S., Duncan, E., Haraldsdottir, E., & Wyke, S. (2019). Mind the gap: Patients' experiences and perceptions of goal setting in palliative care. *Progress in Palliative Care, 27*(6), 291–300.

Boa, S., Duncan, E. A. S., Haraldsdottir, E., & Wyke, S. (2014). Goal setting in palliative care: A structured review. *Progress in Palliative Care, 22*(6), 326–333.

Bornman, J., & Murphy, J. (2006). Using the ICF in goal setting: Clinical application using talking mats. *Disability and Rehabilitation: Assistive Technology, 1*(3), 145–154.

Bovend'eerdt, T., Botell, R. E., & Wade, D. T. (2009). Writing SMART rehabilitation goals and achieving goal attainment scaling: A practical guide. *Clinical Rehabilitation, 23*(4), 352–361.

Bowman, J., Mogensen, L., Marsland, E., & Lannin, N. (2015). The development, content validity and inter-rater reliability of the SMART-goal evaluation method: A standardised method for evaluating clinical goals. *Australian Journal of Occupational Therapy, 62*(6), 420–427.

Brown, S. E., Brady, M. C., Worrall, L., & Scobbie, L. (2020). A narrative review of communication accessibility for people with aphasia and implications for multi-disciplinary goal setting after stroke. *Aphasiology*. https://doi.org/10.1080/0268 7038.2020.1759269.

Bye, R. A. (1998). When clients are dying: Occupational therapists' perspectives. *Occupational Therapy Journal of Research*, *18*(1), 3–14.

Cameron, A., McPhail, S., Hudson, K., Fleming, J., Lethlean, J., & Tan, N. F. E. (2018). The confidence and knowledge of health practitioners when interacting with people with aphasia in a hospital setting. *Disability and Rehabilitation*, *40*(11), 1288–1293.

Carswell, A., McColl, M. A., Baptiste, S., Law, M., Polatajko, H., & Pollock, N. (2004). The Canadian occupational performance measure: A research and clinical literature review. *Canadian Journal of Occupational Therapy*, *71*(4), 210–222.

Carver, C. S., & Scheier, M. F. (2001). *On the self-regulation of behaviour*. Cambridge University Press.

Cott, C. A. (2004). Client-centred rehabilitation: Client perspectives. *Disability and Rehabilitation*, *26*(24), 1411–1422.

Cup, E. H., Scholte op Reimer, W. J., Thijssen, M. C., & van Kuyk-Minis, M. A. (2003). Reliability and validity of the Canadian occupational performance measure in stroke patients. *Clinical Rehabilitation*, *17*(4), 402–409.

Dörfler, E., & Kulnik, S. T. (2020). Despite communication and cognitive impairment—person-centred goal-setting after stroke: A qualitative study. *Disability and Rehabilitation*, *42*(25), 3628–3637.

Fleming, S., Boyd, A., Ballejos, M., Kynast-Gales, S., & Malemute, C. (2013). Goal setting with type 2 diabetes. A hermeneutic analysis of the experiences of diabetes educators. *The Diabetes Educator*, *39*(6), 811.

Gum, A., & Snyder, C. R. (2002). Coping with terminal illness: The role of hopeful thinking. *Journal of Palliative Medicine*, *5*(6), 883–894.

Hammell, K. R. (2013). Client-centred practice in occupational therapy: Critical reflections. *Scandinavian Journal of Occupational Therapy*, *20*(3), 174–181.

Hersh, D., Worrall, L., Howe, T., Sherratt, S., & Davidson, B. (2012). SMARTER goal setting in aphasia rehabilitation. *Aphasiology*, *26*(2), 220.

Hunt, A. W., Le Dorze, G., Trentham, B., Polatajko, H. J., & Dawson, D. R. (2015). Elucidating a goal-setting continuum in brain injury rehabilitation. *Qualitative Health Research*, *25*(8), 1044.

Hurn, J., Kneebone, I., & Cropley, M. (2006). Goal setting as an outcome measure: A systematic review. *Clinical Rehabilitation*, *20*(9), 756–772.

Larsen, E. A., Rasmussen, B., & Christensen, J. R. (2018). Enhancing a client-centred practice with the Canadian occupational performance measure. *Occupational Therapy International*. https://doi.org/10.1155/2018/5956301.

Lawler, J., Dowswell, G., Hearn, J., et al. (1999). Recovering from stroke: A qualitative investigation of the role of goal setting in late stroke recovery. *Journal of Advanced Nursing*, *30*, 401.

Leach, E., Cornwell, P., Fleming, J., & Haines, T. (2010). Patient centered goal-setting in a subacute rehabilitation setting. *Disability and Rehabilitation*, *32*(2), 159–172.

Levack, W. M. M., & Siegert, R. J. (2014). Challenges in theory, practice and evidence. In W. M. M. Levack, & R. J. Siegert (Eds.), *Rehabilitation goal setting: Theory, practice and evidence* (1st ed., pp. 3–19). CRC Press, Taylor & Francis Group.

Levack, W. M. M., Weatherall, M., Hay-Smith, E. J. C., Dean, S. G., McPherson, K., & Siegert, R. J. (2015). Goal setting and activities to enhance goal pursuit for adults with acquired disabilities participating in rehabilitation. *Cochrane Database of Systematic Reviews*, *7*, CD009727.

Lloyd, A., Bannigan, K., Sugavanam, T., & Freeman, J. (2018). Experiences of stroke survivors, their families and unpaid carers in goal setting within stroke rehabilitation: A systematic review of qualitative evidence. *JBI Database of Systematic Reviews and Implementation Reports*, *16*(6), 1418–1453.

Locke, E. A., & Latham, G. P. (2002). Building a practically useful theory of goal setting and task motivation. A 35-year odyssey. *American Psychology*, *57*, 705–717.

McAndrew, E., McDermott, S., Vitzakovitch, S., Warunek, M., & Holm, M. B. (1999). Therapist and patient perceptions of the occupational therapy goal-setting process: A pilot study. *Physical and Occupational Therapy in Geriatrics*, *17*(1), 55–63.

McPherson, K. M., Kayes, N. M., & Kersten, P. (2015). MEANING as a smarter approach to goals in rehabilitation. In R. R. Stiegert, & W. M. M. Levack (Eds.), *Rehabilitation goal setting: Theory, practice and evidence* (1st ed., pp. 105–119). CRC Press; Taylor & Francis Group.

Medical Research Council. (2008). Developing and evaluating complex interventions: New guidance. https://mrc.ukri.org/documents/pdf/complex-interventions-guidance/.

Melton, J., Forsyth, K., & Freeth, D. (2009). Using theory in practice. In E. A. S. Duncan (Ed.), *Skills for practice in occupational therapy* (1st ed., pp. 9–23). Churchill Livingstone.

MRC Population Health Science Research Network. (2014). *Process evaluation of complex interventions*. UK Medical Research Council.

Murphy, J. (2009). Talking mats: A study of communication difficulties and the feasibility and effectiveness of a low-tech communication framework. PhD Thesis. University of Stirling. ISBN 978-1-85769 244 0.

Murphy, J., & Boa, S. (2012). Using the WHO-ICF with talking mats to enable adults with long-term communication difficulties to participate in goal setting. *Augmentative and Alternative Communication*, *28*(1), 52–60.

Murphy, J., Gray, C. M., van Achterberg, T., Wyke, S., & Cox, S. (2010). The effectiveness of the talking mats framework in helping people with dementia to express their views on well-being. *Dementia*, *9*(4), 454–472. https://doi.org/10.1177/1471301210381776.

O'Halloran, R., Hickson, L., & Worrall, L. (2008). Environmental factors that influence communication between people with communication disability and their healthcare providers in hospital: A review of the literature within the international classification of functioning, disability and health (ICF) framework. *International Journal of Language & Communication Disorders*, *43*, 601–632.

Plant, S. E., Tyson, S. F., Kirk, S., & Parsons, J. (2016). What are the barriers and facilitators to goal-setting during rehabilitation for stroke and other acquired brain injuries? A systematic review and meta-synthesis. *Clinical Rehabilitation, 30*(9), 921–930.

Prescott, S., Fleming, J., & Doig, E. (2015). Goal setting approaches and principles used in rehabilitation for people with acquired brain injury: A systematic scoping review. *Brain Injury, 29*(13–14), 1515–1529.

Rose, T. A., Worrall, L. E., Hickson, L. M., & Hoffmann, T. C. (2011). Aphasia friendly written health information: Content and design characteristics. *International Journal of Speech-Language Pathology, 13*(4), 335–347. https://doi.org/10.3109/17549507.2011.560396.

Rosewilliam, S., Roskell, C., & Pandyan, A. (2011). A systematic review and synthesis of the quantitative and qualitative evidence behind patient-centred goal setting in stroke rehabilitation. *Clinical Rehabilitation, 25*(6), 501.

Schwarzer, R. (1992). Self-efficacy in the adoption and maintenance of health behaviours: Theoretical approaches and a new model. In R. Schwarzer (Ed.), *Self-efficacy: Thought control of action* (1st ed., pp. 217–238). Hemisphere Publishing Corp.

Scobbie, L., & Dixon, D. (2014). Theory-based approach to goal setting. In R. R. Stiegert, & W. M. M. Levack (Eds.), *Rehabilitation goal setting: Theory, practice and evidence* (1st ed.). CRC Press; Taylor & Francis Group.

Scobbie, L., Brady, M. C., Duncan, E. A. S., & Wyke, S. (2020). Goal attainment, adjustment and disengagement in the first year after stroke: A qualitative study. *Neuropsychological Rehabilitation.* https://doi.org/10.1080/09602011.2020.1724803.

Scobbie, L., Dixon, D., & Wyke, S. (2009). Identifying and applying psychological theory to setting and achieving rehabilitation goals. *Clinical Rehabilitation, 23,* 321.

Scobbie, L., Dixon, D., & Wyke, S. (2011). Goal setting and action planning in the rehabilitation setting: Development of a theoretically informed practice framework. *Clinical Rehabilitation, 25,* 468–482.

Scobbie, L., Duncan, E. A., Brady, M. C., & Wyke, S. (2015). Goal setting practice in services delivering community-based stroke rehabilitation: A United Kingdom (UK) wide survey. *Disability and Rehabilitation, 37*(14), 1291–1298. https://doi.org/10.3109/09638288.2014.961652.

Scobbie, L., McLean, D., Dixon, D., Duncan, E. A. S., & Wyke, S. (2013). Implementing a framework for goal setting in community based stroke rehabilitation: A process evaluation. *BMC Health Services Research, 13,* 190. https://doi.org/10.1186/1472-6963-13-190.

Siegert, R. J., & Levack, W. M. M. (2015). In *Rehabilitation goal setting: Theory, practice and evidence* (1st ed.). CRC Press; Taylor & Francis Group.

Snyder, C. R., Lehman, K. A., Kluck, B., & Monsson, Y. (2006). Hope for rehabilitation and vice versa. *Rehabilitation Psychology, 51*(2), 89–112.

Stevens, A., Beurskens, A., Köke, A., & van der Weijden, T. (2013). The use of patient-specific measurement instruments in the process of goal-setting: A systematic review of available instruments and their feasibility. *Clinical Rehabilitation, 27*(11), 1005–1019. https://doi.org/10.1177/0269215513490178.

Tennant, A. (2007). Goal attainment scaling: Current methodological challenges. *Disability and Rehabilitation, 15*(29), 1583–1588.

Turner-Stokes, L. (2009). Goal attainment scaling (GAS) in rehabilitation: A practical guide. *Clinical Rehabilitation, 23*(4), 362–370.

Turner-Stokes, L., Williams, H., & Johnson, J. (2009). Goal attainment scaling: Does it provide added value as a person-centred measure for evaluation of outcome in neurorehabilitation following acquired brain injury? *Journal of Rehabilitation Medicine, 41*(7), 528–535.

Wade, D., & de Jong, B. A. (2000). Recent advances in rehabilitation. *BMJ, 320*(7246), 1385–1388.

Wade, D. T. (2005). Describing rehabilitation interventions. *Clinical Rehabilitation, 19*(8), 811–818.

Wade, D. T. (2009). Goal setting in rehabilitation: An overview of what, why and how. *Clinical Rehabilitation, 23*(4), 291–295.

Wade, D. T. (2020). What is rehabilitation? An empirical investigation leading to an evidence-based description. *Clinical Rehabilitation, 34*(5), 571–583.

World Health Organisation. (2001). *International classification of functioning, disability and health (ICF).* Author.

Yang, S., Lin, C., Lee, Y., & Chang, J. (2017). The Canadian occupational performance measure for patients with stroke: A systematic review. *Journal of Physical Therapy Science, 29,* 548–555.

8

Therapeutic Use of Self: A Model of the Intentional Relationship

Renee R. Taylor and Jane Melton

HIGHLIGHTS

- Though significant progress has been made in knowledge development regarding use of self in occupational therapy, research suggests that an increased focus is needed.
- There is still a lack of clarity regarding the exact definition, use, and relevance of therapeutic use of self in occupational therapy.
- Clients possess a number of interpersonal characteristics that, when discovered, can guide therapists' decision making within the relationship.

- An interpersonal event is a naturally occurring communication, reaction, process, task, or general circumstance that occurs during therapy and that has the potential to detract from or strengthen the therapeutic relationship.
- The intentional relationship model provides a means of mapping, interpreting, and responding to client characteristics and to the challenging interpersonal events of therapy by incorporating a variety of perspectives, skills, and approaches.

INTRODUCTION

The intentional relationship model (IRM; Taylor, 2020) defines therapeutic use of self as a therapist's application of empathy and intentionality to the use of six communication modes that are applied thoughtfully to respond to a client's unique interpersonal characteristics and to resolve challenging or poignant interpersonal events emerging in practice. This process requires the therapist to strive toward a fundamental understanding of each client at an interpersonal level, focusing on the client's communication preferences and needs (Taylor, 2020). It requires a personal and subjective investment in the client during which the therapist makes moment-to-moment decisions about how to initiate and respond to the client's reactions to therapy and/or the therapist (Taylor, 2020). The IRM refers to this process as interpersonal reasoning (Taylor, 2020).

A recent survey of practicing occupational therapists within the United States revealed that more than 80% of therapists consider therapeutic use of self to be the most important variable in successful therapy outcomes (Taylor et al., 2009). At the same time, fewer than half of US therapists felt they were adequately trained in this area upon graduation. Additionally, about two-thirds of therapists

felt that there was sufficient knowledge about use of self in occupational therapy (Taylor et al., 2009).

These therapists' perceptions of the importance of therapeutic use of self are supported by other research studies; a growing number indicates that the client–therapist relationship is a key determinant of whether occupational therapy has been successful (Ayres-Rosa & Hasselkus, 1996; Cole & McLean, 2003). In this chapter, we provide an overview of the historical foundations and literature on use of self within the field of occupational therapy. This is followed by a rationale for the introduction of a new conceptual model of use of self and an explanation of the research that has been conducted thus far to support the development of this model. The model and its four components and functions are then described. Ultimately, a case example is presented that illustrates a clinician's use of this model in a practice situation.

HISTORICAL OVERVIEW

The topic of therapeutic use of self has been addressed throughout occupational therapy's history. Recommendations about how therapists should interact with clients have changed as our thinking about practice has evolved over time. A historical account has identified three distinct eras in occupational therapy (Kielhofner, 2004). Each of these eras offers a unique perspective and emphasis on the role of the client–therapist relationship in the therapy process.

The earliest occupational era reflected ideals embraced by the field's founders (Kielhofner, 2004). Initial descriptions of therapeutic use of self came from Europe in the late 1700s during the time of moral treatment (Bing, 1981; Bockoven, 1971). Moral treatment emphasised the facilitation of self-determination through engagement in everyday activities such as arts and crafts, sports, and other pursuits. When more formalised approaches to occupational therapy emerged in the early 1900s, the humanistic approaches of moral treatment were emphasised. Supporters of moral treatment argued that all activity prescriptions should be based on an in-depth understanding of the patient's personality, preferences, and interests (Bing, 1981). Consideration and kindness were put forward as essential interpersonal values. During this era, the therapeutic relationship was viewed as existing solely as a means for encouraging the client to engage in occupation. In creating this relationship, the therapist was to serve in the following roles:

- Expert
- Guide
- Role model
- Motivator through persuasion
- Emulator of the joy of occupation
- Instiller of confidence
- Creator of a positive physical and social milieu

In the mid-20th century, the early occupational era was replaced by a more analytic era labeled the era of inner mechanisms (Kielhofner, 2004). In this era, concern for addressing a client's underlying impairment became the focus. Rooted in the medical establishment, the role of the occupational therapist during this era was to understand the nuances of and correct internal failures of body and mind. The client–therapist relationship was viewed as the central mechanism for change, and understanding of this relationship was largely based on principles borrowed from literature influenced by the psychoanalytic perspective. Often, the relationship was viewed as a means by which to understand a client's unconscious motives, desires, and behaviour toward others and toward occupations. Within the relationship, the therapist's role was to:

- Behave in a competent and professional manner
- Assume an impersonal and objective attitude toward the client
- Instill hope
- Be tactful
- Exert self-control
- Exercise good judgement
- Privately identify with and use emotional reactions to patients in planning how to respond

Within mental health settings, which then comprised a significant amount of occupational therapy practice, it was common to expect that the client would achieve catharsis by acting out unconscious motives and desires within the therapeutic relationship. The therapist then assisted the client in achieving insight into any issues that were viewed to be at the core of the client's pathologic feelings and behaviours. By the 1970s, some believed that occupation had lost its place as the key dynamic of therapy (Kielhofner, 2007; Schwartz, 2003; Shannon, 1977; Yerxa 1967).

In the latter part of the 20th century a new, contemporary era was born, which returned the field to its initial focus on occupation. This era was labeled the return to occupation (Kielhofner, 2004). In part, this new era represented a reaction to what was perceived as an overemphasis on the role of the therapeutic relationship during the era of inner mechanisms. In this contemporary era, the strong focus on the therapeutic relationship has been set aside in favour of a renewed emphasis on occupational engagement as the true mechanism for change and positive outcomes in occupational therapy (Kielhofner & Burke, 1977; Schwartz, 2003; Shannon, 1977; Yerxa, 1967). Similar to the early occupational era, the role of the relationship in the contemporary era is more unidimensional in its focus, which is strictly to facilitate the client's engagement in occupation. The therapist's role is to use a variety of interpersonal strategies to make occupations appealing.

Within this contemporary era there have been three central movements with which the client–therapist relationship has been associated:

- Collaborative and client-centred approaches
- Emphasis on caring and empathy
- Use of narrative and clinical reasoning

Collaborative and client-centred approaches (e.g., Duncan, 2006; Mosey, 1970; Townsend, 2003) have focused on readjusting power imbalances within the therapeutic relationship and on facilitating client control over decision making and problem solving. Generally, these approaches emphasise open communication, orientation toward the client's perspective, recognition of the client's strengths, shared goals and priorities, and a collaborative partnership. There has also been an emphasis on therapist self-awareness. Therapists are encouraged to recognise, control, and correct nontherapeutic reactions, incorporate their own life experiences into an understanding of their client's perspectives, and draw upon their personal reactions to clients to guide their clinical reasoning.

In conjunction with collaborative and client-centred approaches, the contemporary era has also been characterised by an emphasis on empathy and caring within the therapeutic relationship. This can be summarised as an emphasis on the emotional exchange that occurs between client and therapist, on goal-directed activity, and on activities that promote personal growth (Baum, 1980; Devereaux, 1984; Gilfoyle, 1980; King, 1980; Peloquin, 1989a, 1989b, 1990, 1993, 1995, 2002, 2003; Yerxa, 1980). Caring was put forth as a much-needed value, defined as follows (Baum, 1980; Devereaux, 1984; Gilfoyle, 1980; King, 1980; Yerxa, 1980):

- Intimate knowing
- Communicating effectively
- Eliminating the focus on impairment
- Flexibility in adapting to environmental and situational demands
- Harnessing the will of each client
- Believing in the innate potential of the individual
- Using humour
- Connecting at an emotional level
- Using touch to connect
- Restoring personal control through activity

More recently, empathy has been written about extensively and defined as a communication of partnership in the following ways:

- A turning of the soul toward the client
- A recognition of how one is similar to the client and how the client is unique
- An entry into the client's experience
- A connection with the feelings of the client
- The power to recover from that connection and maintain strength to continue therapeutic work

Peloquin (1989b, 1990, 1993) emphasised the roles of art, literature, imagination, and self-reflection. She further argued that the fundamental characteristics required to develop one's therapeutic use of self are well conveyed through reading literature and viewing and doing art (Peloquin, 1989b). She believed that providing therapists with both fictional and nonfictional poems and stories that illustrate empathy and the depersonalising consequences of neglectful attitudes and failed communication could be a powerful motivator for the development of caring (Peloquin 1990, 1993, 1995).

Clinical reasoning and narrative approaches comprise the final general category of contemporary scholarship that includes the client–therapist relationship as a focal point (Clark, 1993; Crepeau, 1991; Jonsson et al., 2001; Kielhofner, 1997; Lyons & Crepeau, 2001; Mattingly, 1991, 1994; Mattingly & Fleming, 1994; Rogers, 1983; Schell, 2003; Schell & Cervero, 1993; Schwartz, 2003; Schwartzberg, 2002). These approaches emphasise the role of therapist understanding and reflection about the unique way in which clients think about and summarise key events in their lives (Kielhofner, 2004). Clinical reasoning approaches incorporate thinking about the relationship as a component of one's overall approach to making sense of assessment findings and developing a treatment plan (Mattingly & Fleming, 1994). This element has been referred to as interactive reasoning (Mattingly & Fleming, 1994), and it has been described as an underground practice in occupational therapy (Fleming, 1991) because relatively little is known about the underlying mechanisms. One exception involves work by Mattingly and Gillette (1991), which resulted in six relationship-building strategies pertinent to clinical reasoning:

- Providing clients with choices
- Individualising treatment
- Structuring therapy activities to maximise the potential for success
- Going outside of the formal therapeutic role and doing special favours or acts of kindness for clients
- Sharing one's personal stories with clients
- Joint problem solving

Narrative approaches (e.g., narrative reasoning) were developed in tandem with clinical reasoning approaches (Kielhofner, 1997; Mattingly, 1994). Narrative approaches seek to organise and make sense of information from clients by encouraging them to present information about themselves through storytelling, poetry, or metaphor. Thinking in story form is thought to allow both the client and the therapist to discover the meaning of the impairment experience according to the client's unique perspective. Therapeutic approaches are then focused toward reconstructing more hopeful narratives to reshape one's life story.

RATIONALE FOR A MODEL OF USE OF SELF

We have seen that occupational therapy's view of the therapeutic relationship has changed and developed throughout history. Early perspectives of the field's first era emphasised the centrality of occupation and the therapist's role in promoting occupational engagement. The second era redefined the therapeutic relationship as a psychodynamic process that, according to some perspectives, replaced occupation as the central dynamic of therapy. With some exception (e.g., Blair & Daniels, 2006) this idea was, in large part, rejected in favour of the contemporary, renewed focus on occupation.

During our contemporary era of heightened occupational focus, the three major themes related to the therapeutic relationship described in the prior section have been introduced: (1) collaborative and client-centred approaches, (2) an emphasis on caring and empathy, and (3) clinical reasoning and use of narrative. These are important themes that offer broad and useful principles related to the therapeutic use of self.

Despite the fact that these approaches coexist with the field's returned emphasis on occupational engagement, they do not directly address the question of how therapeutic use of self can be used specifically to promote both occupational engagement and positive therapy outcomes. Their relationship to an occupationally focused practice is assumed but not made explicit.

In addition, some implicitly assume that, when therapists achieve a reflective, appreciative, and emotionally connected state with clients, a positive therapeutic process will simply emerge. This assumption is a large one that appears to be contradicted in the experience of most practising therapists. Despite the existence of a fairly extensive contemporary literature on collaboration, client-centred practice, caring, empathy, clinical reasoning, and narrative, the vast majority of practising therapists that we surveyed believe occupational therapy does not have sufficient knowledge to support the therapeutic use of self (Taylor et al., 2009). Their perspectives suggest that something is still missing.

To date, there has been no effort to integrate all of the contemporary interpersonal approaches in occupational therapy into a coherent explanation of the therapeutic relationship. Moreover, beyond broad principles, there are few details about how the therapeutic relationship should be approached and managed in light of the central focus on the client's engagement in occupation. Consequently, there is still a lack of clarity regarding the exact definition, use, and relevance of therapeutic use of self in occupational therapy.

These observations were the impetus for developing the conceptual practice model presented in this chapter, the IRM. The model was developed in an attempt to clarify and provide more detailed guidance of how to enact the therapeutic use of self in occupational therapy. Therapeutic use of self involves a highly personal, individualised, and subjective decision-making process. For some therapists, the process is driven by emotional reactions to clients and a perceived reliance on an innate or nurtured intuitive capacity. Others perceive the process as largely rational and grounded in the disciplined application of a set of interpersonal guidelines. Irrespective of such viewpoints, therapeutic use of self is, in large part, a product of the extent to which one possesses a knowledge base and interpersonal skills that can be applied thoughtfully to common interpersonal events in practice. Accordingly, therapeutic use of self is an occupational therapy skill that must be developed, reinforced, monitored, and refined.

The IRM explains therapeutic use of self and its relationship with occupational engagement. Additionally, it provides a means of mapping, interpreting, and responding to the unique and everyday interpersonal events of therapy by incorporating a variety of perspectives, skills, and approaches. The model provides educators, supervisors, students, and clinicians with a common vocabulary with which to discuss and describe the interpersonal phenomena that have an ongoing impact on everyday practice.

THE INTENTIONAL RELATIONSHIP MODEL

The IRM is an empirically based model that was developed over a 3-year period. In part, its concepts were based on practitioner responses to a large-scale ($n = 1000$, response rate 64%) nationwide survey of occupational therapists' knowledge, attitudes, and interpersonal behaviours related to use of self (Taylor et al., 2009). In addition, 12 occupational therapy practitioners from various regions of the world were observed and interviewed using a semistructured interview measure developed by the first author. In each region, these therapists were nominated by their local peers as having exceptional talent in terms of their ability to form successful therapeutic relationships with a wide range of clients. They also participated in an initial introductory interview with the first author to determine their suitability for participation in the formal interview and observation. The insights that emerged from the observation of these expert therapists were critical to the development of this model. The second author is one of the therapists who was selected and studied for her expertise, and her approach to the therapeutic use of self will be used later in this chapter to illustrate some aspects of this model.

Many of the concepts for the IRM have their origins in theory underlying psychotherapy practice models. However, the IRM recognises a fundamental difference between occupational therapy and traditional psychotherapy. Fig. 8.1 portrays the traditional psychotherapy process. In psychotherapy, interpersonal relating between client and therapist is the central focus. The verbal communication between client and therapist is lengthy, intense, highly complex, nuanced, and derived from detailed conceptual models of how psychological change is intended to occur. Interpersonal communication is typically the only activity that occurs during psychotherapy.

In occupational therapy the client–therapist relationship does not and should not pretend to emulate the intensity, duration, and complexity of a traditional psychotherapy relationship.

By contrast, the central focus of occupational therapy is occupational engagement. A diagram of the unique role that the therapeutic relationship plays in occupational therapy is presented in Fig. 8.2.

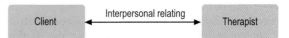

FIG. 8.1 The client–therapist relationship in traditional psychotherapy.

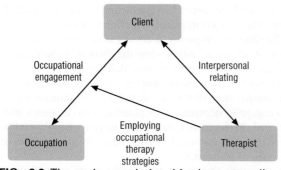

FIG. 8.2 The unique relationship between client, therapist, and occupation in occupational therapy.

As it shows the occupational therapist employs a number of therapeutic strategies, usually rooted in existing models of practice, to facilitate the client's engagement in occupation. Depending on the occupational needs, capacities, and diagnosis of the client, any number of occupational therapy practice models might be employed alone or in combination to promote occupational engagement. However, this main task of promoting occupational engagement through employing the specific methods and strategies of occupational therapy does not exist in isolation of a larger process of relating that occurs between client and therapist.

The IRM explains the relationship between client and therapist that is part of the overall process of occupational therapy. Accordingly, the IRM is intended to complement existing occupational therapy conceptual practice models rather than replace any single model. It explains the detailed and overarching aspects of the client–therapist

relationship, an important aspect of occupational therapy not addressed extensively by other conceptual practice models. Fig. 8.3 shows how the intentional relationship is designed to supplement the use of other occupational therapy conceptual practice models.

As shown, the IRM should complement the usual concepts and strategies of occupational therapy that are directly aimed at facilitating occupational engagement. The model's utility for occupational therapy lies in addressing the otherwise unarticulated aspects of the interpersonal relationship that occur during the therapy process and that influence both occupational engagement and therapy outcomes. The next section defines the elements of this model and provides an explanation of how the elements interact to optimise the circumstances for a successful client–therapist relationship in occupational therapy.

To reiterate, the IRM is not a free-standing model of practice for occupational therapy. If a therapist only utilised this model, the essential work of occupational therapy would not occur. The model was designed to fill a gap in our practical knowledge about how to manage the interpersonal aspects of therapy, particularly the more challenging ones. This model should complement the field's existing methods and models by making the process of establishing a successful relationship with clients easier, clearer, and more straightforward.

Elements of the Intentional Relationship Model

This chapter provides only a basic overview of the IRM. Those who are interested in a more thorough treatment should consult *The Intentional Relationship: Occupational Therapy and Use of Self* (Taylor, 2020). The IRM views the

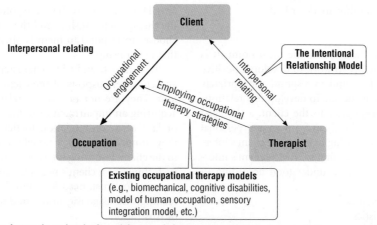

FIG. 8.3 The intentional relationship model as a complement to existing occupational therapy models.

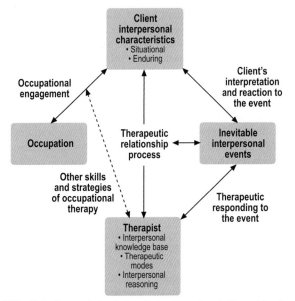

FIG. 8.4 A model of the intentional relationship in occupational therapy.

therapeutic relationship as being comprised of four central elements (Fig. 8.4):

1. The client
2. The interpersonal events that occur during therapy
3. The therapist
4. The occupation

The model explains the requirements for a functional client–therapist relationship, and it incorporates guidelines for responding to common interpersonal events that frequently occur in therapy. In the following section the relevant aspects of each element of the model and their relationships with one another are described.

The Client

According to the IRM, the client is the focal point. It is the therapist's responsibility to work to develop a positive relationship with the client and to respond appropriately when interpersonal events occur. To develop this relationship and respond appropriately to the client, a therapist must work to understand the client from an interpersonal perspective. This involves getting to know the client's interpersonal characteristics. According to IRM, a client's interpersonal characteristics can be understood according to two dimensions:

- Situational characteristics
- Enduring characteristics

Situational characteristics are interpersonal characteristics that are inconsistent with how a client typically and consistently behaves when interacting with others. Instead, they reflect a client's acute emotional reaction to a specific situation. Typically, a client's situational characteristics attract our attention when the client is encountering a situation that is somehow painful, frustrating, or stressful. For most of us, stressful situations result in some negative emotional state that makes it temporarily difficult for us to engage in occupations as planned. Thus a client's situational characteristics are likely to surface when they interfere with the client's ability to engage in the activities of therapy as planned.

A client's situational characteristics are most likely to reveal themselves in therapy when the client is facing a situation where some immediate aspect of the impairment and/or the environment is experienced as stressful. Impairments, particularly when they are new or when there is a medical crisis or exacerbation in severity that disrupts one's usual relationship with the environment, often cause people to experience stress. Therapists are encouraged to assume, on some level, that a client's impairment situation and/or the client's interaction with an unaccommodating or difficult environment will cause the client to be more vulnerable to experiencing a variety of emotional reactions, many of which may be perceived as negative or at least atypical for that individual. For example, feelings of loss are common among newly disabled individuals and they may manifest in terms of sadness, irritability, anxiety, insecurity, or anger. A therapist's interpersonal behaviour, if perceived as insensitive, judgemental, or uncaring, may also serve as a source of stress and cause clients to interact in a manner that is generally inconsistent with their personality. It is important for newer therapists to recognise that these and other acute emotional reactions are normative. In fact they are givens in many health care situations. They bear no reflection on the client's character or personality. However, they do have the potential to play out within the therapy relationship, and the way in which a therapist chooses to respond to them is often vital to the future of that relationship.

By contrast, enduring characteristics are more stable and consistent aspects of the client's interpersonal behaviour. They are not necessarily related to the situation of acquiring an impairment or to the environment's reaction or lack of accommodation to that impairment. Instead, they comprise an interpersonal profile that is idiosyncratic to the client. Enduring interpersonal characteristics include such things as a client's preferred style of communicating, capacity for trust, need for control, general orientation to relating, and usual way of responding to change, challenge, or frustration.

Because they coexist in each client, situational and enduring characteristics are mutually informative. Behaviour that reflects one's acute emotional reaction to a stressful event may temporarily attenuate, alter, or intensify one's interpersonal behaviour in what are usually more stable categories. For example, a client who normally responds to a challenging situation adaptively may become irritated when the therapist recommends a more challenging activity if, earlier in that day, the client underwent a painful biopsy and then discovered that she did not have the funds to pay for transportation after leaving the physician's office. The rationale for distinguishing the two categories of interpersonal characteristics is to help inform therapists' understanding of the client in stressful and nonstressful situations so that therapeutic responses can be appropriately tailored and modulated.

The Interpersonal Events of Therapy

An interpersonal event is a naturally occurring communication, reaction, process, task, or general circumstance that occurs during therapy and that has the potential to detract from or strengthen the therapeutic relationship. In therapy, these events may be precipitated by the following kinds of circumstances:

- Client resistance (e.g., a client refuses or feels unable to participate in some activity)
- Therapist behaviour (e.g., the therapist asks a question that the client perceives as intrusive or emotionally difficult to face)
- Client display of strong emotions in therapy (e.g., an elderly client begins crying during transfer training, or a child client runs up to the therapist and hugs her in the midst of a sensory motor activity)
- A difficult circumstance of therapy (e.g., a client is embarrassed because of losing bladder control or becomes frustrated or fearful in the midst of an activity)
- A rift or conflict between client and therapist (e.g., the client is offended by a comment made by the therapist)
- Differences concerning the aim of therapy (e.g., a client insists on a goal that the therapist believes is not attainable, or the therapist recommends a goal that the client rejects)
- Client requests that test the boundaries or limits of the therapeutic relationship (e.g., the client invites the therapist to attend her wedding)

These, of course, are only a few of the myriad of possible interpersonal events that occur in the course of occupational therapy.

When interpersonal events of therapy occur, their interpretation by the client is a product of the client's unique set of interpersonal characteristics. Sometimes the event may have a significant effect upon the client and other times a client will be unaffected or minimally affected. When such events occur, what is important is that the therapist be aware that the event has occurred and take responsibility for responding appropriately.

Interpersonal events are:
- Inevitable during the course of therapy
- Ripe with both threat and opportunity

Interpersonal events are part of the constant give and take that occurs in a therapy process. They are distinguished from other events or processes in that they are charged with the potential for an emotional response either when they occur or later upon reflection. Consequently, if they are ignored or responded to less than optimally, these events can threaten both the therapeutic relationship and the client's occupational engagement. When optimally responded to, these events can provide opportunities for positive client learning or change and for solidifying the therapeutic relationship. Because they are unavoidable in any therapeutic interaction, one of the primary tasks of a therapist practising according to the IRM is to respond to these inevitable events in a way that leads to repair and strengthening of the therapeutic relationship.

The Therapist

Within the IRM, the therapist is responsible for making every reasonable effort to make the relationship work. Specifically, the therapist is responsible for bringing three main interpersonal capacities into the relationship:
- An interpersonal skill base
- Therapeutic modes (or interpersonal styles)
- Capacity for interpersonal reasoning

This section provides a brief description of each of these interpersonal capacities. The first capacity involves development and application of a wide-ranging fount of knowledge about how to manage the various aspects of one's relationships with other people. The therapist's interpersonal skill base is comprised of a continuum of skills that are judiciously applied by the therapist to build a functional working relationship with the client. The perspective of the model is that, depending on the unique experiences, knowledge, and innate capacities of the therapist, some of these skills will come more naturally while others will require significant effort and practice to develop.

These interpersonal skills are summarised in terms of nine categories:
- Therapeutic communication
- Interviewing skills and strategic questioning
- Establishing relationships with clients
- Families, social systems, and groups
- Working effectively with supervisors, employers, and other professionals
- Understanding and managing difficult interpersonal behaviour
- Empathic breaks and conflicts

- Professional behaviour, values, and ethics
- Therapist self-care and professional development

The first category, therapeutic communication, involves activities such as verbal and nonverbal communication skills, therapeutic listening, assertiveness, providing clients with direction and feedback, and seeking and responding to client feedback. Interviewing skills is another skill set that involves being watchful and intentional about the way in which one approaches the process of asking a client questions. Socratic questioning is a specific approach to questioning born out of cognitive psychology (e.g., Beck, 1995). It involves asking questions in a way that guides the respondent to think more broadly or differently. Establishing relationships with clients includes rapport building, matching one's therapeutic style to the interpersonal demands of the client, managing a client's strong emotion, judicious use of touch, and cultural competence.

Because many clients have caregivers, family members, or other individuals with whom they have regular contact, understanding and working with families, social systems, and groups is an essential aspect of occupational therapy practice. It includes using guiding principles of IRM, in combination with prominent systems theories, to gain the collaboration of partners, parents, other family, and friends to serve the goals of therapy. It also involves understanding the structure, process, and interpersonal dynamics of group therapy.

Another fundamental skill involves knowing how to work collaboratively with supervisors, employers, and other professionals. It involves knowing how to communicate with other professionals about clients both in the presence and in the absence of those clients. Additionally, it requires understanding the power dynamics and value systems that underlie supervisor/student and employer/employee relationships. Understanding and managing clients' difficult behaviour is another category of necessary interpersonal skills required in many practice situations. It involves knowing how to respond effectively to behaviours that involve manipulation, excessive dependency, symptom focusing, resistance, emotional disengagement, denial, difficulty with rapport and trust, and hostility. Responding effectively will help limit the extent to which this behaviour disrupts the goal and process of therapy.

Knowing how to resolve conflicts and empathic breaks (or rifts in understanding between client and therapist) is another fundamental skill set that can salvage a failing relationship or repair minor threats to an otherwise functional relationship. Professional behaviour and ethics encompasses knowledge of how one's own values are consistent or inconsistent with the occupational therapy core values, ethical behaviour and decision making, behavioural self-awareness around clients, being reliable and dependable,

upholding confidentiality, and setting and managing professional boundaries. Therapist self-care incorporates knowing and managing one's own emotional reactions to clients and being accountable to those reactions, a general capacity for self-reflection, an ability to manage one's personal life and seek support when necessary, and the capacity to maintain perspective regarding client outcomes. More information about all of these skills, which comprise a therapist's interpersonal skill base, is provided in Taylor (2020).

The second interpersonal capacity that a therapist brings to the client–therapist relationship is a primary therapeutic mode(s). A therapeutic mode is a specific way of relating to a client. The IRM identifies six therapeutic modes:

- Advocating
- Collaborating
- Empathising
- Encouraging
- Instructing
- Problem solving

A brief definition of each mode and an example of how the second author used the mode in practice is provided in Table 8.1.

Therapists naturally use therapeutic modes that are consistent with their fundamental personality characteristics. For example, a therapist who tends to be more of a listener than a talker and believes in the importance of understanding another person's perspective before making a suggestion would likely use empathising as a primary therapeutic mode in therapy. Therapists vary widely in terms of the range and flexibility with which they use modes in relating to clients. Some therapists relate to clients in one or two primary ways, while others draw upon multiple therapeutic modes depending upon the interpersonal characteristics of the client and the situation, or inevitable interpersonal events, at hand. One of the goals in using the IRM is to become increasingly comfortable utilising any of the six modes flexibly and interchangeably depending upon the client's needs. A therapeutic mode or set of modes defines the therapist's general interpersonal style when interacting with a client. Therapists able to utilise all six of the modes flexibly and comfortably and to match those modes to the client and the situation are described as having a multimodal interpersonal style.

According to the IRM, a therapist's choice and application of a particular therapeutic mode or set of modes should depend largely on the enduring interpersonal characteristics of the client. In addition, certain events or interpersonal events in therapy may call for a mode shift. A mode shift is a conscious change in one's way of relating to a client. Mode shifts are frequently required in response to interpersonal events in therapy. For example, if a client

TABLE 8.1   The Six Therapeutic Modes in Practice

Mode	Definition	Example
Advocating	Ensuring that the client's rights are enforced and resources are secured. May require the therapist to serve as a mediator, facilitator, negotiator, enforcer, or other type of advocate with external persons and agencies	Lobbying to secure adequate resources for the provision of ongoing support and environmental adaptation. This enabled a man with learning disabilities to participate safely in self-care and domestic activities within his own home environment.
Collaborating	Expecting the client to be an active and equal participant in therapy; ensuring choice, freedom, and autonomy to the greatest extent possible	Setting recovery-oriented occupational goals with a man who had been through an inpatient detoxification programme for alcohol misuse. The service user reported that the structured routine for healthy activity choices coupled with feedback to the therapist helped to build him a sense of personal responsibility for achieving the goals.
Empathising	Ongoing striving to understand the client's thoughts, feelings, and behaviours while suspending any judgement; ensuring that the client verifies and experiences the therapist's understanding as truthful and validating	Taking care to fully appreciate the occupational requests and sensitivities of a woman experiencing psychotic symptoms. This approach enabled her to reclaim her values of being a vegan and being very environmentally conscious throughout her therapeutic recovery experience.
Encouraging	Seizing the opportunity to instill hope in a client; celebrating a client's thinking or behaviour through positive reinforcement; conveying an attitude of joyfulness, playfulness, and confidence	Spontaneously responding to a woman attending an occupational therapy group session who, inspired by some background music started to dance. Therapeutic connection was enhanced by this small gesture to join with her joy of the activity.
Instructing	Carefully structuring therapy activities and being explicit with clients about the plan, sequence, and events of therapy; providing clear instruction and feedback about performance; setting limits on a client's requests or behaviour	Enabling a withdrawn woman with little belief in her own abilities to undertake self-care activities. This was achieved by talking the woman through the task, all the while reinforcing verbally the support available with the task if required.
Problem solving	Facilitating pragmatic thinking and solving dilemmas by outlining choices, posing strategic questions, and providing opportunities for comparative or analytic thinking	Allowing a young man with Asperger syndrome to undertake the activities of value to him that also supported his well-being. This involved analysing options and negotiating with his family, who were concerned about his extraordinary choices of some occupations and his neglect of others.

perceives a therapist's attempts at problem solving to be insensitive or off the mark, a therapist would be wise to switch from the problem-solving mode to an empathising mode to get a better understanding of the client's reaction and the root of the dilemma. An interpersonal reasoning process, described in the following paragraph, can be utilised to guide the therapist in deciding when a mode shift might be required and determining which alternative mode to select. Because the interpersonal aspects of occupational therapy practice are complex and require a therapist to possess a highly adaptive therapeutic personality, the IRM recommends that therapists learn to draw upon all six of

the therapeutic modes in a flexible manner according to the different interpersonal needs of each client and the unique demands of each clinical situation.

The third therapist interpersonal competency involves the capacity to engage in an interpersonal reasoning process when an interpersonal dilemma presents itself in therapy. Interpersonal reasoning is a stepwise process by which a therapist decides what to say, do, or express in reaction to the occurrence of an interpersonal dilemma in therapy. It includes developing a mental vigilance toward the interpersonal aspects of therapy in anticipation that a dilemma might occur and a means of reviewing and evaluating options for responding. The six steps of interpersonal reasoning include:

1. Anticipate
2. Identify and cope
3. Determine if a mode shift is required
4. Choose a response mode or mode sequence
5. Draw upon any relevant interpersonal skills associated with the mode(s)
6. Gather feedback

An extensive description and discussion of these steps can be found in Taylor (2020).

The Desired Occupation

Occupational therapy is unique in that the crux of the therapy process is the client's occupational engagement. The final component of the IRM is the desired occupation, which is the task or activity that the therapist and the client have selected for therapy. These desired occupations may include a wide range of tasks and activities such as dressing oneself, driving, shopping, gross motor play, participating in a goal-setting group, completing a craft activity, or engaging in a simulated or modified work task. The selection of the occupation and support for occupational engagement will be primarily informed by other occupational therapy conceptual practice models such as the biomechanical model, the sensory integration model, or the model of human occupation (Kielhofner, 2004).

The primary function of the IRM is to enable the therapist to manage the interpersonal dynamic between the client and the therapist that also occurs as part of the therapy process. This interpersonal dynamic influences the occupational engagement and also serves as an arena in which the emotional reactions that stem from or influence occupational engagement can be positively managed. Thus, according to the model, the therapeutic relationship functions as:

1. A support to occupational engagement
2. A place where the emotions and coping process associated with the client's impairment and its implications for occupational participation can be addressed

Relationships Within the Model

According to the IRM, the client and therapist relationship can be viewed at two different levels or scales:

- The usual therapeutic relationship process that consists of the ongoing rapport and patterns of interaction between client and therapist. This relationship is enduring and it occurs outside of any unusual circumstances or stressors (macro level).
- The therapeutic relationship process that is influenced by interpersonal events of therapy, or the stressors or highlights that have the potential to challenge or enrich

the relationship depending upon how they are responded to and resolved (micro level).

The therapeutic relationship is a socially defined and personally interpreted interactive process between the client and therapist. It is socially defined in that the therapist and the client are engaged in an interaction within publicly understood roles. The therapist is recognised as bringing a certain kind of expertise, ethical guidelines, and values into a relationship. The client is recognised as a person receiving service to address a particular need. The relationship is understood to exist for the sole purpose of achieving an improvement in the client's situation. These parameters are given and provide an important definition of the relationship. Therapist and client are in a particular relationship that can be differentiated from other kinds of relationships such as friendships. At the same time, this relationship has a personal side. The client and therapist are human beings who encounter each other with the same potential range of thoughts and emotions that occur when any two people interact.

Consequently, the therapist's responsibility is to ensure the following:

- Appropriate definitions and boundaries of the therapeutic relationship are sustained
- Positive interpersonal relating such as trust, mutual respect, and honesty characterise the relationship

Sustaining the therapeutic relationship is an ongoing task that does not focus solely on interpersonal events. The everyday therapeutic relationship process that occurs outside of any specific interpersonal events is the macro dimension of the interpersonal process of therapy.

Responding to the immediate events that occur during therapy is the micro dimension. Responding to these interpersonal events of therapy requires that therapists detect the occurrence of an event, read the client's reaction to the event, and decide upon an appropriate way to address the event with the client.

Both the micro and macro scales of therapeutic interaction play a critical role in the overall process of occupational therapy. Moreover, they are interrelated. That is, the nature of the therapeutic relationship will have an influence on how the client interprets and how the therapist responds to interpersonal events and, in turn, interpersonal events and their resolution will either enhance or detract from the therapeutic relationship.

In some cases, the two scales of interaction are difficult to differentiate. For example, some therapy relationships only last for one or two sessions. In these cases, a therapist must work to respond to a client and to interpersonal events with much more vigilance and self-control because a more stable underlying therapeutic relationship does not yet exist. Moreover, the interpersonal events and their resolution during the therapy sessions will be the major determinants of the therapeutic relationship.

However, in most cases, therapy continues over a period of weeks or months, allowing for the development of some kind of predictable pattern or usual way of interacting within the therapeutic relationship. That therapeutic relationship will infuse and be shaped by interpersonal events that occur in the moment-by-moment therapy process. It will also be influenced by characteristics and behaviours that the client and therapist bring to the relationship, as well as by the circumstances surrounding the relationship. These circumstances include such factors as the nature and unfolding of the client's impairment and the context (e.g., school, rehabilitation setting, home, work) in which therapy takes place.

It is the therapist's responsibility to manage and continually strive to fortify the therapeutic relationship and to seek optimal resolutions to interpersonal events in therapy. The stability and success of a therapeutic relationship cannot be assumed. Rather, it begins early in treatment with attempts by the therapist to build rapport, followed by other efforts to develop a relationship that meets the client's immediate interpersonal needs and is appropriate in terms of the circumstances of therapy and the demands of the treatment setting. Recognising and sustaining a successful therapeutic relationship might include such things as:

- Sharing certain interpersonal rituals that facilitate bonding (e.g., paying a visit to a garden or other favourite locale within the client's setting each time before the ending of therapy)
- Witnessing the client enjoying or benefitting from therapy
- Sharing mutual feelings of respect, admiration, or appreciation
- Feeling interested and engaged in the therapy process
- Being open and comfortable digressing during therapy for discussion, venting, or advice-seeking about events in the client's personal life (without interfering with progress toward goals)
- Being able to discuss and overcome the interpersonal events that might otherwise challenge the relationship
- Having a longstanding private joke with a client
- Sharing a certain intensity of eye contact that communicates mutual trust
- Noticing a certain way a client laughs that conveys appreciation of the therapist

These are only a few examples of myriad factors that might contribute to a successful therapeutic relationship. It is the responsibility of the therapist to be vigilant to explore, identify, and sustain those factors that contribute to a relationship that supports positive therapy outcomes.

This is not to say that the client will not make positive contributions to the therapeutic relationship. In most instances, clients will bring important or essential characteristics and behaviours into the therapeutic relationship. However, the fundamental difference is that it is the therapist who must assume the ultimate responsibility for assuring that the relationship is positive. By assuming this responsibility the therapist creates a space in the relationship wherein a client can be vulnerable, distressed, frustrated, or angry without fearing that the relationship will be ruptured. Moreover, this does not mean that the therapist assumes an expert or authoritative stance in the relationship. Rather, it means that the therapist must assume responsibility for the caring within the relationship.

The enduring aspects of the therapeutic relationship are systematically built and fortified as a result of naturally occurring variables in relationship (similar personality styles or interpersonal chemistry or other optimal circumstances and timing) and as a result of the therapist's consistent efforts to build the relationship in the face of the inevitable interpersonal events and challenges that occur. If the therapist's efforts to build a relationship are successful and the client is not particularly sensitive, untrusting, or otherwise vulnerable, the therapeutic relationship becomes stronger over time and is more likely to withstand interpersonal events that would otherwise challenge or strain the relationship.

For any number of reasons, however, the therapeutic relationship may not develop adequately enough to endure threats caused by the interpersonal events that routinely emerge during therapy. Signs that there is difficulty within the therapeutic relationship may include but are not limited to the following:

- Change in affect, attitude, or interpersonal behaviour
- Becoming disengaged from therapy
- Appearing/feeling impatient, irritable, or angry
- Therapy is experienced as "boring"
- The utility of therapy becomes questionable
- Questioning or criticism feels excessive
- Taking therapy "home"
- Dreading or becoming apprehensive about the next appointment
- Having a desire to refer or terminate prematurely
- Conflict with the client
- Client's attendance pattern changes or declines

There are a number of potential reasons why difficulty may emerge within the therapeutic relationship. For example, a client may bring a particular interpersonal history into the treatment relationship that makes it difficult for the therapist to establish rapport in ways that usually work. Conversely, the client may be mistrustful of the therapist because of the circumstances under which he is being seen.

For example, a client may have been mandated by an insurance company to receive an evaluation for work potential and the client perceives that the therapist has tremendous power to influence his life (i.e., whether he continues to receive disability support). Alternatively, a therapist may have a negative reaction to a client because the client reminds the therapist of someone with whom the therapist has had a difficult relationship in the past. General sources of difficulty within the relationship may include but are not limited to the following:

- Client brings a difficult interpersonal history into the relationship or has a diagnosis such as avoidant or antisocial personality disorder
- Circumstances under which the client is being seen are threatening or pressured (i.e., an evaluation is being conducted for the purpose of verifying disability to an insurance company)
- Poor match between client and therapist's interpersonal styles
- Inability to overcome challenges caused by differences in culture, values, or worldview
- Client or therapist reminds the other of someone involved with a past negative experience
- Client or therapist disappoints or fails to meet expectations
- Client or therapist inadvertently says or does something that is perceived as injurious and the situation is not processed and resolved

These and other kinds of obstacles to a more stable enduring relationship with a client are only intensified by inevitable interpersonal events. Examples of events that are likely to further stress an already vulnerable therapy relationship include such things as a therapist's unanticipated absence for a period of time, a common misunderstanding that occurs between client and therapist, a comment or question that is perceived by the client as insensitive or inappropriate, or an unexpected personal crisis that causes the client to regress or temporarily relinquish treatment goals. While these are normal and inevitable examples of difficult aspects of therapy, the way in which the therapist responds to them is a powerful mediator of the final outcome.

Irrespective of the extent to which the therapeutic relationship process is stable and strong, the process of therapeutic responding to interpersonal events is essential to good therapy. If a therapist does not respond adequately to interpersonal events or challenges to the relationship, the process of occupational engagement may suffer and the therapeutic relationship process will quickly erode.

Thus, for the duration of the therapy process, the therapist must engage in a process of interpersonal reasoning, by which a therapist consciously and reflectively monitors both the therapeutic relationship and the interpersonal events of therapy to decide upon and enact appropriate interpersonal strategies. The six steps of this process were presented earlier in this chapter. A full description of the steps of interpersonal reasoning and examples of its application in practice are provided in Taylor (2020).

CASE EXAMPLE

In this section, a case example of how aspects of the IRM can be used in practice is provided by the second author, a practising occupational therapist for the Gloucestershire Partnership National Health Service Trust in Gloucestershire, England, United Kingdom. Jane has been practising for 20 years, and her primary areas of expertise include inpatient and community interventions for adults with severe mental illness and for adults with learning disabilities. Jane also uses the model of human occupation (Kielhofner, 2007) to underpin the formulation of her client's abilities and challenges with regard to their engagement in occupations.

Jane's Interpersonal Challenge: Resolving Power Struggles With Cecile

Cecile is a woman in her 40s who is divorced and lives alone. In the past, Cecile worked in a department store but was fired from her job, which she describes as one of many significant losses in her life. Cecile was referred for occupational therapy during a stay at an inpatient psychiatric unit. Her diagnosis has been difficult to determine, but Cecile has a long history of depression and anxiety with features of both borderline and narcissistic personality disorder.

Before she was referred to occupational therapy, Cecile had been using the psychiatric inpatient unit repeatedly during the previous 3 years. Cecile's behaviour was also characterised by a tendency to lose favour with her health care workers. She often made strong and repeated demands for support and assistance but then became dismissive of any attempts to meet these demands. At times she has been known to become rejecting or subtly hostile toward care workers. Her nonverbal messages matched her verbal communication conveying that she was defensive, hopeless, or angry. She often twisted facts about her care and distorted or ignored attempts at support from family, friends, and caregivers. Her communication was redundant with statements such as "I cannot carry on like this" or "You are not helping me" or "This is not making me better." In therapy, Cecile lacked curiosity and explored new environments only hesitantly. Though she was a highly capable person, she did not take pride in any current achievement nor seek out challenges. She was reluctant to show preferences, engage with others, complete activity, sustain focus, or show that any activity was significant to her. This was particularly true when she was aware that staff were observing her but were not prompting, instructing, or encouraging her. Because of her attitude and behaviors, many health care workers have become weary of providing support and some have refused to work with her.

The Interpersonal Response

Quickly I realised that issues of power were dominating our interactions, and I began to specifically look for interpersonal events that presented power dilemmas. At once Cecile would say something that indicated a desire to change (e.g., "I want to be myself again") and shortly thereafter she would tell me my approach was not working. Because this dynamic occurred repeatedly despite my many efforts to change my approach or incorporate her feedback, I interpreted this pattern's true meaning as "I can say your intervention is not making me better and therefore I am powerful over you—even though I tell you that I want to change." This played out in other ways. For example, we once shared a joke when visiting a local café and Cecile smiled. Because she rarely smiled, I pointed out that I enjoyed seeing her smile. She immediately returned to a masklike expression. On another occasion I was gently questioning Cecile about her interests and achievements, and she quickly became tearful and insisted we stop the conversation.

One of the central tasks of our work together involved understanding this power dynamic as an indication of Cecile's high need for control, which is one of her more consistent and enduring interpersonal characteristics. Knowing this, I then had to work with this dynamic to maximise Cecile's feelings of control so that she could develop other aspects of volition. On some occasions, this meant occasionally giving in to the dynamic and sometimes becoming vulnerable in her eyes. For example, I might use some self-disclosure about how her behavior affects me. I did this with the hope of stimulating her self-reflection about our conversation and raising her awareness of how her use of power in this way affects other people.

On other occasions, I have worked with the power dynamic by standing my ground and providing a rationale for why my approach might assist her. I often validate Cecile's desire for me to see that she is deeply troubled, but I also remind her that if and when she is ready to build strength, I will be there to assist her. On some occasions, we have also agreed to take short, planned breaks from our work together. The reason for these breaks is to give her space from the therapy process, to allow her time to reflect upon the responsibility that she holds within the therapy relationship, and to enable me to reform with ideas and energy to maintain the relationship. Aside from working with the power dynamic in these ways, an overarching aspect of my approach has been to not take any of Cecile's behaviors or comments personally.

The Outcome

Cecile was discharged after an 8-month stay in the hospital. A structured and sophisticated support network was designed and implemented, including regular occupational therapy appointments. Activities were set up and undertaken with the aim of engaging Cecile in making choices, taking control over her activities, regaining interest in past activities, and formulating a pattern within her occupations. Cecile's motivation for doing did not develop any further than what she needed to maintain independent functioning. Importantly, however, it was maintained at the same level, and now after many months since her last hospitalisation, Cecile has not yet felt the need to return to the hospital.

Jane is a very circumspect therapist who has mastered the delicate art of walking on eggshells without breaking them. Her judgement about what people need, particularly when they are feeling vulnerable or threatened, is very precise and a quality that any therapist would admire. This story illustrates that Jane's level of sophistication in managing more difficult interpersonal issues within therapeutic relationships is highly developed. She utilised interpersonal reasoning to recognise inevitable power dilemmas within the relationship and responded to them appropriately by shifting between the empathising and instructing modes to achieve a balance between acceptance-oriented strategies and change-oriented approaches. She was careful to select and time these modes carefully to accommodate Cecile's high need for control within the relationship in a way that allowed her to feel more empowered without feeling the need to dominate or manipulate the relationship.

SUMMARY

In occupational therapy, therapeutic use of self is a fundamental aspect of practice that has significant implications in terms of the course and ultimate outcomes of therapy. In this chapter, we learned that initiating and maintaining a relationship that supports occupational engagement is a complex and dynamic process that must be intentional in order to be maximally responsive to a client's developing interpersonal needs in therapy. The chapter began with a historical overview of prior conceptualisations and approaches to therapeutic use of self throughout the history of our field. A rationale for the need for a conceptual model of practice that uniquely addresses the interpersonal aspects of occupational therapy and does not interfere with other models and approaches to practice was provided. A model that responds to that need, the IRM, was presented. The primary components of the model and their relationships were described. A successful therapeutic relationship was defined according to the model's principles. Finally, a case example was provided by the second author to illustrate application of specific aspects of the model in a practice situation.

REFLECTIVE LEARNING

- In what ways do I currently initiate and maintain therapeutic relationships?
- Which of the six steps of interpersonal reasoning do I find most challenging, and why?
- Which of the six therapeutic modes do I use most?
- Am I missing opportunities to use other therapeutic modes?

REFERENCES

Ayres-Rosa, S., & Hasselkus, B. R. (1996). Connecting with patients: The personal experience of professional helping. *The Occupational Therapy Journal of Research, 16,* 245–260.

Baum, C. M. (1980). Occupational therapists put care in the health system. *American Journal of Occupational Therapy, 34,* 505–516.

Beck, J. (1995). *Cognitive therapy: Basics and beyond.* Guilford Press.

Bing, R. K. (1981). Eleanor Clark Slagle lectureship. Occupational therapy revisited: A paraphrastic journey. *American Journal of Occupational Therapy, 35,* 499–518.

Blair, S. E. E., & Daniels, M. A. (2006). An introduction to the psychodynamic frame of reference. In E. A. S. Duncan (Ed.), *Foundations for practice in occupational therapy.* Elsevier.

Bockoven, J. S. (1971). Occupational therapy—a historical perspective: Legacy of moral treatment—1800s to 1910. *American Journal of Occupational Therapy, 25,* 223–225.

Clark, F. (1993). Occupation embedded in a real life: Interweaving occupational science and occupational therapy. 1993 Eleanor Clarke Slagle lecture. *American Journal of Occupational Therapy, 47,* 1067–1078.

Cole, B., & McLean, V. (2003). Therapeutic relationships re-defined. *Occupational Therapy in Mental Health, 19*(2), 33–56.

Crepeau, E. B. (1991). Achieving intersubjective understanding: Examples from an occupational therapy treatment session. *American Journal of Occupational Therapy, 45,* 1016–1025.

Devereaux, E. B. (1984). Occupational therapy's challenge: The caring relationship. *American Journal of Occupational Therapy, 38*(12), 791–798.

Duncan, E. A. S. (Ed.). (2006). *Foundations for practice in occupational therapy* (4th ed.). Churchill Livingstone.

Fleming, M. H. (1991). The therapist with the three-track mind. *American Journal of Occupational Therapy, 45*(11), 1007–1014.

Gilfoyle, E. M. (1980). Caring: A philosophy for practice. *American Journal of Occupational Therapy, 34*(8), 517–521.

Jonsson, H., Josephsson, S., & Kielhofner, G. (2001). Narratives and experience in an occupational transition: A longitudinal study of the retirement process. *American Journal of Occupational Therapy, 55*(4), 424–432.

Kielhofner, G. & Burke, J.P. (1977). Occupational therapy after 60 years: An account of changing identity and knowledge. *American Journal of Occupational Therapy, 31,* 675–689.

Kielhofner, G. (1997). In *Conceptual foundations of occupational therapy* (2nd ed.). FA Davis.

Kielhofner, G. (2004). In *Conceptual foundations of occupational therapy* (3rd ed.). FA Davis.

Kielhofner, G. (2007). In *The model of human occupation, theory and application* (4th ed.). Lippincott Williams & Wilkins.

King, L. J. (1980). Creative caring. *American Journal of Occupational Therapy, 34*(3), 522–528.

Lyons, K. D., & Crepeau, E. B. (2001). The clinical reasoning of an occupational therapy assistant. *American Journal of Occupational Therapy, 55*(5), 577–581.

Mattingly, C. (1991). The narrative nature of clinical reasoning. *American Journal of Occupational Therapy, 45*(11), 998–1005.

Mattingly, C. (1994). The narrative nature of clinical reasoning. In C. Mattingly, & M. H. Fleming (Eds.), *Clinical reasoning: Forms of inquiry in a therapeutic practice* (pp. 239–269). FA Davis.

Mattingly, C., & Fleming, M. H. (1994). In *Clinical reasoning: Forms of inquiry in a therapeutic practice* (pp. 178–196). FA Davis.

Mattingly, C., & Gillette, N. (1991). Anthropology, occupational therapy, and action research. *The American Journal of Occupational Therapy, 45*(11), 972–978.

Mosey, A. C. (1970). *Three frames of reference for mental health.* Slack.

Peloquin, S. M. (1989a). Moral treatment: Contexts considered. *American Journal of Occupational Therapy, 43*(8), 537–544.

Peloquin, S. M. (1989b). Sustaining the art of practice in occupational therapy. *American Journal of Occupational Therapy, 43*(4), 219–226.

Peloquin, S. M. (1990). The patient–therapist relationship in occupational therapy: Understanding visions and images. *American Journal of Occupational Therapy, 44*(1), 13–21.

Peloquin, S. M. (1993). The depersonalization of patients: A profile gleaned from narratives. *American Journal of Occupational Therapy, 47*(9), 830–837.

Peloquin, S. M. (1995). The fullness of empathy: Reflections and illustrations. *American Journal of Occupational Therapy, 49*(1), 24–31.

Peloquin, S. M. (2002). Reclaiming the vision of reaching for heart as well as hands. *American Journal of Occupational Therapy, 56*(5), 517–526.

Peloquin, S. M. (2003). The therapeutic relationship: Manifestations and challenges in occupational therapy. In E. B. Crepeau, E. S. Cohn, & B. A. Boyt Schell (Eds.), *Willard & Spackman's occupational therapy* (10th ed., pp. 157–170). Lippincott Williams & Wilkins.

Rogers, J. C. (1983). Clinical reasoning: The ethics, science, and art. 1983 Eleanor Clarke Slagle lecture. *American Journal of Occupational Therapy, 37*(9), 601–616.

Schell, B. A. (2003). Clinical reasoning: The basis of practice. In E. B. Crepeau, E. S. Cohn, B. A. Boyt Schell, & M. E. Neistadt (Eds.), *Willard & Spackman's occupational therapy* (10th ed., pp. 131–152). Lippincott Williams & Wilkins.

Schell, B. A., & Cervero, R. M. (1993). Clinical reasoning in occupational therapy: An integrative review. *American Journal of Occupational Therapy, 47*(7), 605–610.

Schwartz, K. B. (2003). The history of occupational therapy. In E. B. Crepeau, E. S. Cohn, B. A. Boyt Schell, & M. E. Neistadt (Eds.), *Willard & Spackman's occupational therapy* (10th ed., pp. 5–13). Lippincott Williams & Wilkins.

Schwartzberg, S. L. (2002). *Interactive reasoning in the process of occupational therapy*. Pearson Education.

Shannon, P. D. (1977). The derailment of occupational therapy. *American Journal of Occupational Therapy, 31*, 229–234.

Taylor, R. R. (2020). In *The intentional relationship: Occupational therapy and use of self* (2nd ed.). FA Davis.

Taylor, R. R., Lee, S. W., Kielhofner, G., & Ketkar, M. (2009). Therapeutic use of self: A nationwide survey of practitioners' attitudes and experiences. *American Journal of Occupational Therapy, 63*, 198–207.

Townsend, E. (2003). Reflections on power and justice in enabling occupation. *Revve Canadienne D'Ergotherapie, 70*, 74–87.

Yerxa, E. J. (1967). Authentic occupational therapy. Eleanor Clarke Stagle lecture. *American Journal of Occupational Therapy, 21*, 1–9.

Yerxa, E. J. (1980). Occupational therapy's role in creating a future climate of caring. *American Journal of Occupational Therapy, 34*(8), 529–679.

9

Problem Solving

Edward A.S. Duncan

HIGHLIGHTS

- The pragmatic focus of occupational therapy lends itself to taking a problem-solving theoretical approach in practice.
- The problem-solving approach is essentially a form of clinical reasoning.
- Using problem-solving theory enables practitioners to form an objective approach to understanding a client's problems.
- The problem-solving approach is essential but suboptimal in its own right. The information it gains must be considered together with the client's perspective when forming shared decisions in practice.

- The problem-solving process is a flexible clinical intervention that can be used with a wide variety of clients.
- Historically part of occupational therapy, emerging high-quality evidence is providing a renewed emphasis on problem solving as an effective approach to practice.
- The problem-solving process helps clients to resolve challenging difficulties and teaches a method of self-care for dealing with other challenges in the future.
- This chapter outlines the problem-solving process and highlights various issues to consider at each stage.

INTRODUCTION

The *Chambers Dictionary* (1994) defines a problem as "a matter difficult to settle or solve" and problem-solving behaviour as "the use of various strategies to overcome difficulties in attaining a goal" (p. 1366). A problem is generally something that is blocking something from being achieved. It can also be something that occurs when a person does not know how to resolve a situation. In other words, "a problem arises when someone wants to do something but either does not know how or is in some way blocked from implementing a known solution. Thus, the problem is the gap that separates individuals from where they are now and where they want to be" (Robertson, 1996, p. 178). The practical nature of occupational therapy has always lent itself to naturally taking a problem-solving approach. Consider the following scenarios:

- A lady has suffered a stroke and is currently in a rehabilitation ward. She is having difficulty getting dressed in the morning and wishes to be able to do so independently so she has control over this when she returns home.

- A husband is having difficulty caring for his wife who has dementia. She frequently gets up at night to go to the toilet. Often her husband finds her wandering around the house disorientated and upset as she cannot find the bathroom.
- A 45-year-old taxi driver has been off work for 3 years with low back pain and depression; he would like to return to work but lacks confidence and doesn't know where to start as he is unable to return to his old job.

Each of these scenarios presents people who are likely to come into contact with occupational therapy and have problems of various forms that they need to resolve.

This chapter is divided into two main sections that present the key ways in which practitioners use problem solving in practice. The first section presents problem solving as a well-established general theoretical approach to practice (Dutton, 2000; Hagedorn, 2001; Roberts, 1996; Robertson, 1996). The second section draws on theory from the cognitive-behavioural frame of reference (see Duncan, 2021) to present how problem solving can also be used as a specific therapeutic intervention.

PROBLEM SOLVING AS A THEORETICAL APPROACH IN PRACTICE

As a theoretical framework for occupational therapy practice, problem solving has long been considered to be a form of clinical reasoning (Paterson & Summerfield-Mann, 2006; Roberts, 1996). Dutton (2000) presented problem solving as the practical manifestation of practitioners' cognitive abilities to break down clients' difficulties and problems into small steps. Robertson (1996) examined problem solving in practice and presented it as a form of cognitive information processing. This approach views problem solving as a rational and logical process that describes how practitioners understand a problem and work to solve it (Robertson, 1996). Whilst occupational therapists often focus on resolving problems, Robertson (1996) emphasised that it is worth initially spending considerable time to conceptualise how the problem is understood as these ideas will shape the future interventions a practitioner will use to resolve the problem.

In some of the earliest theoretical texts from modern-day occupational therapy in the United Kingdom, Hagedorn (2001) argued that the whole occupational therapy process can be viewed in terms of problem solving and suggested that it entailed the following stages:
- Information collection
- Problem identification
- Identification of the desired outcome
- Solution development
- Evaluation and selection
- Development of an action plan
- Implementation and evaluation of results

Opacich (1991) had, however, already outlined a similar series of stages to describe the occupational therapy process; and although Opacich considered these in terms of a clinical reasoning process, Paterson and Summerfield-Mann (2006) suggested they can also be viewed in terms of a problem-solving process. Opacich's (1991) stages are:
- Framing the problem: selecting the theoretical model or frame of reference, considering which assessments to use, etc.
- Delineating the problem: organising assessments to collect information and analysing the findings from assessments that are carried out
- Forming a hypothesis: understanding the findings of the results in light of the selected theoretical perspective and developing a written summary of this
- Developing intervention plans: forming goals for intervention and considering the environment in which the intervention will take place

- Implementing intervention: continual assessment to support, alter, or dismiss the hypothesis that has already been generated

Opacich's (1991) and Hagedorn's (2001) approaches to the occupational therapy problem-solving process have clear similarities. Both approaches are essentially forms of hypothetico-deductive reasoning, which is centered on how a professional builds a hypothesis and forms a sequential series of actions. Unsworth (1999) stated that hypothetico-deductive reasoning is an inadequate clinical reasoning strategy to employ on its own as, by its nature, it excludes the interactions that occur between practitioner and clients in practice. However, it can also be argued that the hypothetico-deductive reasoning of the occupational therapy problem-solving process, whilst inadequate in isolation, is essential for practitioners to form an objective perspective of a client's problem. This understanding can then be shared with clients, and informed by clients' personal experiences, perceptions, preferences, views, and opinions of meaningful others in their life can help form a shared decision about the direction of occupational therapy intervention (Fig. 9.1). Chapter 3 describes the challenges of undertaking shared decision making in practice.

USING PROBLEM SOLVING AS A THERAPEUTIC INTERVENTION

Problem solving in clinical practice is based on the theoretical foundations of cognitive-behavioural therapy. Occupational therapists may find that they use this process intuitively, yet it has a strong theoretical basis (D'Zurilla & Nezu, 2009, 2010). Whilst the problem-solving process originally developed within mental health settings, its applications are broad and should not be considered as an intervention for mental health settings alone (Vignette 9.1). As a therapeutic skill and method of intervention, problem solving has several strengths. It is relatively brief, is applicable to a wide range of issues in differing clinical situations, and aims to empower clients to resolve their own personal issues and challenges without seeking professional assistance in the future.

Problem solving has been identified as being useful for two types of individuals. The first are people who generally cope well but perhaps due to an illness or the nature of the problem they are facing are not currently coping with a specific situation. The second are individuals who generally find it difficult to deal with life or may be said to have generally insufficient coping resources (e.g., strong self-esteem, occupationally involved lives, solution-focused mentality, supportive social network) (Hawton et al., 1994). While the problem-solving process can be used with both groups

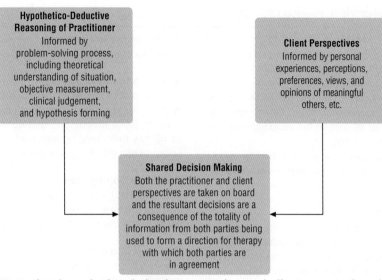

FIG. 9.1 Integrating hypothetico-deductive reasoning and client perspectives in a shared decision-making model of practice.

of individuals, it will likely take longer to instill and be successful with the latter population.

There are various situations in which practitioners may use the problem-solving process outlined in this chapter. A specific situation may arise during a session and the occupational therapist may decide that assisting the client to develop a problem-solving strategy would be useful (e.g., during the break of a social skills group a teenage girl who has anorexia tells her practitioner of her anxiety about going to a friend's sleepover where there will be lots of food). Alternatively, the problems may already be apparent, and the practitioner could introduce the concept of the problem-solving process to a client and agree with the client that it would be useful to focus on problem solving as part of the agreed goals (e.g., discussing discharge and return to work with a client who has had an above-knee amputation). Finally, practitioners may find themselves in crisis situations with clients who they may not know well and who are distressed and would benefit from a problem-solving process to assist them to develop solutions for their immediate issues (e.g., working in crisis teams, or on the duty desk of a community mental health team). Therefore, regardless of the practice setting that one is working in, problem solving is a skill that should be in every occupational therapist's repertoire.

Evidence for the effectiveness for problem solving in occupational therapy has recently grown, which may lead to a renewed focus on its potential. Occupation-based problem solving has been found to have positive impacts in women who have breast cancer (Şahin & Uyanik 2019) and diabetes (Ağce & Ekici, 2020). In the breast cancer study, occupation-based problem solving was found to achieve a reduction of participants' perceptions of cancer-related fatigue and depression and led to perceived benefits in performance, satisfaction, and quality of life (Şahin & Uyanik, 2019). While in the diabetes randomised control trial (Ağce & Ekici, 2020), occupation-based problem solving led to improvements in their self-identified occupational performance problems and developed statistically significant improvements in self-efficacy.

Of course, despite its broad potential for application, problem solving is not the panacea to all situations and is not always an appropriate intervention. There are situations in which problem solving should not be considered. A person who has marked learning difficulties or a severe and enduring mental illness may well be cognitively unable to complete the stages of the problem-solving process (Hawton et al., 1994). Similarly, an individual who has suffered from a stroke or external head injury may (depending on the nature of the event) be unable to complete the stages of the problem-solving process (Fig. 9.2); and while problem solving can be very useful for people experiencing a crisis, in extreme situations (such as in the case of suicidal intent) it is more important to deal with the presenting difficulties, hopelessness, and personal disorganisation (thereby ensuring the person's safety) before attempting to introduce a problem-solving intervention.

VIGNETTE 9.1

Leon is a 43-year-old man. He is married to Eleanor and has one son, Theo (aged 15). Leon was diagnosed with a relapsing/remitting form of multiple sclerosis at the age of 31. Initially he had managed to continue to work in his office; however, he changed his hours to part time last year as he was becoming increasingly tired. Ten months ago Leon suffered a further relapse in his condition and has since been off work completely.

Leon's general practitioner has referred him to see an occupational therapist. The occupational therapist visited Leon at home.

Identifying Problems
In discussion, Leon states that he is having a variety of problems and lists them, in no particular order, as follows:
1. **General weakness:** Leon is now spending almost all of his time in his wheelchair. He is experiencing problems in transferring from his bed to his chair and is having difficulty getting on and off the toilet.
2. **Fatigue:** Leon reports feeling very tired and spending increasing amounts of time in his bed. At times Leon starts a task, but is unable to finish as he lacks stamina. This leaves him feeling frustrated and sad.
3. **Social isolation:** Leon used to enjoy his work. It gave him a sense of purpose, reward, and meaningful social contact. Since he has been off work he rarely leaves his house and has missed contact with others.
4. **Financial problems:** Leon is concerned about his future as his "sick pay" will finish in 2 months and he is unsure how he will cope financially.

Decide Which Goals to Tackle First
In discussion with Leon, it is agreed to refer to social work to assist with his financial concerns and to focus initially on his fatigue.

Agree Goals
Leon wishes to maximise his time awake to look after his self-care and be less tired. Looking after the house is less important to Leon. The following goal is agreed:
1. Leon will have a shower each day before lunch for a week.

Generate Possible Solutions to Meet Goals
Leon considers the following potential solutions to meet his goals:
1. Set his alarm clock for 11 a.m. each day to remind him to have a bath.
2. Go to bed each evening no later than 10:30 p.m. to maximise his energy levels the following day.

3. Promise himself a reward if he manages to achieve his goal for the whole week.

Selecting the Best Strategy
Leon considers that all possible solutions have worth, and in fact they are not mutually exclusive. However, he decides to focus on going to bed no later than 10:30 p.m., as he has been reading some information about energy conservation that his general practitioner had given him.

Develop a Coping Plan
Knowing that he likely to get engrossed with whatever is on TV at the time, he sets a time limit on his broadband so it will cut off the TV at 10:15 p.m. (coping plan).

Putting it Into Action
Leon's occupational therapist encourages him to put his strategy into action as soon as possible. Eleanor thinks Leon's plan is a great idea and says she will encourage him to stick to it. Leon himself acknowledges that going to bed sounds easy, but that he is a creature of habit and enjoys watching American police dramas late at night on digital TV. To manage his strategy he will have to change some habits.

Leon's occupational therapist works with him to develop a wind-down routine for each evening. The aim of this is to help Leon develop new routines and manage his way around the perceived loss of TV. The occupational therapist suggests that Leon could record the programmes he is missing, but Leon dismisses this idea as he says there are so many repeats these days it would not be worthwhile. Instead, Leon decides to switch off the TV at 10 p.m. each evening and spend the last half an hour getting ready for bed. He knows that he has a coping plan that will kick into action if he doesn't switch the TV off himself.

Reviewing the Progress
The practitioner leaves Leon to implement his plan of going to bed earlier and arranges to return in 1 week. When she returns, Leon reports that he had had a shower 6 days out of 7 and that he had managed to get to bed before 10:30 p.m. 4 nights out of 7. On discussion Leon agreed that it was not necessary to think of an alternative strategy at this stage because he could see the benefits that going to bed earlier made on his energy conservation the following day and felt confident that he would be able to at least maintain his performance of the previous week, and potentially improve. Together Leon and his practitioner decided to move on and consider the other issues.

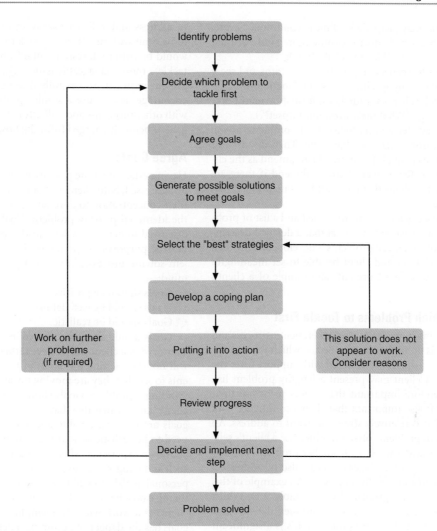

FIG. 9.2 The problem-solving process.

THE PROBLEM-SOLVING PROCESS

Identifying Problems

The identification of client's problems is perhaps the most crucial step of problem solving, and time should be taken to ensure that all the problems are identified and clearly specified. This is a collaborative process between the practitioner and client (Hawton et al., 1994). Identifying problems may seem straightforward—after all, clients are unlikely to be seeing an occupational therapist if they did not have any. Often, however, problem identification is not as straightforward as it may first appear. There can be several reasons for this. Clients can present with problems that are unclearly specified (e.g., "difficulty coping at home" or "unhappy on the ward"). In these situations, it is important that the practitioner helps the client to be more specific about the precise nature of the problem. The aim of this process is to help the client be able to specify exactly what the problem is (e.g., "I am unable to cook dinner for my family and keep the house tidy enough" or "I am finding sharing a living space with strangers very difficult as they want to watch different TV programmes and ask me personal questions I would rather not answer"). Alternatively, clients may present with a range of clinical conditions (depression, anxiety, etc.) but be unable to see how these relate to their personal circumstances or how addressing certain life situations may help their clinical condition. Several strategies can assist clients to become more aware of their underlying problems (Hawton et al., 1994):

- Ask clients to keep a diary of their symptoms and see if these relate to any specific area of life functioning.
- Gently probe clients for further information about how they feel (e.g., "What makes you most upset?").
- Take the first step and try to list clients' problems as you see them, from what they have said. Then discuss this list with the client and change, add, or amend as the client suggests. Remember to ask at the end if there are any other problems that have not been mentioned that should be.

When the steps have been completed and a list of problems has been developed, it is vital that a detailed description of each of the agreed problems is developed. Only then will the practitioner and client be able to set meaningful goals together. Table 9.1 presents an example of a client's problem list.

Decide Which Problems to Tackle First

Problem solving is an empowering therapeutic process and ultimately it is up to the client to decide which issue to address first. This should be achieved with support from the practitioner. A client may present a lengthy problem list, and it is therefore important that clients prioritise their problems. It is also important that clients commence with a problem that is relatively straightforward to address. An early success in problem solving can increase a client's self-belief and, because success with smaller problems can encourage clients that the bigger ones can also be addressed, maintains motivation for the approach. An example of this can be seen in Jack's problem list (see Table 9.1). Whilst Jack is almost certain to view his continued detention in a secure hospital as his main problem, this is a significant and challenging life issue that is likely to take some time

TABLE 9.1   Jack's Problem List

1. Detention in a hospital of high security
2. Frustration at being unable to control his own environment and need for privacy (secondary to problem 1)
3. Difficulty concentrating due to schizophrenia and medication side effects
4. Boredom as unable to carry out activities that he was used to prior to admission and diagnosis of schizophrenia (secondary to problems 1 and 3)
5. Loss of contacts with friends and family
6. Has been unable to discuss personal issues with ward key-worker

to address and will necessarily involve smaller problems to be dealt with first. Helping Jack to achieve his discharge would be better addressed, initially, by supporting him to tackle a more manageable issue (e.g., his boredom) in the present moment. Successfully dealing with that issue may encourage Jack to use a similar problem-solving strategy with other problems and will ultimately support him in his goal of being discharged from the hospital.

Agree Goals

Having established the priority problems that are going to be addressed, both client and practitioner should then turn their concentration to developing detailed goals to address the identified priority problem. Goal setting in general is discussed in detail elsewhere in this book (see Chapter 7). For the purposes of specific goal setting within the problem-solving process, three key aspects should be kept in mind:

- Goals should be positive.
- Goals should be well defined.
- Goals should be realistic.

Goals should always be framed in positive terms (for instance, what a client will achieve rather than what the client will not do). Setting out goals in this way encourages clients to see that they are moving towards a solution and not avoiding a problem. Goals should be well defined so that clients know when they have achieved them; well-defined goals are both observable and measurable. Finally, goals need to be realistic so that they can be achieved. Consider your own experience when you have set personal life goals such as dieting, exercising, etc. Have you ever set unrealistic personal goals? How did you feel when you failed to meet them? Consider what this would be like for some of the clients you work with. To reemphasise, setting unrealistic goals has the danger of becoming a negative experience for clients and is likely to discourage them from developing their problem-solving skills further.

GENERATE POSSIBLE SOLUTIONS TO MEET GOALS

In this stage, the client, with support from the practitioner, lists ways in which goals could be met. Clients should spend some time on this aspect of the problem-solving process to consider how best to meet their goal. It may be that the most immediate solution is not the best; apart from anything else, it may already have been considered by the client and quite possibly tried before. Strategies for developing lists of possible solutions include brainstorming where clients are asked to write down (or dictate if they have difficulties in writing) all the potential tasks that could

TABLE 9.2 Jack's Pros and Cons List, With Likert Scale Weightings	
Goal: Address boredom: Become more involved in activities in current environment	
Potential Solution: Participate three times a week on activities offered to client by occupational therapist	
Advantages	**Disadvantages**
Will distract me from my current situation (4)	I don't like the activities that are being offered (8)
Will sometimes involve getting out of the ward (7)	I don't feel like doing anything (2)
Will keep my multidisciplinary team happy (2)	I feel scared about meeting different people (3)
Will get to meet different people (3)	

Likert scale weighting: 1 = not at all important, 10 = extremely important.

result in the target goal being achieved. Clients should be encouraged to list all potential solutions, however implausible. This can lead to a fairly light-hearted component of the session, where clients let their imagination fly! A side effect of this process is that the generation of extreme solutions can lead clients to consider possibilities they would otherwise have dismissed (Hawton et al., 1994). Once this process has been achieved, clients should list the strengths and weaknesses of each listed solution. Don't dismiss any idea outright.

At times it may appear that there are two or more equally viable solutions. In such cases it can be useful to generate a list of pros and cons for each solution (Table 9.2). This involves assisting a client to generate and list the advantages and disadvantages of each solution. A further step (which may not always be necessary, but further clarifies the importance of items on the list) involves asking the client to weight each listed item. This is achieved by giving Likert scale–style ratings to each item listed. The complete pros and cons list therefore gives further information about the potential of a solution by listing both the number of advantages/disadvantages that would result and their weight in terms of importance to the client.

Selecting the "Best" Strategy

Having developed a list of potential solutions, and where necessary considered their strengths and weaknesses, you then have to decide which strategy is most likely to help solve the problem and/or achieve the goal. It is important to remember, however, that this is a best-guess scenario. That is, it is the best guess of the person involved (and ideally of all involved) that the strategy selected is the most likely to work. It remains a process of trial and error, however, so keep all the potential solutions to hand because the client may yet need to come back and try another!

It is important, however, to choose a strategy that is likely to work. Practitioners should help clients to carefully weigh the options, balancing the potential of a strategy to succeed with consideration of the personal resources that it requires, and whether a specific strategy is achievable

in practice; it may appear the best solution, but if it is not achievable then the client will not be able to carry it out (Fig. 9.3). However, sometimes the "best" strategy can be very apparent; concrete facts or issues can constrain the options available and the selection of a strategy is therefore limited, or other options may carry too much risk to be realistic in practice.

Putting it Into Action

Once clients have chosen their strategy, it is time to put it into action. Often this stage is viewed simplistically and skimmed over in problem-solving literature. However, this is the central moment of the problem-solving process; implementing action to solve problems is challenging. The chances are if this were simple clients would already have solved the problem. The fact that a client seeks help to resolve a problem means that, at some level, it is difficult. Closer consideration of this stage of the problem-solving process is therefore required.

It is important to understand the factors that can influence clients who are about to put their problem-solving plan into action, and consider ways of supporting them

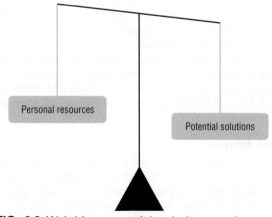

FIG. 9.3 Weighing potential solutions against personal resources.

to ensure their greatest chance of success. To do so, practitioners can draw on both the theory of planned behaviour (Ajzen & Manstead, 2007) and task analysis theory (Hagedorn, 2000).

The Theory of Planned Behaviour

The theory of planned behaviour (Ajzen & Manstead, 2007) is a well-established psychological theory that links attitudes with action (behaviour). It can help to inform some of the aspects that make it more likely that a client will be able to undertake the selected problem-solving strategy:

- Clients should put the selected strategy into action as soon as possible. This is because their intention is more closely related to the behaviour when the time interval between them deciding to do something and doing it is low (Ajzen & Manstead, 2007). In other words, it is relatively easy for clients to say they will do something, but much harder to actually do it; and it gets harder as time passes.
- Clients are more likely to undertake a chosen action if they believe that others who are of importance in their lives (e.g., family) support their action. The theory of planned behaviour describes this as the subjective norm (Ajzen & Manstead, 2007). The subjective norm is the clients' perception of the beliefs of relevant others that they should or should not undertake the chosen strategy. If clients believe they have the social support of family or friends to solve their problems and that they are in support of the chosen strategy, they are more likely to put their plan into action.
- A final factor that increases clients' probability of putting the chosen strategy into practice is their perceived behavioural control of the situation. Perceived behavioural control is a construct that describes a person's perception of the ease or challenge that a particular task brings. The easier they feel it is to achieve, the more likely clients will undertake the strategy (Ajzen & Manstead, 2007). Strategies should therefore appear realistic and achievable in practice.

Putting a problem-solving strategy into action for clients is most likely to be successful therefore when it is done quickly, has the social support of meaningful others in their life, and they believe that what they are about to do is achievable.

Task Analysis

While the selected strategy may be the solution to the problem, it is usually stated in the form of an overall action (e.g., "Go to the gym"). To put the strategy into action requires the task to be broken down into manageable parts, a process known as task analysis. Doing so not only clarifies what has to be carried out, but also makes the task appear more

achievable thereby increasing the amount of perceived behavioural control a client has and consequently increasing the chances that it will succeed! There have been several attempts to describe how this should be achieved. Hagedorn (2000) differentiated task analysis from activity analysis (see Chapter 6) as task analysis focuses on larger-scale activities (e.g., "get fit") whilst activity analysis addresses more focused activities (e.g., "having a bath").

Hagedorn (2000) presented a six-question system of task analysis, a form of action plan, which remains useful to consider when putting the problem-solving process into action:

- What is to be done?
- Who is involved?
- How is it performed?
- Where will it take place?
- When will it be done?
- Why are you doing it (a useful reminder!)?
- These task analysis steps closely resemble a general goal-setting process (see Chapter 7 for a contemporary theory-based approach to goal setting and action planning).
- Developing a coping plan
- As Robert Burns (the 18th-century Scot poet) famously noted in his poem To a Mouse, "…The best laid schemes o' mice an' men / Gang aft a-gley." Or in modern English, "The best laid plans of mice and men often go awry." It is increasingly recognised that whenever one tries to overcome a problem or achieve a goal, barriers (both foreseeable and unforeseeable) will get in the way (Sniehotta, 2009). Coping plans are therefore important to develop. These preempt the challenges that can arise when you try to overcome a problem and describe the actions that you will put into action when such events inevitably occur. Systematic review evidence has shown that developing action plans and coping plans together bring greater benefits to clients than if action plans are developed on their own (Kwasnicka et al., 2013).

Reviewing Progress and Implementing the Next Step

Having put the action and coping plans into practice, both client and practitioner should evaluate how successful they have been. This can normally be easily measured by asking if clients have solved their problem. If the answer to this question is yes, then the process may naturally come to an end; though it can be worth spending some time with clients looking at how to maintain what has been achieved. Alternatively, it may be appropriate to select another problem and commence the process again.

If the problem has not been resolved then the client and practitioner should stop and consider why it did not work and what they can learn from the experience: Was the strategy wrong, or was it not implemented as planned? Is more time required, or more intensity of whatever was being done? It may be that the answer to these questions is that it was indeed the wrong strategy, but it is worth stopping and taking some time to consider why it did not work. If necessary, another strategy can then be selected (taking into account what has been learnt from the last strategy) and the process worked through again. In this way the implementing of strategies to solve problems can be looked on and communicated by the practitioner to the client as a learning process. As part of the learning process it is important to remember and communicate that failure can be an important moment to reevaluate and reflect. Is the problem still perceived as important? Have other priorities emerged?

SUMMARY

Problem solving is a central component of occupational therapy practice. It is used as (1) a theoretical framework to describe the general process and a clinical reasoning approach to occupational therapy and (2) a specific technique based on the cognitive-behavioural frame of reference that is applicable for use with a wide range of clients.

The problem-solving basis of occupational therapy is longstanding. It has been described and presented as a hypothetico-deductive approach (Hagedorn, 2001; Opacich, 1991). This has been criticised as insufficient for occupational therapy practice (Unsworth, 1999). The danger of such criticism is that hypothetico-deductive reasoning may come to be no longer valued within occupational therapy. Instead, this chapter has presented the problem-solving hypothetico-deductive approach as one arm of the decision-making process (see Fig. 9.1) and a central component to the process of shared decision making in practice (see Chapter 3).

The problem-solving process was presented as a useful therapeutic skill and intervention, with a recently emerging evidence base. The aim of working through the problem-solving process is twofold: to help clients resolve problems that have proven too challenging to cope with without support and to help clients learn the process of problem solving so that they are able to implement it without specific structured support in the future. Whilst routinely associated with working in mental health settings, the problem-solving process is in fact useful in a variety of settings with clients with a range of conditions. Whilst the problem-solving process appears intuitively obvious, various factors can be taken into consideration to improve the manner in which this intervention is delivered.

REFLECTIVE LEARNING

- How have you seen problem solving used in practice?
- How could you integrate the concept of coping plans when using a problem-solving process with a client group with which you are familiar?
- What problems are you dealing with yourself just now (we all have them!)? Pick one: not too big, not too small. Challenge yourself to go through the problem-solving process, develop a coping strategy, and put it into practice. What worked? What was hard? The experience of doing this will help you empathise with your clients who are often facing much bigger or longer established challenges.

REFERENCES

Ağce, Z. B., & Ekici, G. (2020). Person-centred, occupation-based intervention program supported with problem-solving therapy for type 2 diabetes: A randomized controlled trial. *Health and Quality of Life Outcomes, 18*(1), 1–14.

Ajzen, I., Manstead, A. S. R. (2007). Changing health-related behaviors: An approach based on the theory of planned behavior. In K. van den Bos, M. Hewstone, & J. de Wit (Eds.), *The scope of social psychology: Theory and applications* (pp. 43–63). Psychology Press.

Chambers Dictionary. (1994). *Problem*. Chambers Harrap Publishers.

Duncan, E. A. S. (Ed.). (2021). The cognitive behavioural frame of reference. In *Foundations for practice in occupational therapy* (5th ed., pp. 141–151). Elsevier/Churchill Livingstone.

Dutton, R. (2000). In *Clinical reasoning in physical disabilities* (2nd ed.). Williams and Wilkins.

D'Zurilla, T. J., & Nezu, A. M. (2009). Problem-solving therapies. In K. S. Dobson (Ed.), *Handbook of cognitive-behavioral therapies* (3rd ed.). Guilford.

D'Zurilla, T. J., & Nezu, A. M. (2010). Problem-solving therapy. In *Handbook of cognitive-behavioral therapies* (pp. 197–225). Guilford.

Hagedorn, R. (2000). *Tools for practice in occupational therapy*. Churchill Livingstone.

Hagedorn, R. (2001). In *Foundations for practice in occupational therapy* (3rd ed.). Churchill Livingstone.

Hawton, K., Kirk, J., et al. (1994). Problem-solving. In K. Hawton, P. M. Salkovskis, & J. W. Kirk (Eds.), *Cognitive behaviour therapy for psychiatric problems: A practical guide* (pp. 406–426). Oxford Medical.

Kwasnicka, D., Presseau, J., White, M., & Sniehotta, F. F. (2013). Does planning how to cope with anticipated barriers facilitate health-related behaviour change? A systematic review. *Health Psychology Review, 7*, 129–145.

Opacich, K. J. (1991). Assessment and informed decision making. In C. Christiansen, & C. Baum (Eds.), *Occupational therapy: Overcoming human performance deficits* (pp. 355–374). Slack.

Paterson, M., & Summerfield-Mann, L. (2006). Clinical reasoning. In E. A. S. Duncan (Ed.), *Foundations for practice in occupational therapy* (4th ed., pp. 315–335). Elsevier/Churchill Livingstone.

Roberts, A. S. (1996). Clinical reasoning in occupational therapy: Idiosyncrasies in content and process. *The British Journal of Occupational Therapy, 59*(8), 372–376.

Robertson, L. J. (1996). Clinical reasoning. Part 1: The nature of problem solving, a literature review. *The British Journal of Occupational Therapy, 59*(4), 178–182.

Şahin, S., & Uyanık, M. (2019). The impact of occupation-based problem-solving strategies training in women with breast cancer. *Health and Quality of Life Outcomes, 17*(1), 1–8.

Sniehotta, F. F. (2009). Towards a theory of intentional behaviour change: Plans, planning, and self-regulation. *British Journal of Health Psychology, 14*(2), 261–273.

Unsworth, C. (1999). *Cognitive and perceptual dysfunction: A clinical reasoning approach to evaluation and intervention.* FA Davis.

10

Group Skills for Practice in Occupational Therapy

Sharan L. Schwartzberg and Mary Alicia Barnes

HIGHLIGHTS

- Essential leader functions build member-to-member interaction to foster group cohesion, which is correlated to successful group outcomes.
- Group structure and process influence group outcomes.
- Effective leadership considers the individual, subgroups, and the group as a whole.

- Groups follow a developmental pattern. Leader skills and activity group processes employed are best geared to the group's phase of development.
- Leaders will make mistakes, and conflict in groups is inevitable. Leaders need to be attuned to group processes and dynamics to effectively address, including being willing to hold a range of group member affect—from anger to love, from pride to shame, from joy to sadness.

OVERVIEW

Groups have been used in occupational therapy since the beginning of practice. There are a variety of skills needed to fulfil the essential functions of the leader role. These skills take into account the individual member's needs, concerns of the group as a whole, the environment, and problematic forces within the group. By employing skills in a strategic manner the leader can be effective in helping both individuals and the group function at their highest levels. The leader must consider the group's phase of development in the types of process intervention and activity suggested as well as potential meaning of leader actions for the group. In early stages of a group, members rely more on the leader for direction to define the purpose of the group and to address feelings that emerge in the group process. As the group matures, the leader becomes less active as members are able to assume the emotional and task roles to support each other and complete the task.

HISTORICAL CONTEXT

Occupational therapists have used groups in their practice from the outset. The types of groups utilised have been influenced by health care delivery systems, needs of individuals and populations, research findings, and shifts in theoretical models for practice. The skills needed for

practice have evolved as research evidence has informed leader understanding as to what might be key mechanisms of change impacting group outcomes. While careful balance of process and product continues in how a leader considers incorporating activity and intentional use of self, key interdisciplinary constructs continue to emerge as essential elements of leader reasoning. The skills for intervention presented in this chapter require reasoning about the needs of the client, the group as a whole, and the context or environment. Leader reasoning is adapted to the type of setting where occupational therapists use groups in their practice. Intervention programmes using groups can include schools, hospitals, outpatient clinics, community agencies, and natural environments such as families, organisations, work teams, and living facilities (Scaffa, 2019a).

LEADERSHIP FUNCTIONS AND SKILLS

Critical Leadership Functions

Yalom and Leszcz (2005) identified four empirically researched significant leadership functions:

1. *Caring*: being a supportive, accepting presence; offering culturally sensitive client-centered self-disclosure; sharing expressions of concern; being genuine; offering a sense of safety within group

2. *Executive functions*: collaboratively creating rules; developing effective norms; helping members to establish goals; maintaining the boundary of time, space, structure, and group routines; stopping process to explore what is happening or intervening when group or member needs redirection

3. *Emotional stimulation* (activation): attending to member affect, expressed or unexpressed in verbal or nonverbal form; confronting group issues or challenging member behavior; modeling emotional risk taking through self-disclosure to facilitate member-to-member interaction to support group and member progress

4. *Meaning attribution*: providing a framework for understanding feelings that emerge within or among group members; clarifying or interpreting what might be happening at the level of the individual, for subgroups, or group as a whole; offering hope and empowering members to identify how change can occur

Composing a Group and Establishing a Group Contract

Before starting a group the leader should assess population and individual member needs. Assessment may include determining member functional capabilities related to motor, cognitive processing, and intra- and interpersonal social-emotional areas. Population-based needs require assessing community resources and the possible impact of disease, disability, or prevention efforts on individuals with problems such as traumatic brain injury, chronic illnesses affecting function, mental illness, and learning challenges.

Once you determine a need for the group exists, leaders need to create a framework addressing the following questions:

1. How many members will you have in the group?
2. Will it be a closed membership or will it allow for new members to join once started?
3. How long will the group meet (start/end times for session and number of sessions)?
4. What will be the group type and purpose?
5. What will be group goals, and how will outcomes be measured?

In beginning a group, the leader frequently presents a group contract to members. This may be discussed in an individual session with the client or in the group as part of its opening routine. Group contracts include (a) expectations for regular attendance and participation (procedures in event of illness or unexpected absence, consequences for lateness and absences, payment depending upon setting), (b) expectations about confidentiality, (c) putting thoughts into words and not actions, and (d) rules about out-of-group socialisation, if any. A group contract helps to promote interpersonal safety and caring by establishing clear boundaries and predictable expectations. Contracts can be written or verbal agreements. The overall aim of the contract is to provide an emotional container so the work of the group can be accomplished.

Selecting Members and Activities for a Group

Once the basic framework is determined, based on the level of member ability and group goals, modality selection is done depending upon group stage and members needs. Modalities can range from educational, activities of daily living, expressive activities, to leisure interest and vocational activities. The performance of occupations is common in occupational therapy groups (Scaffa, 2019b). No matter the modality, the activity is adapted to member need and functioning to support successful participation. Leaders may need to be highly directive in selecting an activity or can facilitate group decision making about their activity programme. If members need a lot of emotional support, the leader may need to take on roles of encourager and mediator while validating the value of the individual to the group's process. It is usually advantageous to work with a co-leader to share in the task and emotional aspects of facilitating a group, especially when members face physical or emotional challenges that impact their ability to function.

Structuring the Overall Group and Individual Sessions

Using formal group protocols can help with assessing needs, session planning, and evaluating group and member progress. These protocols might outline group history, assessments of members and context, general group goals, session plans, and session evaluation methods (Schwartzberg et al., 2008).

Creating the Group

Essential tasks in creating a group include (a) building a cohesive group culture and climate (Burlingame et al., 2018), (b) member selection for group composition, and (c) preliminary group preparation (Vinogradov & Yalom, 1989). These leader activities are modified depending on the setting and programme structure.

Building Group Culture and Climate

It is the leader's responsibility to foster a therapeutic climate and set expectations. In occupational therapy this often involves matching the task or social demand to member ability. The leader must ensure the space is adequate for the activity and accessible to accommodate a range of abilities. Establishing clear norms for procedures such as who has responsibility for setting up and cleaning up the activity is part of building the group culture. An example of the impact of group culture on process and realignment of the dynamics is given in Vignette 10.1.

VIGNETTE 10.1 Building a Group Culture and Climate (by Jenni Guest)

When new facilitators took on an art group for patients with mental illness, they observed members were always late. Members never stayed for the continuous duration of the group, often popping in and out throughout the session, and weekly attendance was sporadic. The new facilitators were concerned about these trends, as it was creating an unsettled climate within the group. When raised for discussion with group members, their comments centred around the behaviour of the previous facilitators, stating the previous leader was never on time, often canceled sessions with no warning, and was always leaving group for a cigarette break or phone call. This highlighted the impact the facilitators' behaviour and attitudes had on how group members saw the group. The new facilitators realised they had to reestablish the group culture. They chose to formally end the original group, taking a short break and starting a new art group. All of this was discussed and agreed upon with current group members. The facilitators asked group members to name the new group, to encourage a climate of ownership and commitment, and ensured group always started on time, with no facilitator breaks.

Member Selection and Group Composition

In selecting group participants, the major challenge is matching individuals so they can function together socially and in performing tasks. Alternatively, the group may have heterogeneous membership to augment learning from others who are different. The leader may decide to compose the group with individuals who are similar to heighten feelings of belonging and to make an easier match between the demands of the task and member functioning.

Preliminary Group Preparation

If at all possible, it is good to meet with a new group member prior to group participation. The aim of preparing the member in advance of the first session is to (1) help the member understand the group purpose, (2) facilitate member identifying personal goals, and (3) discuss potential value for the member of group tasks. This may involve explaining why the group may be helpful, clarifying expectations for participation, and allaying fears regarding group participation. Carefully explaining the nature of the group activities can help avoid member dropoutt. Vignette 10.2 illustrates the impact of lack of preparation on a group member.

Engaging Individual Members and the Group as a Whole

There are many techniques to use for engaging individuals in a group. Bridging activities, communicating with members around group theme, showing and telling members how the activity matches with the group purpose can help members understand group meaning and purpose. Keep in mind, evidence supports the underlying aim of building group cohesion as a moderator of group effectiveness and positive member outcomes (Burlingame et al., 2018).

Bridging

The technique used to bring people in closer emotional connection and to develop a powerful group identity is called bridging (Ormont, 1990). Clients often lack the social skills and emotional or cognitive capacity to easily form emotional and social connections. Using members as bridge builders is most desirable (Ormont, 1990), although it is not always feasible given the level of function of clients. Members may lack insight or emotional attunement to sense the perspective of others. Leader role modeling and facilitating group members becoming bridge builders is a key aspect of leadership. Three methods of

VIGNETTE 10.2 Preliminary Group Preparation (by Jenni Guest)

When observing a music group facilitated by two other occupational therapists, I remember watching the look on a new group member's face when the first activity was introduced. The activity involved listening to a piece of music and then using movement and dance to demonstrate how the music made you feel. This member looked shocked and horrified at the idea of dancing or using movement within a group of people who she did not know. At the end of the session when talking to this client it became clear that her understanding of a music group had been very different than what she had encountered. She thought the group focused on music appreciation and it turned out to be more of an exploratory use of music to express emotions. Sadly, this confusion led to her choosing to not access any group services through the centre.

BOX 10.1   Open-Ended Questioning

Asking one member about how he or she thinks another member feels (Ormont, 1990):

"What do you think Tim feels when you leave the room before we finish the activity?" or "Why might Tim leave before we finish the activity?"

Asking one member about another member's pattern of behaviour (Ormont, 1990):

"What might be happening with Tim when he asks for help on his project from Sarah but doesn't get a reply?"

BOX 10.2   Directed Questioning

Asking a question so that it sounds like an interpretation to invite another member to comment (Ormont, 1990):

"I wonder if you are aware that Tim feels very disappointed when he doesn't get asked to talk about his painting?"

BOX 10.3   Questioning Member About Interaction Taking Place Between Two Others

Asking an important question of a third member to help create a bridge between two other members (Ormont, 1990):

Leader asks John, "What feeling might Tim be keeping from Sarah at this moment?"

leader-initiated bridging are suggested (Boxes 10.1–10.3): (1) asking open-ended questions to the group as a whole, (2) asking direct questions to members, and (3) consulting with another member about what might be happening in an interaction taking place between two other members (Ormont, 1990).

As with any technique, bridging should be used judiciously and not in the following circumstances: (1) when a leader's focusing on an individual will feel traumatic or frightening to the person, (2) at the end of a session with a quiet member, (3) when two members are communicating well and adding leader input is unnecessary, and (4) as a self-protective reaction to feeling challenged as a leader by a difficult group situation. A group leader's wish to have a perfect group or holding unrealistic expectations of oneself (as all-knowing, loving, or powerful) can lead to group therapist shame (Weber & Gans, 2003) and burnout.

Communicating With the Individual in Relation to the Group Theme

Group members may have difficulty understanding how what is occurring in group is relevant to their situation. The leader can take an active role in explaining how the process or content of a session relates to the members' goals or situation. When members are capable, the leader may encourage them to explore the meaning of the themes in relation to their personal life. Comments about themes in the group as a whole, called process commentary (Brown, 2018), should be used prudently. Leaders need to gauge readiness by considering the groups' phase, member ability to comprehend inferences, and desire to be (or not be) the singular focus of the group.

Showing and Telling How the Activity Matches With the Group Purpose

In occupational therapy the group activity, whether it be what Mosey (1970) calls a parallel or cooperative one, has a therapeutic purpose. In a parallel group, members work side by side using materials provided. The leader structures the activity and supports members' social-emotional needs. In a cooperative level group, the leader is in an advisory role. The group is likely to have more consistent attendance, successful outcomes, and client satisfaction when the activity matches the understood purpose of the group. In Vignette 10.3 the group leader introduces an activity that would seem ordinary, perhaps even silly or confusing, without an explanation of its therapeutic value given the group's purpose.

Structuring Process From Formation Stage to Closure Stage of a Group

Groups are known to go through various phases of development (Agazarian & Gantt, 2003). Although there are several configurations of group development, there are broadly five stages of development (Tuckman, 1965; Tuckman & Jensen, 1977):

1. Forming: developing trust and goals
2. Storming: resisting leader authority
3. Norming: finding common goals and developing group expectations
4. Performing: working on group goals
5. Adjourning: separating, consolidating gains, planning for future

In leading a group, the leader assumes a more active role in the forming stage. This may involve setting up the room, the activity, and explaining specific procedures. To facilitate development of trust, the leader needs to maintain the group's boundaries and be consistent in expectations and availability. As the group is able to assume more leadership

---

VIGNETTE 10.3 Show and Tell: How Activity Matches With Group Purpose (by Jenni Guest)

While facilitating a group known as Making Changes, we often used what appeared to be random games and activities as tools to introduce a deeper topic or theme that the group was addressing. When working through a series on self-esteem and confidence I remember using an altered version of Spin the Bottle to introduce the session. It involved the spinning of the bottle and whoever the bottle pointed to, the group member had to compliment or thank them for something they appreciated or had noticed about that member during their time in the group. The member being complimented then had to acknowledge and thank the person for the comment. Each member found this challenging on some level, and there was a high level of laughter.

The purpose of the activity had been threefold: to break the ice at the beginning of session introducing the topic for the week with some fun, to introduce the concept of giving and receiving compliments by identifying good characteristics in those around you, and to allow members to experience being complimented and discuss how members felt and whether people felt comfortable accepting what people had said. The purpose of the activity was only realised when the activity was discussed with group members, providing a discussion platform concerning self-esteem, compliments, and confidence.

---

of itself, shared responsibility emerges for deciding on the activity, materials needed, group process, and preparations for ending the session. In Vignette 10.4 a group leader describes her experience of turning points in variety of groups and their development.

Self-Disclosure

Group leaders must decide how much to share in the group of their own personal reactions and situation. Storytelling is a common technique used in occupational therapy to convey information, develop a personal connection, and establish rapport (Schwartzberg, 2002). Therapists exchange stories with clients to promote alliances and collaborative relationships (Mattingly & Fleming, 1994). They

must make explicit decisions about how much to share based on the best interests of clients. It is wise to take in account varying meanings of leader self-disclosure from cross-cultural perspectives (Dillon, 2019). Vignette 10.5 illustrates the process of clinical reasoning used in leader self-disclosure.

Process Commentary

To enhance members' capability to self-monitor, the leader can summarise observations and then ask members to explain what they see happening in the group (Vinogradov & Yalom, 1989). For example, the leader notes, "I notice that half the group is doing the project at one end of the table and others at the far side of the room talking amongst

---

VIGNETTE 10.4 Structuring Group Process: Forming to Adjourning Stage (by Jenni Guest)

Introducing from the start of a group meeting the idea of group closure can be a useful way of managing the stages of a group. However, this is only appropriate in certain groups, such as those where members have a limited number of sessions (e.g., anxiety management, anger management, and symptom and medication management groups). With more vulnerable group populations or groups that are ongoing, the leader intervenes as individual members terminate.

When starting a new gardening group, an effective way I found of encouraging the group to develop trust and establish goals was for the first group session to be spent at the garden centre. As a group, the members chose the items to use, and we reviewed the purpose of the group. As a leader, my contribution was providing the opportunity,

finances, and transportation. From the start, the group had a sense of purpose, ownership, and began establishing effective communication and trusting relationships.

Whether to mark the closure of a group is something the group needs to decide as a whole, but to acknowledge closure is something leaders have responsibility to ensure happens. One group I was a member in acknowledged the closure through having a photograph taken of the group. It was a way to symbolically take what was gained and learned through the group process away with you. When ending a group because of leaving a post I have found this substantially different and harder, and even attempted to avoid taking responsibility for it. The group took initiative and decided to mark the ending, through sharing cards and what they had gained from being a part of the group.

VIGNETTE 10.5 **Therapist Self-Disclosure (by Jenni Guest)**

When facilitating my first anger management group, the format of the sessions meant that in the last 15 minutes of each session I asked the group to share openly about personal experiences of anger, and dependent on the topic discussed that week on the worksheets, reflect on a specific example. At these moments in the group sessions, I remember being mystified as to why the group dynamics changed so dramatically. The process moved from a talkative and engaged group to unresponsive and disengaged.

During session number 4, I followed the same format of the group; however, when silence descended again in the last 15 minutes, I decided I needed to address the group through reflecting my concerns. At this point, one particular member addressed me directly and asked, "Why each week do you ask us to share with you our experience, when you haven't shared anything personal with us in the last 3 weeks?"

On reflection I could see that his statement was true. I had until that point followed, almost word for word, the predesigned worksheets. Not once had I used a personal illustration to support the topics we had discussed. As a relatively new occupational therapist at the time, I spent the remainder of that week wrestling with the conflict in

my mind between the member's statement and the professional theory I thought I was adhering to of maintaining clear therapist–patient boundaries. However, certain questions remained clear: Why should they share with me, someone who purely sits, listens, and asks them to participate in tasks or answer questions but never discloses any information or completes any of the tasks for oneself? How would I act if I were a group member?

Within the next anger management group session, I decided to start the session differently and opened by reflecting to the group my thought process following the member's question from the previous session. I then continued to introduce, using a personal experience as an example, the topic for discussion. Slowly during that and the subsequent remaining five sessions, the group and I gained comfort and confidence in sharing personal experiences within the group. The group began to discuss these situations and identify with each other, relating similar scenarios they had experienced. My use of client serving, intentional self-disclosure within the group, led the way for other members to share more openly their stories and ultimately allowed the group to evolve into a more effective vehicle to assist members learning and exploring new techniques to managing anger.

---

themselves. I wonder, what do you see happening?" Yalom and Leszcz (2005) explain that through process comments the client may experience the change process as follows:

1. "Here is what your behaviour is like" (p. 180).
2. "Here is how your behaviour makes others feel" (p. 180).
3. "Here is how your behaviour influences the opinions others have of you" (p. 180).
4. "Here is how your behaviour influences your opinion of yourself" (p. 181).

The use of process commentary (Brown, 2018) is very helpful in supporting members to take the initiative in directing their own behaviour rather than relying on the therapist or blaming others.

Reality Testing

Understanding the patterns of one's own behaviour through getting impressions from others is commonly referred to as reality testing. This process can take place through hearing other members' and the leader's observations. Similar to process commentary, reality testing focuses on opportunities in the group for consensual validation of the member's own observations with others in the group (Schwartzberg et al., 2008). Such data can help prevent leaders from intervening based on their own perceptions as an absolute

truth. It is advisable to consider attributional biases, whereby leaders may unconsciously attribute facts about others based on subjective countertransference reactions or adopt misguided evidence-based approaches (Lewis, 2009) due to misperceptions of member or group needs.

Reframing

To create a positive group environment, the leader needs to address potential conflict and increase a sense of support (Vinogradov & Yalom, 1989). By reframing, the leader puts things in a way that emphasises the member's positive intentions, efforts, and contributions. For example, a member in a loud voice demands another member give her supplies to complete an activity. The therapist may say, "Mary, you seem in a big rush and to be putting pressure on John to finish quickly. I know you really want to bring home your project and show your family what you have accomplished in occupational therapy. In this group we have enough supplies for everyone. Is there another member who might lend supplies or do you want to go to cabinet to get your own supplies?" By reframing the situation, the leader again reinforces the member's own capacity to take positive action and thereby defusing what could become a negative interaction in the group. Vignette 10.6 shows

VIGNETTE 10.6 Reframing (by Jenni Guest)

Within a gardening group on an elderly neurorehabilitation unit, I remember being faced with one gentleman who repetitively made statements in group that resulted in other members of group deliberately behaving in a way to isolate or annoy him. Such complaints included not passing him items that he wanted, not talking to him within the group, or choosing to sit next to other people in the group. The member's belief around these situations and scenarios was firmly focused on others' behaviour being deliberately negative towards him. Specifically, he believed people did not want him in the group and this was evidenced by group members never passing him items he asked for when completing activities.

I took the lead on working with the member within the group to look at the situation and try to reframe his belief and thinking around this situation. The phrase, "I appreciate how you feel, but do you think there is another way of looking at that" became one of the most useful phrases. This simple statement acknowledged his feelings and position, whilst also encouraging a time of thinking about the situation and an opportunity to reframe the situation in a more realistic manner.

In truth, some of the origins of the member's frustrations were grounded. He often did not get passed items he asked for in group. When thinking it through we were able to identify the real reason and therefore reframe his belief that ignoring him was a personalised and deliberate act. The true answer was quite simple; he had badly slurred speech and was only able to talk quietly, whilst others in the group were hard of hearing. This was discussed within the group, and a new way of sharing items amongst group members was agreed, thinking about how each member could communicate in a manner to accommodate all members' individual needs.

---

how a member's behavior, when given context or reframed, changes meaning.

Giving Feedback

The process of feedback involves sharing your reaction to another person with a goal of fostering improved ways of relating. For example, the group leader says, "As much as I would like to help you with your project, Fred and I are both occupied. I notice that when someone else in the group needs my help you often also ask for my assistance. I wonder what might be happening for you right now? Sharing attention and taking turns can take some practice. What might the group do to support you right now while you wait?" Feedback is best timed when members are calm, not defensive, and as close to the event as possible. If members appear anxious, angry, or defensive, then it is best to stop the feedback process and try to reframe the situation.

Structured Exercises Versus Open process

The leader needs to think about when it is to the group's advantage to use structured exercises and when it is preferable to listen and attend to themes as well as needs emerging in the session. In settings where there is a quick turnaround for group participation, manualised or predesigned group materials have advantages. The risk in focusing too much on the activity is missing important process themes necessary to successful outcomes for individuals and the group as a whole. For example, the loss of a group member or staff member may be emotionally difficult for a group. To proceed ahead with a preplanned activity could leave members' needs to address feelings and consider a more suitable activity unaddressed as well as endorse avoiding dealing with difficult feelings such as loss.

Leaders need to seek a balance between structure, product, and process. The main question to gauge these choices is: What is in the best interest of the clients and group as a whole? By structuring the group task to the members' level of capability, therapeutic outcomes are more likely. The leader needs to take into consideration the members' cognitive, social, motor, and communication abilities. Environmental factors such as the size of the room, type of furniture, noise level, distractions, and other elements of the physical climate need to be monitored and adjusted to group members' needs. A predictable arrangement of furniture and materials can enhance a sense of safety. Vignette 10.7 illustrates the hazards of overly structuring a group versus group-centred use of structure and open-ended process.

Intervening With Problematic Forces in a Group

It is the leader's responsibility to maintain as cohesive a group as possible. This means addressing diminished group functioning due to subgroups, scapegoating, competitiveness, lateness, absenteeism, boundary violations, or anger occurring in the group. It is the leader's obligation to maintain the safety by reinforcing the contract and stated expectation of the group such as start and end times. By helping members see commonalities and learn to accept difference, possible projections are diminished.

VIGNETTE 10.7   Structured Exercises Versus Open Process (by Jenni Guest)

When asked to provide feedback following a group session, one set of patients described the experience as "the blind leading the blind." In this case the leaders were standing in for other staff and followed the predesigned session plans word for word throughout the group session. However, the rigidity this brought to the group did not allow for the group to take ownership of the material and how they were going to work through it that week. The balance was off between structure and openness.

Even when leaders use structured exercises, they need to react and interact with the group, continuously adapting the materials available to meet the needs of the group and the members.

In one anger management session, this meant only the first activity that had been formally planned was completed. The group discussion that emerged was so productive and relevant for the group it would have been counterproductive to move on to the next item on the plans list.

Encouraging collaboration and communication is helpful in facilitating groups with intercultural conflict, with the leader being mindful of their own attributional style (Okech et al., 2016). Vignette 10.8 illustrates the value of establishing a contract with members around expectations.

The leader's success in intervening is highly dependent on self-awareness and knowing aspects of the member's behaviour that trigger idiosyncratic responses in the leader (Gans & Alonso, 1998). The member's behaviour may also elicit a common reaction from others. By understanding these dynamics, the leader can better modulate responses to and between group members.

Problematic group forces

Problematic behaviours often arise in a group. Rather than see these as destructive elements, called antigroup phenomena (Nitsun, 1996), the leader can mobilise the group to enhance its creative potential.

VIGNETTE 10.8   Establishing a Contract (by Jenni Guest)

During a course on group work, I was involved in setting up a short-term group for children within a preschool. During the preplanning discussion with management it had been emphasised that the philosophy of the centre was to positively reinforce desired behaviour but to not reprimand or discipline children for inappropriate behaviour. On arrival at the preschool and meeting the children, my coworker and I were excited by the prospect of spending time there and optimistic about what we could offer them during our time there. However, it became clear through the first two sessions that this philosophy of only focusing on positive was going to pose a difficulty for us. During the sessions we found ourselves purely crisis managing the behaviour of our group of five children aged 3 to 5, as opposed to leading the activities we had planned. Throughout the group the children wanted to leave and return, interrupting any flow of activity we had managed to establish.

At this point my coworker and I decided we needed to take a proactive stance of establishing a set of ground rules with the children. On reflection I think we had not done this on group commencement because the children were so young. We had assumed as leaders we would enforce our preestablished group rules. How wrong were we? During the next group session, we set out a large piece of paper on the floor and started the session with the children sitting around it. Taking turns around the circle we all put down items on the paper about how we thought the group should run and how our behaviour should be within the group. The children who had been the most challenging were providing some of the most powerful statements, such as "keep our hands to ourselves" and "turn our listening ears on when someone else is talking." It was agreed, or contracted, among the group members that if you decided to attend the group you could only leave and return to the group if you were going to the toilet, otherwise if you chose to leave you had to wait until the next week to come into the group again. It was amazing to watch how the children appeared to enjoy setting themselves rules for the sessions, and during subsequent sessions we started each session revisiting our list and checking if there were any statements that needed to be changed or added. The process probably took less than 10 minutes during that third session, but it set the scene for how the children knew they were to behave when in the group and allowed us to make the most of the limited time the group was together. It also meant on the occasions when behaviour became an issue and jeopardised safety and the purpose of the session, it was possible to discuss the ground rules the child had agreed to and made determining corrective actions for this behaviour much simpler.

SUMMARY

It is the leader's role to compose, plan for, lead, and evaluate a group. Leader reasoning is used to engage individual members and the group as a whole to create therapeutic group contexts for member growth and change. Leader self-awareness and reflection are key to running successful groups.

REFLECTIVE LEARNING

- Think about different groups you have participated in or led. Which have been most successful and why?
- Which groups have you participated in or led that have not gone so well? What would you do differently next time?
- How have you used different leadership roles/functions in groups?
- Thinking of groups you have participated in, can you identify how and when they transitioned through the different stages of Tuckman's group processes?

ACKNOWLEDGMENT

The authors thank Jenni Guest, Occupational Therapist, Oxford, UK, for her case Vignettes and sharing her reflections on practice. Her Vignettes illustrate concepts central to group process and show the value of clinical reasoning. Jenni received her post-professional master's degree from Tufts University, Department of Occupational Therapy, Medford, Massachusetts, United States.

REFERENCES

Agazarian, Y., & Gantt, S. (2003). Phases of group development: Systems-centered hypotheses and their implications for research and practice. *Group Dynamics: Theory, Research, and Practice, 7*(3), 238–252.

Brown, N. W. (2018). Group as a whole process commentary. *Group, 42*(1), 35–48.

Burlingame, G. M., McClendon, D. T., & Yang, C. (2018). Cohesion in group therapy: A meta-analysis. *Psychotherapy, 55*(4), 384–398.

Dillon, N. (2019). Examining the role of therapist self-disclosure in cross-cultural settings. *The Group Circle, 3-4*, 6.

Gans, J. S., & Alonso, A. (1998). Difficult patients: Their construction in group therapy. *International Journal of Group Psychotherapy, 48*(3), 311–326.

Lewis, J. I. (2009). The crossroads of countertransference and attribution theory: Reinventing clinical training within an evidence-based treatment world. *American Journal of Psychoanalysis, 69*(2), 106–120.

Mattingly, C., & Fleming M. H. (Eds.). (1994). Interactive reasoning: Collaborating with the person. In *Clinical reasoning forms of inquiry in a therapeutic practice* (pp. 178–196). FA Davis.

Mosey, A. C. (1970). The concept and use of developmental groups. *American Journal of Occupational Therapy, 24*(4), 272–275.

Nitsun, M. (1996). *The anti-group: Destructive forces in the group and their creative potential.* Routledge.

Okech, J. E. A., Pimpleton-Gray, A. M., Vannatta, R., & Champe, J. (2016). Intercultural conflict in groups. *The Journal for Specialists in Group Work, 41*(4), 350–369.

Ormont, L. (1990). The craft of bridging. *International Journal of Group Psychotherapy, 40*(1), 3–17.

Scaffa, M. E. (2019a). Occupational therapy interventions for groups, communities, and populations. In B. A. Boyt Schell, & G. Gillen (Eds.), *Willard & Spackman's occupational therapy* (13th ed., pp. 436–447). Wolters Kluwer.

Scaffa, M. E. (2019b). Group process and group intervention. In B. A. Boyt Schell, & G. Gillen (Eds.), *Willard & Spackman's occupational therapy* (13th ed., pp. 539–555). Wolters Kluwer.

Schwartzberg, S. L. (2002). *Interactive reasoning in the practice of occupational therapy.* Prentice-Hall.

Schwartzberg, S. L., Howe, M. C., & Barnes, M. A. (2008). *Groups: Applying the functional group model.* FA Davis.

Tuckman, B. W. (1965). Developmental sequence in small groups. *Psychological Bulletin, 63*, 384–399.

Tuckman, B. W., & Jensen, M. A. (1977). Stages of small-group development revisited. *Group and Organization Studies, 2*(4), 419–427.

Vinogradov, S., & Yalom, I. D. (1989). In *Concise guide to group psychotherapy.* American Psychiatric Press.

Weber, R. L., & Gans, J. S. (2003). The group therapist's shame: A much undiscussed topic. *International Journal of Group Psychotherapy, 53*(4), 395–416.

Yalom, I. D., & Leszcz, M. (2005). In *The theory and practice of group psychotherapy* (5th ed.). Basic Books.

11

Record and Report Writing

Lisa McCaw and Jane Grant

HIGHLIGHTS

- Accurate case records and good-quality report writing are essential skills for practice.
- Case records include any material concerning a client. They provide an accurate record of the client's condition over time detailing the assessment, planning and care delivery, and its evaluation. They must demonstrate everything that has been done for or with a client and show practitioners' clinical reasoning.
- Case records can be kept in various formats. Recent developments include client-held records, integrated care pathways, and electronic case records.

- Regardless of practice setting, the occupational therapy process (from initial referral to discharge) must be comprehensively and accurately reported.
- Ensuring good standards of recordkeeping is an important aspect of service quality. Audit can help services to monitor the quality of recordkeeping.
- Current legal issues pertinent to recording and report writing include documenting risk assessment and child protection reports.

INTRODUCTION

Recording and report writing may not initially appear to be the most engaging issue; however, it is a vital and integral component of practice within all settings (Royal College of Occupational Therapists [RCOT], 2018). It is the professional duty of all occupational therapists to maintain accurate and up-to-date records, but relatively little attention has been paid to this subject within the literature.

This chapter outlines the purpose and process of maintaining records and creating reports. Current themes in recording and format of case records are discussed. Aspects of recording and reporting the occupational therapy process are explored and examples are provided. Finally, quality assurance and legal issues in recording and report writing are highlighted.

- The focus of this chapter is on the United Kingdom and its devolved nations' guidelines and standards; however, the principles are valid for good report writing internationally. Although the basic principles are likely to be the same, readers from outside the United Kingdom are advised to read this chapter in line with their national clinical codes and guidelines (e.g., see, Occupational Therapy Australia, 2014).

WHAT ARE RECORDS?

The RCOT (2018) states that "care records include any material that holds information regarding an individual," collected as part of the care provision. Such material can be handwritten, digital, auditory, or visual and would include data held on a computer, a tablet, or a cellphone. Care records include images, auditory, or visual recordings, forms, letters, notes, diary entries, emails, text messages, and duplicate copies.

- In addition, there are less obvious types of information that should be incorporated into case records. Any discussions that take place regarding a person on one's caseload must be recorded. This may include discussions within supervision, team meetings, and telephone calls. If the practitioner is following specific national or local guidelines, procedures, or other standard process, then this should also be demonstrated and recorded in the case record. It is also important to document fully all activity, including frequent and repetitious activities; otherwise, the information cannot be proven to have occurred. Individuals' responses to interventions should always be recorded. Similarly, if a planned intervention does not occur, perhaps due to nonattendance, this should be recorded with an explanation, if possible. Recording such information demonstrates that any disruption to care and intervention is unavoidable and not due to practitioner disorganisation or lack of competence (RCOT, 2018).

PURPOSE OF RECORDS

Staff members working in health and social care setting are required to adhere to various recordkeeping standards. According to the RCOT (2018), case records can serve multiple purposes, including to:

- Provide a chronological and accurate record of the occupational therapy process (assessment, decision making, planning, treatment, and outcomes of care provided).
- Highlight problems and changes in the service user's condition at an early stage.
- Provide a record of the service user's goals, preferences, and choices.
- Document consent.
- Protect the best interests of the service user by supporting evidence-based care of high quality and ensuring that rationale for care is documented.
- Facilitate good communication between all involved.
- Clearly demonstrate your role and practice as an occupational therapist.
- Provide legal documents that may be used as evidence in a court of law or enquiry.
- Provide continuity of information as many different health and social care professionals can be involved in the treatment of a single individual.
- Clinical records are also valuable documents to audit the quality of care provided (Mathioudakis, 2016).

Professional and Legal Requirements

The RCOT (2021) professional standards for occupational therapy practice, conduct, and ethics require registrant occupational therapists to keep high-quality records to "protect the welfare of those who access the service" (p. 24).

It is each occupational therapist's professional responsibility to ensure that case records are fit for purpose and processed in accordance with legislation (RCOT, 2021). Records of care provide evidence that an occupational therapist has met duty of care within the practice. Documenting the evidence that supports the practice, where available, is also a key professional requirement (RCOT, 2021).

As well as a professional requirement, good recordkeeping is also a regulatory requirement. The Health and Care Professions Council (HCPC) is the regulatory body for UK occupational therapists. As part of HCPC's "Standards of Conduct, Performance and Ethics" (2018), all registrants must keep full, clear, and accurate records for everyone

cared for, treated, or given a service. Records must be completed promptly and as soon as possible after providing care, treatment, or other services. Records must be kept secure by protecting them from loss, damage, or inappropriate access (HCPC, 2016).

- Failure to keep records in a competent manner may result in investigation of competency or misconduct. If not accurately recorded, an event or activity cannot be proven to have occurred; therefore the practitioner may be regarded as unfit or unsafe to practice. Potential recordkeeping failures include incomplete or missing entries, inaccurate terminology, and lack of clarity or succinct language. Competency may also be challenged if records are not completed in a timely manner, do not document clinical reasoning, demonstrate poor completion of assessments, and fail to identify goals, interventions, and outcomes. In addition, records must connect the intervention with the care plan, indicate whether the goals were met, have clearly documented risk assessment and actions taken, record any meetings or communications with others, and identify any referrals made (HCPC, 2013).
- In delegating tasks to another practitioner or student, it is the responsibility of the occupational therapist to ensure that the individual is competent to undertake the task, which includes recordkeeping (RCOT, 2018).

CONTENT AND QUALITY OF RECORDS

Occupational therapy case records have two purposes: (1) to provide a clinical record of interventions with people and (2) (and only infrequently) to enable evidence of occupational therapy practice to be presented as evidence in court proceedings. The Professional Standards for Occupational Therapy Practice ("Standards") require that practitioners in all settings (a) provide comprehensive and accurate records that demonstrate practice is appropriate and meets the duty of care and (b) justify accounts of all they plan or provide for service users (RCOT, 2021).

Records must demonstrate all occupational therapy activity and include everything that has been planned, done, or occurs with or on behalf of a service user. This must also include professional and clinical reasoning. Occupational therapists need to demonstrate the outcomes of the care they have provided. This may include problems and actions taken to resolve them (RCOT, 2021).

The RCOT (2018) provides clear guidance for occupational therapists and occupational therapy services in relation to keeping records. Its checklist for keeping records states that records should:

- Clearly identify the client by name, address, and date of birth on all records kept

- Document details of all key people involved in the client's care, both professionals and family/carers
- Document all referral details, including date and source of referral and reason for referral when given
- Document any social, medical, or rehabilitative history
- Document, date, and time all assessments made, methods used, and resulting outcomes
- Document and date the views and wishes of the client about goals or treatment plans, and any time frames suggested
- Document the consent and nature of consent given to intervention
- Document, date, and time all interventions planned and carried out in connection with the client, and the resulting outcomes
- Document and date all reviews, and alterations to goals, treatment plans, or time frames
- Document all interventions or decisions made by members of the multidisciplinary team when it impacts the occupational therapy care given, including decisions taken in clinical supervision
- Incorporate in the records all correspondence, telephone conversations, and reports related to the client's care
- Document and date interventions or contact with family and carers and any outcomes
- Document all information and advice provided to the client and family/carers
- Document all discharge, closure, or transfer details
- Document the destination of onward referrals or care transfers and any information that needs to be considered in handover (with the knowledge and consent of the service user)

Signing and Countersigning

When signing a care record or making a digital entry the therapist is verifying the accuracy and is identifying oneself as the person responsible for the activity in the entry and for the entry itself.

It is a professional requirement for occupational therapists to ensure that they sign and print their name in a clear and legible manner. The therapist's designation should also be recorded. For digital entries, all therapists should use their own individual username and password, which should not be shared with colleagues.

Occupational therapists are no longer required to countersign entries made by occupational therapy students or assistants unless local policy states otherwise.

Use of Acronyms and Abbreviations

In their guidance on recordkeeping, the RCOT (2018) highlights that abbreviations and acronyms are useful when trying to record in a concise way, especially if it can be assumed that the other members of the multidisciplinary team will understand the terms used. However, it should be remembered that clients have the right to access their records upon request and should be able to read and understand what is written in them. In addition, the use of certain terms and acronyms may change over time and are likely to differ across different service providers.

Timing and Dating Entries

It is necessary to record the date and time of the care provided to each service user. This allows the therapist to document and demonstrate that the care was appropriate and proceeded as planned (or not). In addition, it allows the frequency of intervention to be monitored and outlines a time frame to monitor individuals' progress or deterioration. It is important to remember that this may serve as a vital piece of evidence should case records be examined later. Retrospective entries must state the time and date that the individual was seen in addition to the time and date of the actual entry. An explanation should be recorded if there is a considerable delay in making the entry (RCOT, 2018). Attention should be paid to variations that may occur with digital systems to ensure that accuracy is maintained.

Timely Recordkeeping

To reduce the likelihood of inaccuracies or omissions in recordkeeping, it is important that records are completed in a timely manner, preferably as soon after the event as possible (RCOT, 2018).

Confidentiality and Information Sharing

Practitioners should be aware of the responsibilities they have when it comes to confidentiality and sharing of information. The RCOT (2021) highlights that confidentiality is a legal and ethical duty; however, this duty is not absolute. Central to the primary consideration of maintaining confidentiality is the requirement to ensure individuals' well-being or protection, or the well-being and protection of the wider community. Written records are data, and therefore UK practitioners are duty bound to adhere to the latest versions of the UK General Data Protection Regulation (UK GDPR) and to the Data Protection Act (Great Britain Parliament, 2018).

Practitioners must carefully consider when and with whom they should share individuals' information. Guidance on how to do this can be drawn from the Caldicott Principles (Department of Health, 2013). These principles emerged from a 1997 review of client-identifiable information within the National Health Service (NHS) in England, chaired by Dame Fiona Caldicott. This review explored how patient information was being used and highlighted the potential risk to confidentiality. Several recommendations were made regarding information passing between organisations for reasons other than direct care, research, or as a legal requirement. The aim was to ensure that client information is only shared for valid reasons and that the minimum necessary information was shared (Department of Health, 2006a). Following the review, the Caldicott committee developed six principles that should be followed when sharing client information. In 2013 a seventh principle was added to the list:

- Principle 1: Justify the purpose(s) for using confidential information.
- Principle 2: Only use confidential information when absolutely necessary.
- Principle 3: Use the minimum information that is required.
- Principle 4: Access to confidential information should be on a strict need-to-know basis.
- Principle 5: Everyone must understand their responsibilities.
- Principle 6: Understand and comply with the law.
- Principle 7: The duty to share personal information can be as important as the duty to have regard for patient confidentiality.

Gaining and Documenting Consent

Consent is when a person gives express permission for any sort of intervention, care, or service. For consent to be informed it must be based on a clear understanding of action, of the information given, and of the implications and consequences that arise from this action (RCOT, 2018). Standard 1 of HCPC's "Standards of Conduct, Performance and Ethics" (2018) highlights the importance of making sure that practitioners gain consent from service users or other appropriate authorities before they provide care, treatment, or other services. Once consent for assessment or intervention is obtained, it should be recorded and regularly confirmed. The nature of consent given (e.g., verbally, in writing, through a guardian or advocate, or by other means) should also be recorded. All written consent forms should be kept in the client's records. Consent should also be gained before a student observes or provides an intervention, and again the consent and nature of the consent should also be documented.

There are times when documenting consent may be difficult or inappropriate (e.g., when working with children or adults who may experience the impaired capacity to make informed decisions). Consent relating to people under the age of 16 should always be sought from the person who has the relevant parental responsibility. However, some children under the age of 16 can give consent themselves, provided they can fully understand the information that is provided. This is known as the Gillick principle or having

Gillick competence: when a young person would like to receive an intervention but doesn't want parents or carers to know, is seeking support in confidence regarding substance abuse, or has strong views about future living arrangements that may conflict with parents or carers (Griffith, 2016).

Even when people lack ability to provide informed consent, they should always be involved as much as possible about making decisions about themselves. Practitioners should ensure they consider clients' relevant circumstances, if they would be able to give consent at a future date if a decision was postponed, what their beliefs, values and wishes are, and what the views of their close family members are. Guidance on making decisions for people who lack capacity in the United Kingdom are drawn from devolved legislation (Department of Health, 2005, 2016; Scottish Government, 2016).

Correcting Errors

It is important that any errors noted are corrected immediately and initialed. Information should not be added or altered at a later date; if any additions are essential, these should be noted as a separate or supplementary note or entry, dated, and signed. Correction fluid should never be used to correct errors; instead, they should be scored out with a single line so that the original text is still legible.

FORMAT OF CASE RECORDS

Case records may be kept in a variety of different ways, some of which are outlined later. Current developments in recordkeeping include the integration of case records across services, the move from paper-based records to electronic systems, and patient-held notes. Regardless of such innovations, the same standards of recordkeeping should be applied across all types of records.

One example of a specific recordkeeping system used in some services is problem-orientated medical records. This system was introduced in 1968 by Lawrence Weed, an American physician, in an attempt to provide a more logical and clearer way of communicating information about an individual to another clinical professional (NHS Information Authority, 1999). Within problem-orientated medical records, practitioners are encouraged to write records using a specific format called SOAP: subjective-objective-assessment-plan. This type of recordkeeping is frequently found in physical health settings and is based on a problem-solving approach that aims to gather information, appraise it, plan an action, and evaluate an outcome. The SOAP system can be useful as it enables the reader to gain a quick understanding of a client's functioning. However, it has been criticised as being too mechanistic and based predominantly on a medical model that does not fit with a holistic, client-centred philosophy of occupational therapy (Blijlevens & Murphy, 2003). In their critical review of the SOAP note-writing structure within their service, Blijlevens and Murphy (2003) stated that people for whom SOAP notes were used "appeared to be regarded as made up of damaged body parts that needed to be restored to enable that person to perform fundamental activities in their home," and the notes did not reflect "who the client was in terms of their meaningful occupations and in what context these normally occurred" (p. 4). As an alternative, they proposed that recordkeeping should take a more client-centred approach—that is, a goal-setting approach known by the acronym COAST (Gately & Borcherding, 2012). The COAST format is an alternative method of documenting treatment goals. COAST supports practitioners to consider all aspects of goal setting, including:

- Client: What will the client perform?
- Occupation: What occupation?
- Assist level: With what level of assistance/independence?
- Specific condition: Under what conditions?
- Timeline: By when?

A commonly used alternate structured method of recording goals is the SMART format (Berge & Renger, 2017), though this system also has limitations (see Chapter 7):

Specific: Provide a clear statement of the objectives
Measurable: How will change be measured?
Achievable: Is the goal achievable? Do you have the required support and resources?
Realistic (or Relevant): How does the goal fit in with the overall objective and how meaningful or useful is it?
Timely: Provide an agreed date for achieving the goal setting

Electronic Case Records/Integrated Digital Case Records

The contemporary occupational therapist is required to be digitally literate. The trend toward the introduction of electronic case records is now well established, but implementation has been fraught with challenges and expense. Within England, the development of electronic patient records has been part of health policy since 2010. However, delivering on this target has been and remains highly challenging. The latest iteration of relevant legislation (NHS, 2019) covering electronic patient records in England requires all hospital records to be digitised by 2023. At the time of writing, it seems unlikely this target will be met.

A key development across the four nations of the United Kingdom in recent years has been the development of integrated health and social care services. The aim of this integration is to streamline the experience for people, make more effective use of resources, and improve communication between the historically separate health and social care services. This integration is now well established, but streamlining the use of multiple different recordkeeping systems between the different agencies remains challenging in many areas. As the College of Occupational Therapists (2014) noted, "Many therapists will have experience of having to change the case management systems that they use to record interventions and outcomes… (and) therapists may have experienced frustration with the headings and outcomes included in the new systems with the differences between systems and/or a lack of options relevant to occupational therapy" (p. 2).

Patient-Held Records

Patient-held case records refer to records that are held and controlled by people receiving services rather than by the services themselves. To date, patient-held records are most established in the community for those requiring antenatal services, cancer care, and care for long-term conditions (RCOT, 2018). Patient-held records may be particularly useful for those receiving care from a variety of professionals. In addition, it is thought that they may allow individuals to be more active participants in their care (e.g., being able to have the information that shows what has worked or been unhelpful in the past). This information may be useful in mental health settings when discussing issues such as relapse. It has been suggested that patient-held records also reduce any possible coercive elements of treatment (Henderson & Laugharne, 2000); however, possible difficulties exist. These include confidentiality issues, reliability of the client to carry the information and keep records safe, and duplication of the information (Warner et al., 2000). Practitioners are advised to follow local policy regarding whether duplicate records should be retained by the professional. If policies restrict the keeping of such records, it is the responsibility of that organisation or authority to accept any possible consequences.

Patient-held records do not appear to be universally beneficial. They have been suggested as a cost-efficient way of improving the care and outcome for those experiencing severe mental illness (Henderson & Laugharne, 1999); however, Warner et al. (2000) found that patient-held shared case records had no significant effect upon mental state or satisfaction of mental health service users. The uptake of the scheme was low by both staff and individuals, and it appeared that those experiencing a psychotic illness were less likely to use the records. In relation to the use of patient-held records in palliative care, a study by Cornbleet et al. (2002) found no significant evidence to support the introduction of such a scheme. There appeared to be no improvement in information giving or sharing, or to the degree to which the family was involved in decision making. However, most individuals who had a record found it to be of some benefit. A realist review of the benefits and challenges of patient-held records for children and young people with complex needs found that people were more engaged, had improved self-advocacy, and felt empowered. However, service providers needed to have sufficient knowledge about patient-held records, and organisations needed to ensure that staff understood the benefits of the system, to ensure good implementation and use in practice (Diffin et al., 2018).

RECORDING AND REPORTING THE OCCUPATIONAL THERAPY PROCESS

Referral

A documented system for prioritising and recording referrals should be used. It is each practitioner's responsibility to record or retain the referral details in the appropriate occupational therapy records (RCOT, 2018). This should include the source and date of referral. Practitioners must also inform the referring agency should the referral be declined and provide a justification for this decision. If the referral is considered inappropriate, it may be recommended that the client's details are passed on to an alternative service. Should this occur, informed consent (see earlier) must be documented (RCOT, 2018).

Assessment

Occupational therapists use many different types of assessments (see Chapter 5). If a standardised assessment is used, the aims and procedures must be clearly stated. Any variation during the assessment that would affect the standardised process must be recorded. The type of assessment used will depend on the area of practice and needs of the individual. Examples may include but are not limited to a comprehensive initial assessment, home visit assessments, workplace/vocational assessments, dressing assessments, and kitchen assessments.

All assessments, whether standardised or nonstandardised, interview or observational, should be recorded. A description of each person's individual factors, circumstantial or environmental aspects, and features of the activity that allow or impinge upon performance should be documented. The therapist's confidence in the assessment results should also be included (American Occupational Therapy Association, 2003). Should other factors that could affect the results (e.g., an individual's tiredness) exist, they should also be documented.

Well-developed electronic case records/integrated digital case records should contain electronic templates for every commonly used assessment tool, enabling occupational therapists to directly enter assessment data into the individual care record, ensuring high-quality data recording (College of Occupational Therapists, 2014).

Recording Progress

Efficient reporting should be organised and comprehensible. It should provide descriptive characteristics of the individual and the context in which the assessment or intervention occurred. Documentation is particularly useful for sharing small, gradual, and hard-to-detect changes. Evidence should be recorded either quantitatively or qualitatively (Tickle-Degnen, 2000). By documenting a clear relationship between the assessment outcomes, goals, and proposed intervention plan, practitioners can also educate others regarding the varied scope of occupational therapy interventions (Kyle & Wright, 1996).

Various factors need to be considered when documenting individuals' progress (or lack of) as a result of occupational therapy. Reports should clearly indicate what, if any, progress has been made. When using narratives in progress notes, practitioners should emphasise how progress is being made in relation to the intervention plan, which will have been jointly developed with the individual and his or her goals. Because safety issues are particularly important, these issues should be routinely documented. Any adverse incidents or near misses should also be documented and recorded in the organisation's specific risk reporting documentation.

Documenting Clinical Reasoning

Studies by Harman et al. (2009) and Davis et al. (2008) found that practitioners reported difficulty in translating evidence-based interventions into clinical documentation. Practitioners' clinical reasoning and decision making should be driven by evidence-based practice and should always be described when recording an individual's progress. Describing clinical reasoning and decision making enables other readers to clearly understand not only what was done, but also why it was done, and what the expected next steps will be. While these issues are important in all recordkeeping, they are particularly relevant when practitioners are required to demonstrate effectiveness to third-party payers.

Neidstadt (1996) suggested that mostly pragmatic and procedural reasoning styles are used within medical-, physical-, and health-oriented environments. However, narrative reasoning engages the individual in a life history storytelling process that ultimately places the practitioner in a better position to understand the client's subjective experiences, values, and goals for the future. By gathering and reporting this information, practitioners ultimately build a picture of the person through what this person does. As a result, meaningful client-centred goals can be established (Neidstadt, 1996).

Reflecting theory within documentation is a powerful method of communicating professional reasoning and rationale. Not only does it enable communication of the aims, interventions, and outcomes of therapy, but it can also enhance professionalism and credibility. However, it can be difficult to effectively communicate profession-specific information clearly within documentation. It is therefore important that care is taken to record complex professional reasoning and theory in language that can be clearly understood by an individual who is not necessarily from the same professional background.

All assessment results should be recorded and comprise all decisions made, including not to continue intervention either by the individual receiving occupational therapy or relevant other. It is important to remember that assessment results are shared jointly with the individual and practitioner and that, within the bounds of legality (see earlier), it is the individual's choice to share the information with relevant others or to withhold consent.

Goal Setting and Intervention Plans

Following an initial screening and subsequent assessment, collaborative goals are established (see Chapter 7 for further information) and should be recorded. Any needs or goals that cannot be addressed must also be recorded and reasons for this documented.

Without clear client-centred goals (see Chapter 7) it is not possible to evaluate the impact of occupational therapy intervention. Occupational therapists should record each individual's assessed needs and subsequent goals and intervention plan. It is crucial that goals be clearly documented and client centred, as well as clear and reviewable to provide a means for evaluating therapy. Goal setting is itself a complex task and has been described in detail elsewhere (see Chapter 7).

Reassessment/Alteration to Intervention Plans

In addition to documenting a clear intervention plan, all subsequent occupational therapy interventions and contacts must be documented. Because assessment and evaluation of interventions are ongoing, any changes to them should also be recorded.

Discharge Planning

When considering discharge or transfer from the service, practitioners should assess progress made toward agreed goals and record the level of support or assistance needed in any areas of functioning. They should also make recommendations for future support or interventions if appropriate and propose any follow-up or further assessment needed. The discharge process will vary according to local service requirements. Any plans for an individual's discharge, case closure, or transfer of care should be recorded within their intervention plans (RCOT, 2018). While practitioners usually write a short informative report when an individual is discharged, the depth and requirement for these reports will vary depending on local service policies and practice.

ENSURING STANDARDS OF RECORDKEEPING

Ensuring good standards of recordkeeping is an important aspect of service quality. Undertaking documentary audits enables organisations to evaluate and monitor the services they provide and allows the identification of potential areas of documentary risk, inefficiency, or ineffectiveness providing opportunities to take any necessary action to improve quality of services. The involvement of individuals who receive intervention in the audit process is now actively encouraged to gain their views as recipients of care. Participation in audit is now a clinical governance requirement, and several audit tools are available to assist services in this process.

LEGAL ISSUES IN DOCUMENTING AND REPORT WRITING

Practitioners should also consider their involvement in documentation that is not occupational therapy specific. These may include involvement in risk assessment and risk management, child protection reporting, and legal reports for court.

Risk Assessment and Child Protection

Occupational therapists are required to continually balance enabling individuals to achieve their desired goals with keeping them as safe as possible. While risk needs to be continually assessed, risk itself should not be allowed to become another barrier to enabling individuals to achieve their desired goals (RCOT, 2018). Within the context of balancing risk and goal achievement, practitioners must assess the possibility of any health and safety risks and clearly document the outcomes of any risk assessment and shared decision making that is carried out. Contingency plans should be developed for risks that cannot be eradicated, and any decisions made, based upon their assessment, should be documented. For example, practitioners should ensure that appropriate risk management policies and incident reporting procedures have been developed. Practitioners should always work to enable individuals to achieve their goals as safely as possible. We are, however, living in an increasingly litigious society where occupational therapists are concerned about the possibility of being sued if something goes wrong. Almost 20 years ago, Mandelstam (2005) described a reduction of practitioner decision-making confidence due to worries of legal action. There is no reason to suggest that this reduction in confidence has reduced. This can lead to inaccurate perceptions of risk and overly defensive individual and organisational practices.

It is important for occupational therapists working with children and young people to be aware of their possible involvement in scenarios involving child protection issues. Each nation has a framework of legislation, guidance, and practice to identify children who are at risk of harm, take action to protect those children, and prevent further abuse from occurring. As with all other areas of practice, issues concerning child protection should be carefully documented.

Court Reports

It is important to remember that professional practice notes provide a record of interventions carried out with individuals and may, on rare occasions, be used as evidence in court proceedings. In court, the approach to documentation is, "If it is not recorded, it has not been done" (Lynch, 2009, p. 45). This underlines the importance of timely and accurate documentation.

Sometimes occupational therapists are called upon by court as expert witnesses. As expert witnesses of fact, practitioners may be asked to produce a statement or a report. Statements include personal details and professional background, and should provide a coherent, chronological record of events. Technical jargon should be fully explained. Reports should be logical, factual, and truthful. Records and notes may be required. The content of the report will differ depending on the specific case. The guidelines produced by the College of Occupational Therapists (2013) provide a useful example of how to structure a court report.

SUMMARY

This chapter has provided an overview of the key aspects of recording and report writing. Although guidelines produced by professional bodies are available, variations in national and local procedures exist and should be referenced. This chapter provides essential information and guidance to effectively and accurately record clinical information and create reports. It should be treated as an initial introduction to the topic, equipping readers to develop further skills and continue their reading, reflection, and action regarding recording and report writing.

REFLECTIVE LEARNING

- Consider the following:
  - How careful am I in my accuracy and timeliness of recordkeeping?
  - Do I describe my clinical reasoning and decision making in my clinical documentation? How could I improve this?
  - How could I improve my recordkeeping practice?
- Undertake an audit of your recent case records. If you work in a team, you could share records within your team and randomly select a sample of each other's recent case records. Then, using a structured audit tool (such as provided by RCOT [2018]), audit the adherence of your records to the standard provided. Use the findings of this exercise as a reflective exercise and discuss how your report writing could be further improved.

REFERENCES

American Occupational Therapy Association. (2003). Guidelines for documentation of occupational therapy. In K. M. Sames (Ed.), *Documenting occupational therapy practice*. Pearson Prentice Hall.

Bjerke, M. B., & Renger, R. (2017). Being smart about writing SMART objectives. Evaluation and program planning, 61, 125–127.

Blijlevens, H., & Murphy, J. (2003). Washing away SOAP notes: Refreshing clinical documentation. New Zealand Journal of Occupational Therapy, 50(2), 3–8.

College of Occupational Therapists. (2004). *COT/BAOT briefing: 28 service user involvement*. Author.

College of Occupational Therapists. (2013). *Acting as an expert witness: A guide for occupational therapists*. Author.

College of Occupational Therapists (2014) Managing information: A 10-year strategic vision for occupational therapy informatics. London: COT.

Cornbleet, M. A., Campbell, P., Murray, S., Stevenson, M., & Bond, S. (2002). Patient-held records in cancer and palliative care: a randomized, prospective trial. Palliative medicine, 16(3), 205–212.

Davis, J., Zayat, E., Urton, M., Belgum, A., & Hill, M. (2008). Communicating evidence in clinical documentation. *Australian Occupational Therapy Journal*, 55(4), 249–255.

Department of Health. (2005). *Mental Capacity Act*. HMSO.

Department of Health. (2006a). *The Caldicott guardian manual*. Department of Health, UK Council of Caldicott Guardians.

Department of Health. (2006b). The records management: NHS code of practice. www.dh.gov.uk/en/Managingyourorganisation/Informationpolicy/Recordsmanagement/index.htm.

Department of Health. (2016). *Mental Capacity Act (NI)*. HMSO.

Diffin, J., Byrne, B., & O'Halloran, P. (2018). The use of patient-held records by children and young people managing a health condition: A realist review of the literature. *BMJ Supportive & Palliative Care*, 8, 378.

Gateley, C. A., & Borcherding, S. (2012). Documentation manual for occupational therapy: Writing SOAP notes. Thorofare, NJ: Slack.

Great Britain Parliament. (2018). *Data Protection Act 2018*. London Stationary Office. www.legislation.gov.uk/ukpga/2018/contents/enacted.

Griffith, R. (2016). What is Gillick competence? *Human Vaccines & Immunotherapeutics, 12*(1), 244–247.

Harman, K., Bassett, R., Fenety, A., & Hoens, A. (2009). "I think it, but don't often write it": The barriers to charting in private practice. *Physiotherapy Canada, 61*(4), 252–258.

Health and Care Professions Council. (2013). *Standards of proficiency.* Occupational Therapists Health Professions Council.

Health and Care Professions Council. (2018). *Standards of conduct, performance and ethics. Your duties as a registrant.* Author.

Henderson, C., & Laugharne, R. (2000). Patient held clinical information for people with psychotic illnesses. The Cochrane Database of Systematic Reviews, (2), CD001711–CD001711.

Kyle, T., & Wright, S. (1996). Reflecting the model of human occupation in occupational therapy documentation. *Canadian Journal of Occupational Therapy, 63*(3), 192–196.

Lynch, J. (2009). *Health records in court.* Radcliffe Publishing.

Mandelstam, M. (2005). *Occupational therapy: Law and good practice.* College of Occupational Therapists.

Mathioudakis, A., Rousalova, I., Gagnat, A. A., Saad, N., & Hardavella, G. (2016). How to keep good clinical records. Breathe, 12(4), 369–373.

National Health Service. (2019). The NHS long term plan. https://www.longtermplan.nhs.uk/.

National Health Service Information Authority. (1999). *Briefing paper: Problem orientated medical record (POMR) and SOAP.* Author.

Neidstadt, M. (1996). Teaching strategies for the development of clinical reasoning. *American. Journal of Occupational Therapy, 50*(8), 676–684.

Newell, S. (2001). Clinical risk assessment for an occupational therapy inpatient group programme. *British Journal of Occupational Therapy, 64*(4), 200–202.

Occupational Therapy Australia. (2014). *Code of ethics.* Author.

Royal College of Occupational Therapists. (2015). *Ethics and conduct.* Author.

Royal College of Occupational Therapists. (2018). In *Keeping records: Guidance for occupational therapists* (4th ed.). Author.

Royal College of Occupational Therapists. (2021). *Professional standards for occupational therapy practice, conduct and ethics.* Author.

Scottish Executive. (2006). *Hidden harm. Next steps. Supporting children—working with parents.* Author.

Scottish Government. (2016). Adults with Incapacity (Scotland) Act 2000.

Tickle-Degnen, L. (2000). Monitoring and documenting evidence during assessment and intervention. *American Journal of Occupational Therapy, 54*(4), 434–436.

Warner, J. P., King, M., Blizard, R., McClenahan, Z., & Tang, S. (2000). Patient-held shared care records for individuals with mental illness: randomised controlled evaluation. The British Journal of Psychiatry, 177(4), 319–324.

Evidence-Based and Research Skills for Practice

12

Finding and Appraising the Evidence

Edward A.S. Duncan and M. Clare Taylor

HIGHLIGHTS

- The chapter provides an overview if the development of evidence-based occupational therapy.
- The nature of evidence within evidence-based occupational therapy is discussed.

- Guidance is provided on how to effectively search for evidence.
- An introduction is given on how to appraise the evidence you find and use it in everyday practice.

OVERVIEW

The aim of this chapter is to explore ways of both locating and evaluating the evidence that underpins practice. Developing the skills of evidence-based, or evidence-informed, occupational therapy is vital in today's political climate. Without a sound appreciation of the evidence, or lack of evidence, to support occupational therapy interventions and actions, practitioners will be unable to justify the rationale for these interventions and actions.

The chapter will begin by reminding the reader of the background and context of the use of evidence in practice, and how evidence-based practice has evolved into evidence-informed practice. The main focus of the chapter will be on exploring both the nature and sources of evidence with practical examples of searches. Having located some evidence, the next step is to appraise the rigour and value of that evidence; this process will then be discussed. Finding and appraising evidence is often difficult for the busy practitioner, however, so the chapter will therefore discuss ways of including appraisal into everyday practice.

A BRIEF HISTORICAL CONTEXT ON THE USE OF EVIDENCE IN OCCUPATIONAL THERAPY

The understanding and use of evidence, both within occupational therapy and within health and social care more generally, has a long history (Boaz & Davies, 2019). The need to find and appraise evidence is central to modern-day occupational therapy practice. The terms *evidence-based practice* and *evidence-informed practice* are probably very familiar to most readers. However, it is worth spending a little time reviewing these definitions, to provide a context for the remainder of the chapter.

Prior to the 1980s evidence was not as central to occupational therapy practice. Indeed, research to generate evidence was largely absent. This is equally true for many of the allied health professions. Evidence-based practice within allied health and occupational therapy, in particular, has its roots in the evidence-based medicine movement, which began at McMaster University in Canada in the 1980s (Taylor, 2007), linked to the use of a problem-based approach to the teaching of medicine. By the mid-1990s evidence-based medicine had been defined as "the conscientious, explicit and judicious use of current best evidence in making decisions about the care of individual patients" (Sackett et al., 1996, p. 71).

By the late 1990s evidence-based practice had begun to seep into the consciousness of the occupational therapy profession, especially in the United Kingdom and Canada, with special issues of both the *British Journal of Occupational Therapy* (College of Occupational Therapists, 1997) and the *Canadian Journal of Occupational Therapy* (Canadian Association of Occupational Therapists, 1998) as well as books (e.g., Law, 2002; Taylor, 2007) and articles (e.g., Brown & Rodgers, 1999; Bennett & Bennett, 2000) on the implementation of evidence-based practice in occupational therapy. It is also worth noting that the 1997 Casson Memorial Lecture in the United Kingdom (Eakin, 1997), the 2000 Eleanor Clarke Slagle Lecture in the United States (Holm, 2000), and the 2001 Sylvia Docker Lecture in Australia (Cusick, 2001) all explored evidence-based practice and evidence-based occupational therapy and encouraged practitioners to find and use evidence to support their everyday practice.

This interest in evidence-based occupational therapy also led to the development of a number of definitions of evidence-based occupational therapy, one of the best known of which defines it as: "Client-centred enablement of occupation, based on client information and a critical review of relevant research, expert consensus and past experience" (Canadian Association of Occupational Therapists et al., 1999, p. 267).

However, the essence of evidence-based occupational therapy is probably best expressed by Cusick (2001): "When we practice with evidence, it means we should ask ourselves the following question: 'am I doing the right thing in the right way with the right person at the right time in the right place for the right result—and am I the right person to be doing it?'" (p. 267).

In more recent years, an argument has formed that practitioner's practice should be evidence informed rather than evidence based. Glasziou (2005) noted that patients' values and preferences are often missed within narrow interpretations of evidence-based practice. Such narrow definitions also give little space for clinical experience. While many people advocate that evidence-based practice always accounted for the perspective of both the individual client and the professional, this nuanced difference in description is important and has become broadly accepted. Within the United Kingdom, as members of the Health Care Professions Council (HCPC), occupational therapists are professionally bound to practice in an evidence-informed manner (HCPC, 2018).

Regardless of whether it is described as evidence based or evidence informed, the challenge for the evidence-based occupational therapist is to find and appraise the relevant evidence. However, the challenge does not end once the evidence has been located. The evidence may indicate that a particular intervention has been shown to be effective. The evidence may also show that there is little or no evidence to support the effectiveness of a chosen intervention, and evidence-informed occupational therapy then needs the courage to change practices that may be long established, to ensure that occupational therapy is seen as an effective and relevant profession. Thus evidence-informed occupational therapy is a way of thinking critically about every intervention and action and, as such, is just one of the tools of clinical reasoning and reflective practice. However, because of the use of up-to-date best evidence, evidence-informed practice is a powerful tool.

Why Is Appraisal of Evidence Important?

While the principles of evidence-informed occupational therapy and a questioning approach to the value of our interventions and activities as practitioners might appear to be a valuable philosophy, and very useful in the abstract, we must also remind ourselves of the reasons that evidence-informed occupational therapy is vitally important for all practitioners.

Evidence-informed practice has been established into health and social care policy for some time, example, professional practice at both statutory (HCPC, 2018) and professional levels (College of Occupational Therapists, 2003, 2005). However, for many practitioners there has been a resistance to this drive for evidence-informed occupational therapy. Dubouloz et al. (1999) found that occupational therapists were slow to integrate research evidence into their clinical decision making. However, this has changed in recent years with evidence-based practice being viewed as useful and important by occupational therapists internationally (Bennett et al., 2003; Garcia et al., 2020; Lindström & Bernhardsson, 2018).

THE STAGES OF EVIDENCE-INFORMED OCCUPATIONAL THERAPY

While evidence-informed occupational therapy can be described as a way of thinking about practice, it is also a problem-solving process that mirrors both the research process and the occupational therapy process. Sackett and Rosenberg (1995) originally articulated the five stages of evidence-based practice:

1. To convert our information needs into answerable questions
2. To track down, with maximum efficiency, the best evidence with which to answer these questions
3. To appraise the evidence critically (i.e., to weigh it up) to assess its validity (closeness to the truth) and usefulness (clinical applicability)
4. To implement the results of this appraisal in our clinical practice
5. To evaluate our performance

While other chapters focus on stages 4 and 5 (see Chapters 14 and 5, respectively), this chapter focuses on the first three stages of this process:

- Asking a question
- Finding the evidence
- Appraising the evidence

However, the process of evidence-informed occupational therapy should not be viewed as a one-off activity; it should run parallel to the process of clinical reasoning and can be applied at each stage of the occupational therapy process to ensure that every action from initial assessment to final evaluation is effective and based on sound reasoning and evidence. Bennett and Bennett (2000) developed a framework that shows how evidence-informed practice can be used at every stage of the occupational therapy process. Rappolt (2003) developed a model of what they called an evidence-based person-centred process (but would now also be described as evidence informed), which integrates three strands of evidence (from the client, from research, and from professional expertise) into the occupational therapy process.

Asking Good Questions

The first stage of the evidence-informed occupational therapy process is to identify and articulate a question that will guide the search for evidence to be appraised. Because of the original medical focus of evidence-based practice, questions are often thought of as clinical questions relating to diagnosis, prognosis, or treatment (Rosenberg & Donald, 1995) and are phrased in terms of the following:

What is the evidence for the effectiveness of x (the intervention) for y (the outcome) in a patient with z (the problem or diagnosis)?

This might fit very nicely into medical practice when thinking about whether treatment with aspirin and warfarin will reduce the risk of stroke in an elderly lady with hypertension, but how can it relate to the complexities of occupational therapy practice?

Herbert et al. (2005) expanded the application of the clinical question to include the following:
- Effects of intervention
- Patients' experiences
- Course of the condition, or the life course of a particular patient group (prognosis)
- Accuracy of diagnostic tests or assessments

While broadening the idea of the clinical question beyond assessing the potential effectiveness of an intervention, this approach still does not address the totality of occupational therapy practice. However, if we adopt Cusick's (2001) approach of asking the right questions, we can use an evidence-informed approach to all stages of the occupational therapy process; for example:
- Am I the right person? Does this person need to be seen by someone with occupational therapy skills?
- What are the right skills needed to work with this person?
- Am I doing the right thing? Not only is this the right intervention, but also is this the right assessment tool?
- Am I doing it in the right way and for the right reasons? What is the most effective model or frame of reference?
- Do I have all of the relevant information that I need to plan this intervention properly?
- Am I doing it with the right clients? Do all patients/clients with this problem need to be seen by an

occupational therapist, or just those with other particular problems?
- Am I doing it at the right time? Should I see this client in the morning or the afternoon?
- Should I see them everyday or just once a month?
- Is it being done in the right place? Would I be better working with this patient/client in his or herr own home rather than in hospital?

The Anatomy of a Well-Built Question

The task for the evidence-informed occupational therapist is to devise a question. This question will arise from practice, possibly by asking oneself one of the "right" questions outlined earlier or by articulating or reflecting on a particular incident or client to develop a scenario to help you to develop the final evidence-informed question.

Having identified and articulated a scenario, it is then possible to refine this information further to create and structure a specific evidence-based question. The clearer the structure of the question, the more focused and, hopefully, successful the search for evidence.

As noted, an evidence-based question usually consists of a number of elements:
- Problem
- Intervention
- Outcome

Richardson et al. (1995) refer to these elements as the anatomy of a well-built question and add a further element: a comparative intervention. The inclusion of a comparative intervention is common practice in the context of evidence-based practice where the effectiveness of drug *x* may be compared with that of drug *y*. The inclusion of a comparative intervention may be perceived as having less relevance to many for occupational therapy, although it may be of value in the context of some questions, and the comparator could also be usual practice.

This approach is commonly referred to as PICO (*p*roblem, *i*ntervention, *c*omparative intervention, *o*utcome). Table 12.1 illustrates the elements can easily be applied to occupational therapy especially if the elements are renamed:
- Person; rather than problem
- Action; rather than intervention
- Comparative action; rather than comparative intervention
- Application

This structure can then be applied to any scenario, as Box 12.1 illustrates.

Searching for the Evidence

Having articulated the evidence-based question, the next task is to search for and locate the evidence to address this question. However, before we can embark on the search it

TABLE 12.1   Elements of a Well-Built Question

Person
Describe your client/patient/client group and her/his/their problem. This may be a diagnosis, a functional problem, or an occupational performance problem. The description should also include all key information (e.g., age, sex, occupational status).

Action
Describe the main action or activity of interest. This may be an intervention or assessment undertaken by the occupational therapist, but it could also be a task/activity/strategy used by the client.

Comparative Action (If Applicable)
Describe the comparative or alternative action/intervention/assessment/task. This may also take the form of alternative approaches to the intervention (e.g., group or individual sessions, different frequency of intervention).

Application
Describe what you hope to achieve, what effect the action may have on your client/patient/client group, or how you hope to apply the action.

is necessary to understand what constitutes evidence in occupational therapy.

What Do We Mean by Evidence?

Sackett & Wennberg (1997) definition of evidence-based practice talks about the need to use best evidence to support the decision-making process. However, the nature of best evidence is perhaps the most contentious and debated area within the concept of evidence-based practice (Sackett & Wennberg, 1997; Taylor, 2007). The traditional view, drawn from evidence-based medicine, has been to adopt a hierarchy, or levels, of research evidence. Table 12.2 outlines the hierarchy of evidence for evidence-based medicine.

The question for the evidence-based occupational therapist is, Which of this long list might be the best evidence to use to address a particular evidence-based question? As Sackett (1998), Sackett and Wennberg (1997), and Taylor (2007) argue, the nature of the best evidence depends on the type of evidence-based question being asked. Table 12.3 gives an overview of the types of research evidence that might be appropriate for the different types of evidence-based question.

Having established a list of the potential types of research evidence to address a particular question, the evidence-informed occupational therapist's next task is to decide whether there is a particular order or hierarchy of the types of evidence, to ensure that the best evidence is found.

BOX 12.1   Identifying a Scenario

Scenario 1
The stroke unit where you are working is keen to use "constraint induced therapy" as an intervention. You are unsure of the potential value of this approach, especially in relation to other more established intervention approaches, and decide to explore the literature to find out what evidence exists to demonstrate the effectiveness of constraint induced therapy.

Scenario 2
You have been asked to cofacilitate a fatigue management group for people living with multiple sclerosis (MS). The central philosophy of the group is self-help and impairment and to use strategies that are informed by experience as well as research evidence. You identify some relevant anecdotal knowledge but want to adopt a more evidence-based approach. You decide to collect evidence from a range of sources to inform your planning of the fatigue management group. You also hope that the evidence will give you ideas about assessing the outcomes and the success of the group.

TABLE 12.2   Types of Research Evidence

- Systematic reviews of randomised controlled trials
- Controlled clinical trials
- Nonrandomised experimental studies
- Single case design studies
- Cohort studies
- Cross-sectional studies
- Longitudinal studies
- Correlational studies
- Qualitative research studies
- Systematic reviews of qualitative research
- Surveys
- Delphi studies
- Consensus studies

TABLE 12.3 Levels of Evidence Within Evidence-Based Medicine
• Randomised controlled trials
• Nonrandomised experimental studies
• Nonexperimental studies
• Descriptive studies
• Respected opinion
• Expert discussion

TABLE 12.4 Appropriate Research Evidence for Particular Types of Questions
Effectiveness of interventions
Systematic reviews of randomised controlled trials (RCTs)
RCTs
Other experimental designs (e.g., controlled clinical trials)
Single-subject design studies
Client's experiences and perceptions
Qualitative research studies
Systematic reviews of qualitative research
Descriptive research studies (e.g., surveys)
Appropriateness of assessments
Cross-sectional studies
Measurement studies
Prognosis and life course of a particular condition or group of people
Cohort studies
Longitudinal studies
Qualitative research studies
Correlational studies

Developing a hierarchy of the most appropriate evidence for the effectiveness of interventions is relatively straightforward. The hierarchy, outlined in Table 12.3, was developed to show the value and weighting of evidence for the effectiveness of interventions, with systematic reviews of randomised controlled trials (RCTs) seen as the most rigorous and reliable form of evidence. Similar hierarchies have been developed for the following:

- Therapy/prevention/aetiology/harm questions
- Prognosis questions
- Diagnosis questions
- Differential diagnosis/symptoms questions
- Economic questions (Phillips et al., 2009)

The appropriateness of a similar hierarchy for qualitative research is much more questionable, with many authors (e.g., Barbour, 2001; Pawson et al., 2003) arguing that, while it is possible to critically appraise the rigour and strength of a particular qualitative study, it is neither possible nor appropriate to locate different types of qualitative studies within a hierarchy.

The identification of the best evidence is a complex task. Using specific types of research evidence to address particular evidence-informed questions may seem the most useful approach (Table 12.4). However, it may also act as a constraint to the development of a broad perspective on the best evidence with which to answer evidence-informed questions. Certainly an RCT or a systematic review should provide powerful evidence for the effectiveness of a particular intervention; it may not, however, be the only evidence required for clinical reasoning and decision making. Pawson et al. (2003) argue, from a social care perspective, that evidence should include:

- Organisational knowledge
- Practitioner knowledge
- Service-user knowledge
- Research knowledge
- Policy knowledge

Evidence from research may only give a partial answer to any evidence-informed question. The research evidence must be balanced with information from clients about their values and perspectives, as well as the therapist's experiential knowledge. The intervention or action decision will also be influenced by contextual factors such as service priorities and resources, as well as local and national policies. Evidence can therefore be understood in terms of pieces of a complex jigsaw, which together provide the best evidence to answer any evidence-informed question.

Structuring a Search

Having clarified the elements of the evidence-informed question, the next stage in the process is to use these elements to provide a clear structure for the task of searching for some evidence, which will then be appraised for its value in the context of the evidence-informed question.

Once the evidence-informed question has been articulated, there is often a temptation to go straight to the Internet to find some evidence. However, if you start searching without sufficient thinking and planning, your search will probably be very frustrating and ultimately unsuccessful. It is much more useful to spend some time thinking about the structure of your search so that any time spent at the computer or in the library is usefully spent and might also result in the successful location of some relevant and valuable evidence.

Developing a search strategy consists of a number of stages:

- Articulating a clear question, which can then be used to identify key words and search terms

- Identifying the most relevant information sources, which might include specific databases (see later for further discussion of databases) or library collections
- Identifying the types of evidence that are most appropriate for the question

Identifying the key words and search terms is an important task if the search is to be successful. It is always useful to look at the search terms and key words that you have identified and then to think of synonyms or alternative terms, as well as different spellings (many terms have different spellings depending on whether the usage is English or American).

Most databases do not readily understand natural language, the colloquial language that we use every day. However, the majority of databases have a thesaurus of accepted terms and key words. Databases use what are known as Boolean operators to help the searcher refine the search question. Operators can be used to focus the search. The most common Boolean operators are:

- AND: used to combine two search terms to find articles that contain both terms
- OR: allows you to use alternative terms to broaden a search
- NOT: used to exclude articles with particular unwanted terms, to narrow a search

It is also sensible to set limits to any search to avoid being swamped by information that is inappropriate, irrelevant, or inaccessible. Common limits are the language the article is written in, the age of the article, and the type of article.

Table 12.5 provides a summary of the pointers to assist in structuring a search and Box 12.2 illustrates how the questions identified in the previous scenarios can be developed into search strategies.

Where to Look

Rather than wandering vaguely around the library randomly selecting interesting-looking books and journals, the evidence-informed occupational therapist should focus on the most appropriate resources in the search for relevant evidence. Bibliographic indexes and databases have been developed to help the practitioner locate the most suitable information. However, many databases are only available by subscription, so it is worth checking with your library to see which databases you might be able to access. The databases most relevant to occupational therapy are identified in Table 12.6.

Databases have different areas of focus. MEDLINE, PubMed (the free access version of MEDLINE), and EMBASE have a very medical focus, whilst CINAHL and AMED focus more on allied health. ASSIA, PsychLit, and SocioFile draw heavily on social science literature; ERIC has an educational focus. A number of specific databases now exist. These databases, unlike general databases, employ quality checks and so will only include citations for work that meets their standards for good evidence. There

---

TABLE 12.5   Structuring the Search

Improving the Search Terms

- Use synonyms and both English and American terminology (e.g., learning difficulty/learning disability/mental retardation).
- Use English and American spellings (e.g., paediatrics/pediatrics).
- Be sure to spell words correctly.
- Use quotation marks for collections of words that collectively have a specific meaning (e.g., "occupational therapy").
- Use an asterisk (*) or $ (the truncation symbol) to find all terms beginning with a subject (e.g., alcohol* will retrieve articles related to alcohol, alcoholic, alcoholics, and alcoholism).
- Use Boolean operators (AND, OR, NOT) to expand or limit the search (e.g., "occupational therapy OR physiotherapy" will retrieve all articles related to occupational therapy and physiotherapy individually, whereas "occupational therapy AND physiotherapy" will retrieve only those articles that relate to combinations of occupational therapy and physiotherapy; "occupational therapy NOT physiotherapy" will exclude articles that include reference to physiotherapy.

Setting Limits

- Limiting your search to English language–only references means that you avoid identifying a potentially useful reference only to find that you need a translator as the original paper is in German or Japanese.
- Limiting your search to papers published in the last 5 years will mean that you only access "current" evidence, not something that was published in 1960, which may have since been refuted, although sometimes historical evidence might be of value.
- Limiting your search to include only research papers, which means that any opinion pieces or other nonresearch evidence will be excluded.

BOX 12.2 Developing an Evidence-Informed Question

Scenario 1

Person: people experiencing hemiparesis, especially upper limb involvement, following a stroke

Action: constraint induced therapy

Comparative action: all other current approaches to stroke intervention

Application: improved upper limb (UL) function, independence in activities of daily living (ADL), increased meaningful occupational behaviours

Evidence-Informed Question

What is the evidence for the effectiveness of constraint induced therapy, in comparison to existing approaches to stroke rehabilitation, in improving UL function/independence in ADL or increasing meaningful occupational behaviours in clients who experience hemiparesis following stroke?

Scenario 2

Person: people experiencing fatigue as a consequence of MS

Action: living with fatigue; fatigue management

Comparative action: not relevant for this question

Application: guidelines for facilitating a fatigue management group

Evidence-Based Question

What information can be derived from a range of evidence into the experience of living with MS-related fatigue, to facilitate a fatigue management group?

TABLE 12.6 Examples of Databases Relevant to Occupational Therapy

- ASSIA
- BIDS
- CINAHL
- EMBASE
- ERIC
- MEDLINE
- PubMed
- PsychLit
- SocioFile
- Cochrane Library
- DARE
- Campbell Collaboration
- OTDBase
- Google/Google Scholar

are also a number of occupational therapy-specific databases that may be of value. OTSeeker (www.otseeker.com; Bennett et al., 2003; McCluskey et.al 2006; McKenna, 2004, 2005) is a particularly valuable resource as it also incorporates an evidence-based approach and does not require a subscription. Web-based search engines (e.g., Google, Google Scholar) are also databases, although they are less rigorous in what they include than more specific databases; this can have advantages as grey literature is more readily discoverable on Google Scholar.

Appraising the Evidence

Once suitable research evidence has been identified and located, the job is not finished. Research evidence should not be accepted at face value. While many journals use a rigorous process of peer review and critical evaluation prior to the publication of any article, it does not mean that a published piece of research is flawless or that it can be applied to any practice situation. Box 12.3 outlines two examples of situations in which you may require to search and appraise the evidence.

Having located relevant research evidence, the next stage is to critically appraise the evidence. Critical appraisal can be defined as "the ability to read original and summarised research, to make judgements on its scientific value and to consider how its results can be applied in practice" (Taylor 2003, p. 102).

Critical appraisal provides a structured framework to assess the value and trustworthiness of a piece of research within the context of practice. The structure of the critical appraisal process allows the evidence-informed occupational therapist to review not only the findings of the research but the whole research process, too. Critical appraisal should give the reader the opportunity to identify both the strengths and the weaknesses of a particular research paper. The weaknesses of the research should be weighed and evaluated carefully but should be viewed in the context of whether the facts make you question the conclusions of the researchers. Critical appraisal should be positive rather than negative and viewed with an open mind and the ability to challenge your own, as well as the researcher's, ideas and assumptions.

Adopting a critical appraisal approach to reading the research evidence will encourage the reader not to ignore, or skip over, the complicated sections of a research paper, such as the results section. Skipping over parts of an article may lead to misinterpretation of findings or erroneously accepting (or rejecting) the author's conclusions. Critical appraisal is often more interesting if it is not a solitary activity, so that the findings and ideas can be discussed and ideas and comments can be challenged and reviewed. Journal clubs are useful as a way of sharing critical appraisals of

---

BOX 12.3   Developing Search Strategies

Scenario 1

Evidence-Based Question

What is the evidence for the effectiveness of constraint induced therapy, in comparison to existing approaches to stroke rehabilitation, in improving UL function/independence in ADL or increasing meaningful occupational behaviours in clients who experience hemiparesis following stroke?

Types of Evidence

The question focuses on the effectiveness of an intervention, so the search needs to look for systematic reviews and randomised controlled trials (RCTs)

Keywords

"Constraint induced therapy" OR "constraint induced movement therapy" AND stroke

Limits

English language only

Scenario 2

Evidence-Based Question

What information can be derived from a range of evidence into the experience of living with MS-related fatigue, to facilitate a fatigue management group?

Types of Evidence

The question focuses on people's experiences of dealing with illness as well as the effectiveness of an intervention, therefore a range of evidence, including both qualitative research studies and RCTs/systematic reviews, will be sought.

Keywords

"Multiple sclerosis AND fatigue OR fatigue management"

Limits

English language only

---

research literature, though they do not necessarily increase evidence-informed practice (Wenke et al., 2018).

The Key Questions

Critical appraisal is a process of asking a series of structured questions about the rigour and applicability of the research. Any critical appraisal, irrespective of the type of research being appraised, is structured around three essential questions:

- How rigorous/valid/trustworthy is the research?
- What are the findings?
- Can the findings be applied to my particular context and question?

These questions can be broken down further to explore the research in depth. The first group of questions addresses the rigour of the research and helps the reader to appraise how good the research is. The second group of questions helps the reader to focus on the research findings and to assess the significance, both statistical and clinical, or strength of the findings. The final group of questions gives the reader the opportunity to explore whether the research and its findings can be used in the context of practice (i.e., does the research give any evidence to support or challenge current practice?).

Appraising Different Types of Evidence

While the three questions outlined earlier give an overall structure to any critical appraisal, they have to be adapted to suit different types of research methodology. Critical appraisal methods have developed considerably over recent years. Some standardised measures have become internationally recognised best practice. The GRADE approach to appraising controlled studies, systematic reviews, and guidelines is now internationally recognised as best practice (Goldet & Howick, 2013). A similar appraisal approach, the GRADE-CERQual, has been developed for appraising findings from qualitative evidence synthesis, including guidelines (Lewin et al., 2018). Critical appraisal is usually best facilitated through an appraisal checklist, which will outline the key questions for a particular research type. The Critical Appraisal Skills Programme is an international organisation that provides an up-to-date set of well-developed critical appraisal checklists (www.casp-uk.net).

Including Appraisal in Everyday Practice

Evidence-informed occupational therapy is not about doing research; it is about using research evidence to underpin interventions and actions within everyday practice. The challenge is to find space in the busy workweek to search for and appraise the relevant research evidence. The chapter will now explore a number of ways that appraisal of evidence can be incorporated into everyday practice.

Journal Clubs

Journal clubs have been a regular feature of medical education and practice for many years (Linzer, 1987). They usually consist of people presenting an overview of a paper they had read and then attempting to stimulate discussion. However, with the advent of evidence-based medicine, the format of journal clubs began to change (Sackett et al., 1997), and evidence-based journal clubs began to be established (Phillips & Glasziou, 2004). Evidence-based journal clubs also developed not only among medical practitioners but also for groups of occupational therapists, nurses, and other allied health professionals (Bannigan & Hooper, 2002; McQueen et al., 2006; Sherratt, 2005).

Evidence-informed journal clubs provide an opportunity for a group of like-minded colleagues to meet to discuss and appraise the relevant research evidence linked to a clear evidence-based question, probably using an appraisal checklist as a way of structuring and recording their discussions.

Journal clubs are a useful way of both promoting and recording evidence of continuing professional development. They enable participants to maintain and enhance their critical appraisal skills and their knowledge of the research base for practice. They also provide an opportunity to review and reflect on current practice. The outcome of a journal club discussion might be to implement changes to current interventions or actions, or to enhance confidence in the value of those interventions and actions. The journal club can provide a valuable opportunity for groups of colleagues to explore issues, share ideas, consider different perspectives, and participate in shaping and developing departmental policy and practice. Specific guidelines for establishing a journal club are beyond the scope of this chapter but can be found in a number of publications (e.g., Phillips & Glaszious, 2004; Sherratt, 2005; Taylor, 2007). Over time, approaches to journal clubs have evolved, and digital engagement has revolutionised how journal clubs can be delivered (McGlacken-Byrne et al., 2020).

As the focus of this chapter is on evidence-informed occupational therapy, it is appropriate to outline the evidence for the value of journal clubs in changing practice. A systematic review that investigated just this question (Harris et al., 2011) concluded that the evidence to support journal clubs as a means to change practice is unclear. In a more recent evaluation of journal club approaches, several participants responded that they updated a guideline or adopted a new therapy. Interestingly, fewer respondents stated they stopped an existing therapy, though this may be due to the studies that were reviewed (Wenke et al., 2018). Journal clubs would appear, at face value, to be useful activities both for developing an evidence-informed awareness and culture within a department and for helping ensure that practice is evidence informed.

Evidence-Based Reflection and Use of Single-Subject Research Designs

In the discussion on the nature of evidence earlier in the chapter it was noted that experience is often reported as the main source of evidence used by practitioners when making decisions about interventions and actions as part of the clinical reasoning process. All practitioners use clinical experience to guide their reasoning process. Without recourse to evidence, however, there is a danger that their practice heuristics (mental shortcuts) may lead to biases in their perceptions and decision making.

With care and balance, reflection on action may provide useful tools to help the evidence-based occupational therapist articulate the experiential evidence used in practice (see Chapter 4). The process of reflection involves describing an event and then looking at the decision-making and reasoning process, which underpin the actions taken within that event. The event concerned can be any interaction with a client. To use these reflections to develop an evidence-based case study the following topics should be addressed:

- Description of a case study or incident
- Reflection on action and articulate experiential evidence
- Explore and appraise the research evidence
- Synthesis and dissemination

It is not always possible to find evidence for the area of practice you are interested in (though see Chapter 15 for further information on how you can develop your research skills in practice). What can you do when that happens? Undertaking a large-scale research study may feel outside the scope of what you can achieve. However, with careful consideration and thought, it is possible to appraise the evidence of your practice interventions by careful collection and analysis of data from the individuals you work with. Doing this requires learning about the single-subject research design. Single-subject research designs are an underexplored aspect of occupational therapy practice appraisal and evidence development. There is growing recognition of the value that single-subject research design studies can have in health care. These include testing new interventions for which there is little or no evidence, determining intervention effects, and comparing different combinations of interventions (McDonald & Nikles, 2021). Single-subject research design studies are not case studies but carefully considered experimental designs (Krasny-Pacini & Evans, 2018). Single-subject research designs (also known as n = 1 studies) allows therapists to evaluate the impact of an intervention on a single client. Despite having a long history and being proposed in occupational therapy literature as far back as the 1980s (Campbell, 1988), their use in occupational therapy has never really been maximised. Used in isolation they have relatively little strength. However, single case series design can be used where the outcomes of multiple cases are combined. While not as rigorous as controlled studies, single case series designs provide a feasible means (with appropriate ethical and governance approvals) for clinicians to undertake rigorous research on the effectiveness of interventions that do not yet have sufficient evidence. Their outcomes could be used both to support practice and provide the rationale for further robust evaluation using larger, more complex effectiveness methodologies.

SUMMARY

This chapter focused on how to use evidence to inform occupational therapy practice. It began by outlining the nature of evidence-informed evidence and discussed ways of searching for evidence. An introduction to critically appraising a research paper was given before concluding by presenting a number of ways of incorporating critical appraisal into everyday practice. Finally, an introduction into the potential of using single-subject research designs to find evidence for your practice was provided. Single-subject research designs provide a feasible method of generating and appraising evidence from practice, where published studies in your area of interest are lacking.

REFLECTIVE LEARNING

- What do I know about the evidence base for my current/preferred practice area? How up to date is it?
- What are the burning practice questions in my area that I need evidence for?
- How familiar am I with critical appraisal tools? Choose a recent quality occupational therapy peer-reviewed academic paper that interests you. Choose the appropriate critical appraisal tool from www.casp-uk.net and appraise the paper. Ideally share your findings with a colleague, or another student, or in a blog.
- How can I join a journal club—either in person or online?
- How could I use single-subject research design in my practice if evidence for my work is lacking?

REFERENCES

Bannigan, K., & Hooper, L. (2002). How journal clubs can overcome barriers to research utilisation. *British Journal of Therapy & Rehabilitation, 9*(8), 299–303.

Barbour, R. S. (2001). Checklists for improving rigour in qualitative research: A case of the tail wagging the dog? *British Medical Journal, 322*(7294), 1115–1117.

Bennett, S., & Bennett, J. W. (2000). The process of evidence-based practice in occupational therapy: Informing clinical decisions. *Australian Occupational Therapy Journal, 47,* 171–180.

Bennett, S., Hoffmann, T., McCluskey, A., McKenna, K., Strong, J., & Tooth, L. (2003). Evidence-based practice forum-Introducing OTseeker-(Occupational therapy systematic evaluation of evidence): a new evidence database for occupational therapists. *American Journal of Occupational Therapy, 57*(6), 635–638.

Boaz, A., & Davies, H. (Eds.). (2019). *What works now?: Evidence-informed policy and practice.* Policy Press.

Brown, G. T., & Rodgers, S. (1999). Research utilization models: Frameworks for implementing evidence-based occupational therapy practice. *Occupational Therapy International, 6*(1), 1–23.

Campbell, P. H. (1988). Using a single-subject research design to evaluate the effectiveness of treatment. *American Journal of Occupational Therapy, 42*(11), 732–738.

Canadian Association of Occupational Therapists. (1998). Special edition on evidence-based practice. *Canadian Journal of Occupational Therapy, 65*(3).

Canadian Association of Occupational Therapists, Association of Canadian Occupational Therapy University Programs, Association of Canadian Occupational Therapy Regulatory Organizations, & the Presidents' Advisory Committee. (1999). Joint position statement on evidence-based practice. *Canadian Journal of Occupational Therapy, 66,* 267–269.

College of Occupational Therapists. (1997). Special edition on evidence-based practice. *British Journal of Occupational Therapy, 60*(11).

College of Occupational Therapists. (2003). *Professional standards for occupational therapy practice.* Author.

College of Occupational Therapists. (2005). *Code of ethics and professional conduct.* Author.

Cusick, A. (2001). OZ OT EBP 21C: Australian occupational therapy, evidence-based practice and the 21st century. *Australian Occupational Therapy Journal, 48*(3), 102–117.

Dubouloz, C. J., Egan, M., Vallerand, J., & von Zweck, C. (1999). Occupational therapists' perceptions of evidence-based practice. *The American Journal of Occupational Therapy, 53*(5), 445–453.

Eakin, P. (1997). The Casson memorial lecture 1997: Shifting the balance—evidence-based practice. *British Journal of Occupational Therapy, 60*(7), 290–294.

Garcia, J., Copley, J., Turpin, M., Bennett, S., McBryde, C., & McCosker, J. L. (2020). Evidence-based practice and clinical reasoning in occupational therapy: A cross-sectional survey in Chile. *Australian Occupational Therapy Journal.*

Glasziou, P. (2005). Make it evidence informed practice with a little wisdom. *BMJ, 330*(7482), 92.

Goldet, G., & Howick, J. (2013). Understanding GRADE: An introduction. *Journal of Evidence-Based Medicine, 6*(1), 50–54.

Harris, J., Kearley, K., Heneghan, C., Meats, E., Roberts, N., Perera, R., & Kearley-Shiers, K. (2011). Are journal clubs effective in supporting evidence-based decision making? A systematic review. BEME Guide No. 16. *Medical Teacher, 33*(1), 9–23.

Health Care Professions Council. (2018). *Standards of proficiency, occupational therapists.* Author.

Herbert, R., Jamtvedt, G., Mead, J., et al. (2005). *Practical evidence-based physiotherapy.* Churchill Livingstone.

Holm, M. B. (2000). The 2000 Eleanor Clarke Slagle lecture: Our mandate for the new millennium: Evidence-based practice. *American Journal of Occupational Therapy, 54,* 575–585.

Humphris, D. (2005). Types of evidence. In S. Hamer, & G. Collinson (Eds.), *Achieving evidence-based practice* (2nd ed.). Baillière Tindall.

Krasny-Pacini, A., & Evans, J. (2018). Single-case experimental designs to assess intervention effectiveness in rehabilitation: A practical guide. *Annals of Physical and Rehabilitation Medicine, 61*(3), 164–179.

Law, M. (Ed.). (2002). *Evidence-based rehabilitation.* Slack Incorporated.

Lewin, S., Booth, A., Glenton, C., Munthe-Kaas, H., Rashidian, A., Wainwright, M., & Noyes, J. (2018). Applying GRADE-CERQual to qualitative evidence synthesis findings: Introduction to the series. *Implementation Science, 13,* 2.

Lindström, A. C., & Bernhardsson, S. (2018). Evidence-based practice in primary care occupational therapy: A cross-sectional survey in Sweden. *Occupational Therapy International,* 2018:5376764.

Linzer, M. (1987). The journal club and medical education: Over one hundred years of unrecorded history. *Postgraduate Medical Journal, 63,* 475–478.

McCluskey, A., Lovarini, M., Bennett, S., McKenna, K., Tooth, L., & Hoffmann, T. (2006). How and why do occupational therapists use the OTseeker evidence database?. *Australian Occupational Therapy Journal, 53*(3), 188–195.

McDonald, S., & Nikles, J. (2021). N-of-1 trials in healthcare. *Healthcare, 9,* 330.

McGlacken-Byrne, S. M., O'Rahelly, M., Cantillon, P., & Allen, N. M. (2020). Journal club: Old tricks and fresh approaches. *Archives of Disease in Childhood-Education and Practice, 105*(4), 236–241.

McKenna, K. (2004). In practice. OT seeker: Facilitating evidence-based practice in occupational therapy. *Australian Occupational Therapy Journal, 51*(2), 102–105.

McKenna, K. (2005). Australian occupational therapists' use of an online evidence-based practice database (OTseeker). *Health Information & Libraries Journal, 22*(3), 205–214.

McQueen, J., Nivison, C., Husband, V., & Miller, C. (2006). An investigation into the use of a journal club for evidence-based practice. *International Journal of Therapy and Rehabilitation, 13*(7), 311–317.

Pawson, R., Boaz, A., Grayson, L., et al. (2003). *Knowledge reviews 3: Types & quality of knowledge in social care.* SCIE & The Policy Press.

Phillips, B., Ball, C., Sackett, D., Badenoch, D., Straus, S., Haynes, B., Dawes, M. and Howick, J., 2009. Oxford centre for evidence-based medicine-levels of evidence (March 2009). https://www.cebm.ox.ac.uk/resources/levels-of-evidence/oxford-centre-for-evidence-based-medicine-levels-of-evidence-march-2009

Phillips, R. S., & Glasziou, P. (2004). What makes evidence-based journal clubs succeed? *Evidence Based Medicine, 9,* 36–37.

Rappolt, S. (2003). The role of professional expertise in evidence-based occupational therapy. *The American Journal of Occupational Therapy, 57*(5), 589–593.

Richardson, W. S., Wilson, M. C., Nishikawa, J., et al. (1995). The well-built clinical question: A key to evidence-based decisions (editorial). *ACP Journal Club, 123,* A12–A13.

Rosenberg, W., & Donald, A. (1995). Evidence based medicine: An approach to clinical problem-solving. *BMJ, 310,* 1122–1126.

Sackett, D.L. (1998). Shamanism (was: Pre-test probability). *Evidence-Based Health.* http://www.mailbase.ac.uk/lists/evidence-based-health/1998-03/0066.html.

Sackett, D. L., & Wennberg, J. E. (1997). Choosing the best research design for each question. *BMJ, 315,* 16–36.

Sackett, D. L., Richardson, W. S., Rosenberg, W., et al. (1997). *Evidence-based medicine: How to practice & teach EBM.* Churchill Livingstone.

Sackett, D. L., & Rosenberg, W. M. C. (1995). On the need for evidence-based medicine. *Journal of Public Health, 17*(3), 330–334.

Sackett, D. L., Rosenberg, W. M. C., Gray, J. A. M., et al. (1996). Evidence-based medicine: What it is and what it isn't. *BMJ, 312,* 71–72.

Sherratt, C. (2005). The journal club: A method for occupational therapists to bridge the theory-practice gap. *British Journal of Occupational Therapy, 68*(7), 301–306.

Taylor, M. C. (2003). Evidence-based practice: informing practice and critically evaluating related research. In G. Brown, S. A. Esdaile, & S. E. Ryan (Eds.), *Becoming an advanced practitioner* (pp. 90–117). Butterworth-Heinemann.

Taylor, M. C. (2007). In *Evidence-based practice for occupational therapists* (2nd ed.). Blackwell Publishing.

Wenke, R. J., Thomas, R., Hughes, I., & Mickan, S. (2018). The effectiveness and feasibility of TREAT (tailoring research evidence and theory) journal clubs in allied health: A randomised controlled trial. *BMC Medical Education, 18*(1), 1–14.

13

Implementation Science

Katrina Bannigan

HIGHLIGHTS

- Implementation science is related to the fourth stage of the evidence-based practice process—implementing the findings of critical appraisal into practice—and previously the work related to this was known by terms such as research utilisation, knowledge transfer, knowledge exchange, and knowledge management.
- Implementation science—the scientific study of methods to promote the systematic uptake of research findings into routine practice—is now an area of scholarship within it is own right reflecting the fact that this a highly skilled and complex area of practice and research.
- Implementation science is underpinned by six key concepts—strategies, context, outcomes, fidelity,

adaptation, and sustainability—and a range of theoretical approaches are used to inform this work.
- The key theoretical approaches to implementation used in occupational therapy are outlined; The knowledge to action model, the consolidated framework for implementation research, and the integrated-PARIHS framework.
- Deimplementation (i.e., stopping using practices that are not evidence based and regarded as low-value care) is an emerging area of implementation science.
- Implementation science in occupational therapy is explored through vignettes and the practical actions that are required at professional, organisational, and individual levels to increase implementation in occupational therapy.

OVERVIEW

The topic featured in this chapter has evolved considerably since the last edition of this book, so the title of the chapter has changed from "Knowledge Exchange" to "Implementation Science." This chapter will set implementation science in the context of evidence-based practice, consider what implementation science is before reporting on six vignettes that provide an indication of the contemporary use of implementation science in occupational therapy, and the implications for the practice of implementation science. The aim is to provide a good understanding of implementation science, its relevance to occupational therapy, and its import to your work. The vignettes used in this chapter have been developed from the literature and are based on the experience of implementation science of occupational therapists working in practice. They show how closely related theory and practice are. This chapter has been written in the expectation that you will also make links between its content and the content of the chapters on using theory in practice (see Chapters 2, 3 and 4), Finding and Appraising

the Evidence (see Chapter 12), Improvement Science in Practice (see Chapter 14), and Leadership Skills (see Chapter 18) because each informs and supports the other.

IT'S TRICKIER THAN WE INITIALLY THOUGHT

In the era of evidence-based practice it is accepted that health and social care should be underpinned by accurate, up-to-date research to achieve the best outcomes for those accessing services (see Chapter 12). This means the improved health and well-being of society is dependent on high-quality research, which is why so much money is invested in health and social care research across the world. For example, in the United Kingdom more than £1.5 billion are spent on medical research a year (Clark, 2020), and the United States spends nearly $200 billion a year (Research America, 2019). As such, it is expected that research should always be used before other sources when making decisions in practice (Aveyard & Sharp, 2017). As evidence-based practice is an indisputable part of practice, it would imply that research findings are routinely used in practice. This is not the case.

The problem is when evidence-based practice was first introduced there was an excessive focus on critical appraisal, which distorted perceptions of the process. It fostered the sense that just having high-quality research findings was enough to change practice, but the reality is "evidence rarely spreads by itself" (Nilsen & Birken, 2020, p. 2). At the time the previous edition was being written, the complexity of translating research findings into everyday practice was starting to be recognised. It was accepted that, although important activities (diffusion: a passive process of research awareness raising, which is largely uncontrolled or unplanned and dependent on the individual seeking out information [Lomas, 1993]; and dissemination: a targeted process of raising awareness of research messages [National Health Service Centre for Reviews and Dissemination, 1999]) had limitations and neither led to the uptake of research findings into practice (in terms of changing practice), they are passive processes. The chapter in the previous edition explained that knowledge exchange would only happen if more active steps—involving collaboration, interaction, mutual learning, and problem solving—were adopted to bring researchers and practitioners together to develop processes tailored to the settings in which practitioners work (Bannigan, 2009). Implicit in these developments was the understanding that knowledge exchange is as much a social process (i.e., focused on people) as a technical process (i.e., focused on research). This acknowledgement of the practical, and very human, issues involved meant a wider range of knowledge needed to be drawn upon (e.g., change management and communication skills) (Bannigan, 2007). We cannot ignore the fact that the existence and/or publication of research findings does not lead to changes in practice, no matter how high quality the research findings, the effect size achieved, or well packaged they are. Even the use of clinical guidelines is not guaranteed to change practice (Restall et al., 2020).

This is problematic because the significant constraints on resources in the health and social sector mean an investment in research is only an investment if ultimately it shapes and changes practice. Implementation is the point at which research findings stop being research findings and become practice. The oft-cited observation that it takes on average 17 years for research to be implemented into practice (Nilsen & Birken, 2020) suggests we are not currently experiencing a good return on investment in health and social care research. In the previous edition, when this chapter was called knowledge exchange, the focus was on using research findings to inform practice. The term knowledge exchange was used in preference to knowledge transfer or research utilisation, which reflected

the then state of the discipline; it was struggling to define itself (Bannigan, 2007). In the intervening years the term implementation science has been settled upon as the name for this discipline, and implementation science is a fully accepted area of expertise and, as can be seen from the definition (see later), the discipline has a sharper focus. That this aspect of the evidence-based process has become a recognised area of scholarship in its own right is an acknowledgement that it is a highly skilled and complex area of practice and research. The discipline of implementation science is necessary to effectively enhance the adoption of evidence into practice and so evidence-based occupational therapy (Juckett et al., 2019).

Implementation Problems Are Unique, Complex, and Wicked

The existence of implementation science also emphasises that what we do in terms of implementation, as with all activity in health and social care, should be evidence based (van Achterberg et al., 2008). Implementation is far from straightforward (Bannigan, 2007), and implementation problems have been described as unique, complex, and wicked (Greenhalgh, 2020). Therefore we need to be well informed about the best evidence to effectively navigate solutions to achieve implementation. The reality is there is no one-size-fits-all solution and "there are many wrong answers to the question of how to 'do' implementation, there is rarely a single right answer" (Greenhalgh, 2020, p. xxiv). The complexity of translating research-based knowledge into practice, whilst also recognising the values of the people we work with as well as our values as occupational therapists, is well recognised (Metzler & Metz, 2010).

WHAT IS IMPLEMENTATION SCIENCE?

In the first issue of the *Implementation Science Journal* (Box 13.1) implementation science was defined as "the scientific study of methods to promote the systematic uptake of research findings and other evidence-based practices (EBPs) into routine practice, and, hence, to improve the quality and effectiveness of health services" (Eccles & Mittman, 2006, para 2). Essentially the purpose of implementation science is to bridge the gap between what is known and what is actually done (World Health Organization, 2004). Even though the terminologic tangle of the past is resolving, implementation research is used interchangeably with implementation science (Nilsen & Birken, 2020). A significant change in the scope of implementation science has been the additional focus on deimplementation—that is, "abandoning practices that are not evidence-based, usually referred to as low-value care" (Nilsen et al., 2020, para 1). (Low-value care refers to

BOX 13.1   Implementation Science Journals

There are three main implementation science journals: *Implementation Science, Implementation Research and Practice,* and *Implementation Science Communications.* They are all available online (there is no print version)

- *Implementation Science:* https://implementation-science.biomedcentral.com/
- *Implementation Research and Practice:* https://us.sagepub.com/en-us/nam/implementation-research-and-practice/journal203691
- *Implementation Science Communications:* https://implementationsciencecomms.biomedcentral.com/

They publish research relevant to increasing the uptake of research findings in routine practice, organisations, and policy. They cover implementation science across the full spectrum of health care services and settings and are interdisciplinary in their perspective. *Implementation Science* and *Implementation Science Communications* have papers focused on occupational therapy. *Implementation Research and Practice* is a newer journal, and the papers published to date are relevant to occupational therapy. They are peer reviewed, which means all the papers included in the journal have been fully peer reviewed. As they are open access, it means readers have full text access to the content without charge.

interventions that have been shown to be of low or no clinical benefit.) Many of the precepts outlined in the previous edition still stand. For example, Lomas (2007) described "human interaction as the engine that drives research into practice" (p. 130), and this has not changed. What has changed is that our understanding of implementation is starting to crystalise. It recognised that there are foundational theoretical concepts in implementation science as well as theoretical approaches to implementation science (Rapport et al., 2017). Nilsen and Birken (2020) have systematised the underpinning knowledge into six key concepts: strategies, context, outcomes, fidelity, adaptation, and sustainability. Each of these concepts is considered in turn before focussing on deimplementation and theoretical approaches.

Strategies

Strategies are the actions (or steps) taken to achieve implementation, sometimes called implementation interventions (Leeman & Nilsen, 2020), and include activities such as audit and feedback, care pathways, conferences, educational materials, educational meetings, guideline reminders, and local opinion leaders. A full taxonomy of health system interventions is available from https://epoc.cochrane.org/epoc-taxonomy. In their scoping review, focused on the strategies and factors related to the uptake of older adult occupational therapy interventions into practice, Juckett and Robinson (2018) suggest the following:

> *Clinic or organisational team leaders seeking to integrate research into practice may consider using strategies such as workshops, follow-up consultations from experts, fidelity vignettes, peer mentoring, and standardised training modules to enhance the implementation process related to older adult interventions (p. 6).*

Laver (2017) has also called for an increase in the use of patient-mediated interventions for implementation in occupational therapy because, as well as being low cost and more likely to increase implementation, they are compatible with the profession's philosophy.

It has long been recognised that active multicomponent strategies are more likely to be effective than single component strategies, but how strategies should be combined and under what circumstances is not clear cut (Leeman & Nilsen, 2020). Robust research is needed to determine what combination of strategies contribute best to achieving effective implementation. A systematic review of implementation in rehabilitation found most of the included studies used a multicomponent implementation strategy and that education-related components were the most frequently used strategy regardless of whether it was a single or multicomponent intervention (Jones et al., 2015). Neither single nor multicomponent implementation strategies were shown to be effective, but this lack of effect may be attributable to methodological issues. One challenge was the reporting of the implementation interventions as poor when assessed against the WIDER recommendations (see later) for reporting behavioural change interventions (Jones et al., 2015).

Ideally before an implementation project is started it should be well planned—intervention mapping techniques can help to ensure that strategies are selected that have strong underpinning logic (see Leeman & Nilsen, 2020 for more details)—and documented in an implementation plan (Rapport et al., 2017). Without quality documentation it is hard to assess effectiveness of implementation interventions (Jones et al., 2015). The implementation interventions must be specified in detail (Blase et al., 2012). Rapport et al. (2017) refer to the process whereby an actionable plan is appropriately and successfully executed as "effective implementation" (p. 118).

Context

It is the interaction between research findings (evidence), context, and implementation interventions that determines whether implementation will be successful or not (Eriksson et al., 2017). This means context is an important part of the implementation process; it has an active role to play and is not just "a back cloth to action" (Dopson & Fitzgerald, 2005, p. 102). As context shapes implementation, and the context for practice is unique (Greenhalgh, 2020), thinking about and taking into account context is an integral part of planning an implementation project (Nilsen, 2020). Lockwood et al. (2016) have argued "facilitation of evidence implementation must be localised and context driven, nuanced to the immediate environment and those who work in it" (p. 323). If there needs to be an understanding of how the evidence being implemented fits the context, researchers cannot do this alone (Verhagen, 2020). For implementation to be dynamic and iterative, widespread communication and increased collaboration between knowledge producers and users, typically separated by mandate and funding structures, is needed to ensure that knowledge products are relevant, meaningful, and sensitive to context (White et al., 2013). This is why Eriksson et al. (2017), when designing an implementation plan for a client-centred activity of daily living intervention (Table 13.1), described the importance of partnership with practitioners and researchers. Practitioners understand the real-world practice context in a way researchers never can and so are equal partners in the process of implementation. This highlights just how close research and practice (context) are: One cannot exist or be understood independently of the other.

Outcomes

Successful implementation, like any other area of life, can only be judged if there are data to demonstrate what has changed and outcomes data are needed to inform this judgement. Again, as with the key concepts already discussed, this means outcomes are an important part of implementation planning because, if you understand what outcomes are desired, it provides a direction for implementation activity (Lockwood et al., 2016). A challenge within occupational therapy is "less is understood about how to conduct [implementation] research and measure implementation outcomes" (Juckett et al., 2019, p. 2).

To understand whether implementation has been effective there are a range of considerations that need to be made. It has been proposed by Proctor et al. (2011) that there is a taxonomy of implementation outcomes, which includes measuring the following:

- **Acceptability**: Is the implementation perceived as acceptable within the practice setting?
- **Adoption**: Has there been uptake of the implementation within the practice setting?

- **Appropriateness**: Does the implementation fit the practice setting?
- **Feasibility**: Was the practice setting able to use the innovation being implemented?
- **Fidelity**: Is the implementation being delivered in the practice setting as intended?
- **Implementation cost**: How much did it cost to implement within the practice setting?
- **Penetration**: What was the level of integration of the innovation being implemented within the practice setting?
- **Sustainability**: Was the practice setting able to maintain the innovation being implemented?

The measures used in an implementation project should be clearly articulated as part of the implementation plan, alongside the strategies used and contextual factors already described.

Fidelity

Fidelity is referred to in different ways in the literature (i.e., implementation fidelity, fidelity of implementation, fidelity, treatment fidelity, treatment integrity, intervention fidelity; Breitenstein et al., 2010). "Implementation fidelity is the degree to which an intervention is delivered as intended" (Breitenstein et al., 2010, p. 164). It recognises that the same outcomes are unlikely to be achieved in an implementation site if there is no fidelity to the way the evidence was produced initially. This is why fidelity is a key concept and another essential part of implementation planning. As fidelity measures are correlated with achieving implementation, this involves identifying the core components of the intervention being implemented and identifying measures that will demonstrate that these were achieved during implementation (Blase et al., 2012). There are three components of this:

- **Adherence**: How well practitioners conform to the core components of the intervention?
- **Competence**: How skilfully the practitioners executed the core components of the intervention?
- **Context**: An assessment of contextual factors that may have an impact on fidelity (Breitenstein et al. 2010).

Pyatak et al. (2019), in their study of the implementation of Lifestyle Redesign for diabetes in primary care, provided an example of how implementation fidelity has been measured in an occupational therapy study. They measured therapist fidelity to the Lifestyle Redesign manual by reviewing electronic medical records to check how far the documentation of the occupational therapy provided reflected the domains in the Lifestyle Redesign manual. They found 100% fidelity, which suggests that the intervention people received in the study was Lifestyle Redesign (i.e., the occupational therapists adhered to the

TABLE 13.1		**Vignettes of Implementation Science in Occupational Therapy**		
Reference	**Practice Focus**	**Implementation Focus**	**How Were Occupational Therapists Involved?**	**Key Implementation Message(s)**
Allen et al. (2020)	Stroke rehabilitation	A complex, shared decision-making (SDM) intervention using cognitive orientation to daily occupational performance (CO-OP)	Implementation activity: engaging leadership figures, implementation facilitators worked with individual sites to develop site-specific implementation goals and plans, implementation support period ended with site-specific CO-OP consolidation sessions As a member of an interprofessional team of stroke rehabilitation clinicians across five sites participated in • Two-day training workshop to learn the theory and application of the CO-OP approach in clinical practice • Four-month support period encouraged to use CO-OP in their practice with the support of facilitators • Ten (two from each site) became site champions and gathered feedback before attending a focus group A semistructured focus group (n = 8) was conducted approximately 3 months after support period ended Data were analysed by the researchers using iPARIHS	Context-specific facilitation is key to integrating a novel, complex intervention into interprofessional practice, particularly interventions that require significant shifts in clinical practice from clinician-directed decision making to SDM Facilitators should lay out a framework for training, communication, and implementation that is structured but still provides flexibility for iterative learning and active problem solving within the relevant practice context More research on the long-term effects of SDM approaches on clinical practice and patient outcomes in stroke rehabilitation
Colquhoun et al. (2020)	Various departments in acute care, inpatient, and outpatient occupational therapy	To understand what beliefs influence the use of the Canadian Occupational Performance Measure (COPM) in occupational therapy practice	Potential participants received information regarding the study during a staff meeting The interviews (n = 15) were face-to-face and lasted approximately 30–45 min The interview guide was based on the theoretical domains framework (covers 14 domains of behaviour change)	Six domains were most relevant to the use of the COPM: Social influences Social professional role and identity Beliefs about consequences Beliefs about capabilities Skills Behavioural regulation This can be used to inform our understanding of the use of this measure in occupational therapy practice and identify potential targets for behaviour change interventions aimed at increasing the use of the COPM by occupational therapists

(Continued)

TABLE 13.1		Vignettes of Implementation Science in Occupational Therapy (*Cont.*)		
Reference	Practice Focus	Implementation Focus	How Were Occupational Therapists Involved?	Key Implementation Message(s)
Culph et al. (2020)	Dementia (reablement)	The implementation of the care of people with dementia in their environments (COPE) program from the perspective of the professionals involved	Implementation strategies: planning; educating; restructuring; quality management COPE: up to 10 consultations over approximately 4 months delivered primarily by an occupational therapist, with consultation from a registered nurse Two forms of data collection • Interviews to explore the experience of implementing an evidence-based program into the Australian health care system • Draw a simple diagram of their organisation to visualise the implementation context and to demonstrate their perception of the strength of the relationships with different members of their organisation, by drawing a dotted line for a weak relationship, a single solid line for a relationship, and three solid lines for a strong relationship	Additional preparation work is required of organisations to consider relationships in their strategies for implementation Strong trusting relationships with managers were instrumental in advocating for the need for reablement programs and the occupational therapy professional role in dementia care Large teams of occupational therapists were seen to be beneficial in supporting each other in case complexities Relationships between occupational therapists and nurses were often missing or perceived as weak relationships A conducive physical environment contributed to stronger more collaborative relationships
Jutzi et al. (2020)	Stroke rehabilitation	CO-OP	Implementation intervention used the KTA No direct involvement in the data collection because an audit of medical records was used	Training in a top-down approach may lead to increased and more specific client-centred occupation-based goal setting Even when client-centred occupation-based goals are present, occupational therapists do not consistently record matching top-down treatment plans Documented top-down treatment plans lack the details needed to understand what treatment occurred, but these details are usually provided for bottom-up treatment plans

(*Continued*)

			TABLE 13.1	Vignettes of Implementation Science in Occupational Therapy (*Cont.*)

Reference	Practice Focus	Implementation Focus	How Were Occupational Therapists Involved?	Key Implementation Message(s)

Restall et al. (2020)	Paediatric rehabilitation (constraint induced movement therapy [CIMT])	The factors that influence implementation of clinical practice guidelines (CPG) using the case of CIMT	Stakeholders had been brought together to promote uptake of the guideline, but the process of implementation had got stuck
			A CIMT CPG was circulated to all participants prior to the focus group
			Focus groups with therapists who had, or were likely to have, children in their caseload for whom CIMT has been shown to be applicable
				Insights about potential ways to unstick CPG uptake in paediatric rehabilitation, such as:
				  Consistency between guidelines and relevance to practice context
				  Room for "art and science" in clinical decision making
				  Education and information exchange
				  Using motivators to seek out guidelines
				  "Right blend of child and parent and commitment"
				  Structure of the guideline
				  Confidence in the CIMT guideline
				  Challenges of managing multiple stakeholders
				  Suggest using a combination of knowledge (known as mindlines)

Schell et al. (2020)	Developmental coordination disorder (DCD)	Integration of DCD evidence into frontline practice	KTA framework used to describe activities that occurred during the knowledge translation process Implementation activities: information dissemination; education; addition of DCD to a neurodevelopmental assessment clinic; and development of a community of practice. Outcome evaluation methods included surveys, interviews, referral tracking, and database creation	Knowledge translation strategy implementation resulted in increased knowledge among clinicians and community stakeholders Process standardisation, increased referrals querying DCD, established knowledge brokers, and practice change Predetermined and systematic implementation strategy design is essential for embedding evidence into frontline practice

iPARIHS, Integrated–promoting action on research implementation in health services framework; *KTA,* knowledge to action model.

manual; Pyatak et al., 2019). This outcome does not provide any insight into how skilfully the occupational therapist executed the skills associated with the domains of the Lifestyle Redesign manual. Contextual factors were not explicitly discussed in the context, but timeliness and efficiency were discussed in the paper, and these may inform this discussion.

Adaptation

Adaptation is a key concept in implementation because "constant adjustments in practices, organisations, and systems are made on purpose to realise and improve recipient benefits. Adaptation is not done once; it is a continual goal-orientated process" (Fixen et al., 2019, p. 24). Constant adjustments are needed in response to barriers and/or facilitators that may arise during the process of implementation to ensure the project does not derail. Eriksson et al. (2017) highlighted an issue in their implementation study that may have merited adjustment. Managers agreed to services being involved in their project, which meant some occupational therapists expressed frustration because they did not feel fully informed about what was involved in the project. This was problematic because, if an adjustment was not made, it could have had a negative impact on the occupational therapists' openness to learning about, and motivation to engage with, the intervention and perhaps decrease the likelihood of implementation. Part of the planning process should involve ensuring that resources are available to monitor the process and then be able to respond to any issues that arise requiring adjustment.

Sustainability

Sustainability focuses on the ability of an implementation project to maintain momentum. From an implementation planning perspective this means to begin with the end in mind—that is, to consider what it will take to ensure that an implementation plan will be successful and not fizzle out without achieving an embedded change in practice. This involves what Blase et al. (2012) describe as a two-pronged approach involving a consideration of (1) the financial sustainability (time and resources) and (2) programmatic sustainability (the infrastructure and monitoring). In reality,

> Sustainability is an ongoing and vigilant overlay at every point in the implementation journey. The goal is to ensure the long-term survival and improvement of the intervention and its continued benefits … in the context of a changing organisational environment and fluctuating systemic conditions.
>
> **Blase et al., 2012, p. 21**

Theoretical Approaches in Implementation Science

Theory is also important because, as Nilsen (2020) pointed out, "Poor theoretical underpinning makes it difficult to understand and explain how and why implementation succeeds or fails, thus restraining opportunities to identify factors that predict the likelihood of implementation success" (p. 8). There are too many theoretical approaches in implementation science to be covered here (consult Nilsen [2020] for a definitive overview of the topic and the theoretical approaches). The three theoretical approaches are introduced here—the knowledge to action (KTA) model, consolidated framework for implementation research (CFIR), and integrated–promoting action on research implementation in health services (integrated-PARIHS) framework—because they seem to be the ones most used in the occupational therapy and wider allied health professions literature. However, Colquhoun et al.'s (2010) scoping review found limited evidence of the use of implementation theory in occupational therapy. That there are illustrative examples in this chapter suggests this has changed, but it is important to be mindful of the need to use theory. Before outlining the theoretical approaches, it is worth noting Greenhalgh's (2020) words of caution:

> … a theoretical approach is—at best—nothing more than a suggested way of organising your thoughts about a complex topic or issue…Organising your thoughts is an important step in addressing an implementation task, but an implementation theory, model or framework will not actually do the work of implementation. Nor will it take the pain or the politics out of the process, or make impossible things possible or hard things easy, or unhappy teams happy (p. xxii).

The Knowledge to Action Model

The KTA process model, developed by Graham et al. (2006), specifies the steps involved in implementation and thus can be used as a practical guide (Nilsen, 2020). There are two components of the KTA:

1. **Knowledge creation**: a process involving the identification of and knowledge and tailoring it to context
2. **Action cycle**: a process involving the activities needed to achieve implementation, which may need adapting to the local context (see Graham et al. [2006] for a detailed overview of the steps involved)

This model, like others, assumes a degree of linearity between the two components (Nilsen, 2020). There is now an increased recognition of the need for a more sophisticated approach to implementation (hence the inclusion of facilitation in the integrated-PARIHS model). The KTA has been used in occupational therapy by Townley et al. (2018), who used it to introduce evidence-based feeding and swallowing interventions to paediatric settings. They developed an evidence-based handbook (knowledge creation) for other occupational therapists to use the action cycle to explore implementation into their practice setting (Townley et al., 2018). A citation analysis identified that the KTA has also been used for implementation projects focused on unilateral spatial neglect poststroke and best practice in paediatrics (Field et al., 2014).

The Consolidated Framework for Implementation Research

The CFIR, developed by Damschroder et al. (2009), is described as a determinant framework in that its purpose is to explain what influences implementation outcomes (Nilsen, 2020). The framework is what it says it is: a consolidation of existing implementation theories; it has brought together existing knowledge and removed duplication and redundant concepts (Damschroder et al., 2009). The resultant framework has five domains, made up of constructs associated with effective implementation:

1. **Intervention characteristics**: intervention source, evidence strength and quality, relative advantage, adaptability, trialability, complexity, design quality and packaging, and cost
2. **Outer setting**: patient needs and resources, cosmopolitanism, peer pressure, and external policies and incentives
3. **Inner setting**: structural characteristics, networks and communications, culture, and implementation climate
4. **Characteristics of the individuals involved**: knowledge and beliefs about the intervention, self-efficacy, individual stage of change, individual identification with organisation, and other personal attributes
5. **The process of implementation**: planning, engaging, executing and reflecting, and evaluating

Examples of how the CFIR has been used to support implementation activity in occupational therapy include it being used as a theoretical framework to support the charting of data in a scoping review of stroke rehabilitation (Juckett et al., 2020), as a template to extract data in a systematic review of the facilitators and barriers to implementing patient-reported outcome measures (Briggs et al., 2020), and in data analysis of a qualitative study of the implementation of upper limb stroke rehabilitation (Connell et al., 2014). This demonstrates that CFIR is widely applicable in the field of implementation science.

Promoting Action on Research Implementation in Health Services: The Integrated-PARIHS Framework

The PARIHS framework, originally developed by Kitson et al. (1998), is another determinant framework, so it is not a theory as such because it focuses on what influences implementation—typically barriers and facilitators—rather than how the change takes place (Nilsen, 2020). It was revised, taking into account gaps in the theory, new knowledge, and the findings of evaluations of its use in practice. It is now called the integrated-PARIHS (iPARIHS) framework (Harvey & Kitson, 2015) and it is built on the premise that there are four key determinants—characteristics of the evidence (innovation), context, recipients, and facilitation—that shape implementation (Nilsen, 2020). In essence, iPARIHS

> *…positions facilitation as the active ingredient of implementation, assessing and aligning the innovation to be implemented with the intended recipients in their local, organisational and wider system context. Facilitation is operationalised through a network of novice, experienced and expert facilitators applying a range of enabling skills and improvement strategies to structure the implementation process, engage and manage relationships between key stakeholders and identify and negotiate barriers to implementation within the contextual setting.*
>
> ***Harvey & Kitson, 2015, p. 11***

Warner and Townsend (2012) suggested that occupational therapists could use PARIHS to explore the factors that impinge on their ability to apply occupation-based knowledge to practice or to develop a facilitation strategy to implement evidence into practice. PARIHS was used in an implementation study to develop an understanding of the evidence and context for family-centred care for older adults (Warner & Stadnyk, 2014); it was used to structure the data collection and guide discussions. A citation analysis identified that the PARIHS has also been used for implementation projects focused on perceptions of implementing client-centred intervention, clinical reasoning, the use of theory, and stroke rehabilitation (Bergström et al., 2020).

Deimplementation

As intimated earlier, deimplementation is a relatively novel concept in implementation science. It has been estimated that 10% to 30% of all health care practices have little or no benefit to the patient (Nilsen et al., 2020). This is a pervasive problem, which has resource implications for health and social care. Anecdotally in health and social care it is acknowledged that the challenges associated with stopping using an intervention are as difficult as implementation. This may be why Davidson et al. (2017) have called for a distinct discipline:

> De-implementation science, as it might be called, would appropriately recognise and identify problem areas of low value and wasteful practice, carry out rigorous scientific examinations of the factors that initiate and maintain such practices, and then employ evidence-based interventions to extinguish these practices (pp. 463–464).

A recent scoping review (Nilsen et al., 2020) identified 10 theories that have been used to understand deimplementation, but only half of these were specifically for deimplementation. Thus they cautioned about assuming that theories are interchangeable between implementation and deimplementation. Only one study on deimplementation in occupational therapy was identified, and it focused on adopting best practices in home care services and stopping using untested practices (Guay et al., 2019). It is anticipated that deimplementation will be the area of implementation science to see the most growth between now and the next edition of this book.

IMPLEMENTATION SCIENCE AND OCCUPATIONAL THERAPY

Having established that implementation science is a rapidly evolving area of scholarship (Slavin, 2012), the next step is to provide an indication of the current state of the art in occupational therapy. A rapid review of CINAHL identified six occupational therapy implementation projects that were published in 2020. They have been summarised as vignettes (see Table 13.1).

There is evidence of implementation science in occupational therapy. There are considerably more vignettes than the last edition. The rapid review identified 24 projects over the last 5 years, but constraints on space meant only the vignettes from the last year could be reported (see Table 13.1). Some areas of practice feature more prominently (e.g., stroke rehabilitation), and this likely reflects the availability of evidence to implement in practice but also suggests implementation requires more attention within occupational therapy. Others concur with this (Donnelly et al., 2016; Juckett et al., 2019), and the challenges associated with this are reflected upon in the next section.

The Implications for Practice of Implementation Science

This part of the chapter focuses on the implications for implementation science for us as occupational therapists,

whether we are students or working as occupational therapists, regardless of whether we are working in practice or management or academia. Intrinsically, **research** should be developed with its end use in mind (Bennett, 2017). This means successful implementation is not just about researchers but contingent on the following:

- **People we work with**: This requires not simply knowing who the end users may be, but extends to co-creation of knowledge:

> Integrated knowledge translation' where researchers and knowledge-users work together to shape the research process both prior to the commencement of research and beyond its completion … is not a new idea; however, true involvement of consumers in co-creation of research and its translation is now increasingly valued.
>
> *Bennett, 2017, p. 349*

- **Practitioners**: It is important to understand what influences the process of practitioners implementing research into practice (Eriksson et al., 2017) because they are an integral part of the process.

Juckett et al. (2020) reviewed the barriers and facilitators in stroke rehabilitation, and whilst they identified barriers and facilitators to implementation, their overall conclusion was the need for effective implementation strategies that promote implementation by occupational therapists still requires attention. This suggests profession-wide initiatives as well as organisational-level and individual-level activities are needed to promote implementation (Grajo et al., 2020).

Profession-Wide Initiatives

Just as the occupational therapy profession needed to embrace evidence-based practice, it now needs to take action to forward the implementation science agenda (Juckett et al., 2019). Profession-wide initiatives were identified:

- **Implementation across international boundaries**: Occupational therapists working in Australia and the Asia Pacific region have been encouraged to consider implementation beyond their own national boundaries, but this will be dependent on developing research partnerships (Mackenzie & McKinstry, 2018). These partnerships are about collaboration and sharing skills because different countries will require tailored implementation projects to reflect their context (Mackenzie & McKinstry, 2018).
- **Occupational therapy journals**: Journals, such as the *Australian Occupational Therapy Journal* (Brown & Robinson, 2019) and *Canadian Journal of Occupational Therapy* (Zur, 2016), are making stringent efforts to

ensure the work published in our journals is more implementation friendly. For example, they are including new sections such as "Implications for Practice" (Brown & Robinson, 2019) and "CJOT: Evidence for Your Practice" (Zur, 2016).
- **National surveys**: These have been used to understand research use in practice by occupational therapists. For example, Nott et al. (2020) surveyed **occupational therapists** working with adults experiencing neurocognitive impairments and suggested that the use of specialist cognitive interventions in practice is not keeping pace with the growing evidence base; in line with Juckett et al.'s (2020) observations, Nott et al. 2020 identified the need for more effective implementation strategies in occupational therapy.

A call for incorporating implementation science into the occupational therapy curriculum to build capacity (Grajo et al., 2020) was identified, but no developments in relation to this could be found.

Organisational Initiatives

A range of organisational initiatives have been suggested. The type and nature of implementation activities varied according to the type of organisation (Donnelly et al., 2016) but will require support from service managers and organisational leaders. The organisational initiatives identified were:
- **Shape the organisational culture in occupational therapy services** (including academic settings) to encourage implementation of research findings in practice, such as conference papers and publications and collaboration between academia and practice. The aspiration should be for university departments to directly link research and practice, such as giving practitioners more access to resources (Grajo et al., 2020).
- **Provide collaborative mentoring**, rather than individual mentoring, to support practitioners and academics to engage in implementation science (Baldwin et al., 2017).
- **Facilitate communities of practice**—formalised social learning systems—to support implementation (Grajo et al., 2020).
- **Survey occupational therapy teams** to determine what perceived barriers and facilitators influence practitioners' adoption of research findings (Juckett & Robinson, 2018).

Individual Activities

From an individual occupational therapist's perspective implementation is not something we can ignore; it is an ethical imperative to be able to use research findings in our everyday practice (College of Occupational Therapists, 2015). This means we have a personal responsibility to narrow the gap between research and practice by doing the following:
- **Start a conversation**: At its simplest this is what implementation is about (Lomas, 2007) and, as not engaging is not an option, if you do not have the confidence to engage in implementation some of the organisational-level initiatives, such as the mentoring programmes (see earlier), can help to overcome this.
- **Do not reinvent the wheel**: Make use of preexisting resources, such as the *Recommendations to Improve Reporting of the Content of Behaviour Change Interventions* (WIDER), a framework to identify and describe the essential components for detailed reporting of implementation (Albrecht et al., 2013).
- **Specific activities for academics** include (a) collaborating with implementation scientists and practitioners to increase the uptake of research findings; (b) plan, document, and evaluate implementation activities to develop evidence for what works; and (c) designing education to prepare students for the challenges of implementation in practice (Grajo et al., 2020).
- **Specific activities for practitioners** include (a) developing the search and appraisal skills needed to use research, and (b) engage in organisational initiatives such as mentoring and communities of practice

SUMMARY

This chapter focused on implementation science in the context of delivering high-quality health and social care. It has been explained how implementation science emerged from evidence-based practice. The nature of implementation science was explained—in terms of the key concepts and the key theoretical approaches used in occupational therapy—which collectively highlighted the importance of planning, documenting, and evaluating implementation plans to ensure implementation success. Given the continuing gaps in knowledge about implementation in occupational therapy, initiatives to increase implementation were explored at profession-wide, organisational, and individual levels.

REFLECTIVE LEARNING

- How do the key concepts of implementation fit with the theoretical approaches to implementation science?
- Do any of the vignettes of implementation in occupational therapy apply to your area of practice? Thinking about your response, what would be the barriers and facilitators you would need to address to be able to implement the findings in your service?

- To what extent do you think there are aspects of occupational therapy practice that could be regarded as low value and so should be considered for deimplementation?
- Within the scope of your current role, what initiatives or activities could you contribute to, to increase the focus on implementation in occupational therapy?

REFERENCES

Albrecht, L., Archibald, M., Arseneau, D., & Scott, S. D. (2013). Development of a checklist to assess the quality of reporting of knowledge translation interventions using the Workgroup for Intervention Development and Evaluation Research (WIDER) recommendations. *Implementation Science, 8*, 52. https://doi.org/10.1186/1748-5908-8-52.

Allen, K. M., Dittmann, K. R., Hutter, J. A., Chuang, C., Donald, M. L., Enns, A. L., Hovanec, N., Hunt, A. W., Kellowan, R. S., Linkewich, E. A., Patel, A. S., Rehmtulla, A., & McEwen, S. E. (2020). Implementing a shared decision-making and cognitive strategy-based intervention: Knowledge user perspectives and recommendations. *Journal of Evaluation in Clinical Practice, 26*(2), 575–581. https://doi.org/10.1111/jep.13329.

Aveyard, H., & Sharp, P. (2017). In *A beginner's guide to evidence-based practice in health and social care* (3rd ed.). McGraw-Hill Education Open University Press.

Baldwin, J. A., Williamson, H. J., Eaves, E. R., Levin, B. L., Burton, D. L., Oliver, T., & Massey, O. T. (2017). Broadening measures of success: Results of a behavioral health translational research training program. *Implementation Science, 12*(92). https://doi.org/10.1186/s13012-017-0621-9.

Bannigan, K. (2007). Making sense of research utilisation. In J. Creek, & A. Lawson-Porter (Eds.), *Contemporary issues in occupational therapy: Reasoning and reflection* (pp. 189–216). John Wiley.

Bannigan, K. (2009). Knowledge exchange. In E. A. S. Duncan (Ed.), *Skills for practice in occupational therapy* (pp. 231–248). Elsevier.

Bennett, S. (2017). Knowledge translation in occupational therapy. *Australian Occupational Therapy Journal, 64*(5), 349–1349. https://doi-org.gcu.idm.oclc.org/10.1111/1440-1630.12433.

Bergström, A., Ehrenberg, A., Eldh, A. C., Graham, I. D., Gustafsson, K., Harvey, G., Hunter, S., Kitson, A., & Rycroft-Malone, J. (2020). The use of the PARIHS framework in implementation research and practice—a citation analysis of the literature. *Implementation Science, 15*, 68. https://doi.org/10.1186/s13012-020-01003-0.

Blase, K. A., Van Dyke, M., Fixsen, D. L., & Wallace, F. B. (2012). Implementation science: Key concepts, themes, and evidence for practitioners in educational psychology. In B. Kelly, & D. F. Perkins (Eds.), *Handbook of implementation science for psychology in education* (pp. 13–36). Cambridge University Press.

Breitenstein, S. M., Gross, D., Garvey, C. A., Hill, C., Fogg, L., & Resnick, B. (2010). Implementation fidelity in community-based interventions. *Research in Nursing & Health, 33*(2), 164–173. https://doi.org/10.1002/nur.20373.

Briggs, M. S., Rethman, K. K., Crookes, J., Cheek, F., Pottkotter, K., McGrath, S., DeWitt, J., Harmon-Matthews, L. E., & Quatman-Yates, C. C. (2020). Implementing patient-reported outcome measures in outpatient rehabilitation settings: A systematic review of facilitators and barriers using the consolidated framework for implementation research. *Archives of Physical Medicine & Rehabilitation, 101*(10), 1796–1812. https://doi.org/10.1016/j.apmr.2020.04.007.

Brown, T., & Robinson, L. (2019). Implementation science and AOTJ's role in bridging the occupational therapy best practice—Actual practice gap. *Australian Occupational Therapy Journal, 66*(2), 127–129. https://doi.org/10.1111/1440-1630.12576.

Clark, D. (2020). Public expenditure on medical research in the United Kingdom (UK) 2013–2019. Statista. https://www.statista.com/statistics/298897/united-kingdom-uk-public-sector-expenditure-medical-research/#:~:text=In%20the%20year%202015%2F16,totaled%201.6%20billion%20British%20pounds.

College of Occupational Therapists. (2015). Code of ethics and professional conduct. https://www.rcot.co.uk/practice-resources/rcot-publications/downloads/rcot-standards-and-ethics.

Colquhoun, H. L., Islam, R., Sullivan, K. J., Sandercock, J., Steinwender, S., & Grimshaw, J. M. (2020). Behaviour change domains likely to influence occupational therapist use of the Canadian Occupational Performance Measure. *Occupational Therapy International*. https://doi.org/10.1155/2020/3549835.

Colquhoun, H. L., Letts, L. J., Law, M. C., MacDermid, J. C., & Missiuna, C. A. (2010). A scoping review of the use of theory in studies of knowledge translation. *Canadian Journal of Occupational Therapy, 77*(5), 270–279. https://doi.org/10.2182/cjot.2010.77.5.3.

Connell, L. A., McMahon, N. E., Harris, J. E., Watkins, C. L., & Eng, J. J. (2014). A formative evaluation of the implementation of an upper limb stroke rehabilitation intervention in clinical practice: A qualitative interview study. *Implementation Science, 9*, 90. https://doi.org/10.1186/s13012-014-0090-3.

Culph, J., Clemson, L., Scanlan, J., Craven, L., Jeon, Y.H., & Laver, K. (2020). Exploring relationships between health professionals through the implementation of a reablement program for people with dementia: A mixed methods study. *Brain Impairment*, 1–13. https://doi.org/10.1017/BrImp.2020.2.

Damschroder, L. J., Aron, D. C., Keith, R. E., Kirsch, S. R., Jeffrey, A. A., & Lowery, J. C. (2009). Fostering implementation of health services research findings into practice: A consolidated framework for advancing implementation science. *Implementation Science, 4*, 50. https://doi.org/10.1186/1748-5908-4-50.

Davidson, K. W., Ye, S., & Mensah, G. A. (2017). Commentary: De-implementation science: A virtuous cycle of ceasing and desisting low-value care before implementing new high value care. *Ethnicity & Disease, 27*, 463–468. https://doi.org/10.18865/ed.27.4.463.

Donnelly, C. A., Cramm, H., Mofina, A., Lamontagne, M., Lal, S., & Colquhoun, H. (2016). Knowledge translation activities in occupational therapy organizations: The Canadian landscape. *The Open Journal of Occupational Therapy, 4*(2). https://doi.org/10.15453/2168-6408.1189.

Dopson, S., & Fitzgerald, L. (2005). The active role of context. In S. Dopson, & L. Fitzgerald (Eds.), *Knowledge to action? Evidence-based health care in context* (pp. 79–103). Oxford University Press.

Eccles, M. P., & Mittman, B. S. (2006). Welcome to implementation science. *Implementation Science, 1*, 1. https://doi.org/10.1186/1748-5908-1-1.

Eriksson, C., Erikson, A., Tham, K., & Guidetti, S. (2017). Occupational therapists' experiences of implementing a new complex intervention in collaboration with researchers: A qualitative longitudinal study. *Scandinavian Journal of Occupational Therapy, 24*(2), 116–125. http://dx.doi.org/10.1080/11038128.2016.1194465.

Field, B., Booth, A., Ilott, I., & Gerrish, K. (2014). Using the knowledge to action framework in practice: A citation analysis and systematic review. *Implementation Science, 9*, 172. https://doi.org/10.1186/s13012-014-0172-2.

Fixen, D. L., Blase, K., & Van Dyke, M. K. (2019). *Implementation practice and science*. Active Implementation Network.

Graham, I. D., Logan, J., Harrison, M. B., Straus, S. E., Tetroe, J., Caswell, W., & Robinson, N. (2006). Lost in knowledge translation: Time for a map? *Journal of Continuing Education in the Health Professions, 26*, 13–24. https://doi.org/10.1002/chp.47.

Grajo, L. C., Laverdure, P., Weaver, L. L., & Kingsley, K. (2020). Becoming critical consumers of evidence in occupational therapy for children and youth. *American Journal of Occupational Therapy, 74*(2), 1–7. https://doi.org/10.5014/ajot.2020.742001.

Greenhalgh, T. (2020). Foreword. In P. Nilsen, & S. A. Birken (Eds.), *Handbook of implementation science* (pp. xxii–xxiv). Edward Elgar Publishing Limited.

Guay, M., Ruest, M., & Contandriopoulos, D. (2019). Deimplementing untested practices in homecare services: A preobservational-postobservational design. *Occupational Therapy International*. https://doi.org/10.1155/2019/5638939.

Harvey, G., & Kitson, A. (2015). PARIHS revisited: From heuristic to integrated framework for the successful implementation of knowledge into practice. *Implementation Science, 11*, 33. https://doi.org/10.1186/s13012-016-0398-2.

Jones, C. A., Roop, S. C., Pohar, S. L., & Scott, S. D. (2015). Translating knowledge in rehabilitation: Systematic review. *Physical Therapy, 95*(4), 663–677. https://doi.org/10.2522/ptj.20130512.

Juckett, L. A., & Robinson, M. L. (2018). Implementing evidence-based interventions with community-dwelling older adults: A scoping review. *American Journal of Occupational Therapy, 72*(4), 1–9. https://doi.org/10.5014/ajot.2018.031583.

Juckett, L. A., Robinson, M. L., & Wengerd, L. R. (2019). Narrowing the gap: An implementation science research agenda for the occupational therapy profession. *The American Journal of Occupational Therapy, 73*(5). https://doiorg.10.5014/ajot.2019.033902.

Juckett, L. A., Wengerd, L. R., Faieta, J., & Griffin, C. E. (2020). Evidence-based practice implementation in stroke rehabilitation: A scoping review of barriers and facilitators. *American Journal of Occupational Therapy, 74*(1), 1–14. https://doi.org/10.5014/ajot.2020.035485.

Jutzi, K. S. R., Linekwich, E., Hunt, A. W., & McEwen, S. (2020). Does training in a top-down approach influence recorded goals and treatment plans? *Canadian Journal of Occupational Therapy, 87*(1), 42–51. https://doi.org/10.1177/0008417419848291.

Kitson, A., Harvey, G., & McCormack, B. (1998). Enabling the implementation of evidence based practice: A conceptual framework. *Quality in Health Care, 7*, 149–158. http://dx.doi.org/10.1136/qshc.7.3.149.

Laver, K. (2017). Patient-mediated interventions are an under-utilised approach to increasing knowledge translation in occupational therapy. *Australian Occupational Therapy Journal, 64*(2), 89–90. https://doi.org/10.1111/1440-1630.12388.

Leeman, J., & Nilsen, P. (2020). Strategies. In P. Nilsen, & S. A. Birken (Eds.), *Handbook of implementation science* (pp. 235–258). Edward Elgar Publishing Limited.

Lockwood, C., Stephenson, M., Lizarondo, L., Den Hoek, J., & Harrison, M. (2016). Evidence implementation: Development of an online methodology from the knowledge-to-action model of knowledge translation. *International Journal of Nursing Practice, 22*, 322–329.

Lomas, J. (1993). Diffusion, dissemination, and implementation: Who should do what? *Annals of the New York Academy of Sciences, 70*(3), 226–237. https://doi.org/10.1111/j.1749-6632.1993.tb26351.x.

Lomas, J. (2007). The in-between world of knowledge brokering. *British Medical Journal, 334*, 129–130. https://doi.org/10.1136/bmj.39038.593380.AE.

Mackenzie, L., & McKinstry, C. (2018). Knowledge translation in the context of the Asia Pacific region. *Australian Occupational Therapy Journal, 65*(3), 165–167. https://doi.org/10.1111/1440-1630.12487.

Metzler, M. J., & Metz, G. A. (2010). Translating knowledge to practice: An occupational therapy perspective. *Australian Occupational Therapy Journal, 57*(6), 373–379. https://doi-org.gcu.idm.oclc.org/10.1111/j.1440-1630.2010.00873.x.

National Health Service Centres for Reviews and Dissemination. (1999). Getting evidence into practice. *Effective Health Care, 5*(1). Royal Society of Medicine Press. https://www.york.ac.uk/media/crd/ehc51.pdf.

Nilsen, P. (2020). Overview of theories, models and frameworks in implementation science. In P. Nilsen, & S. A. Birken (Eds.), *Handbook of implementation science* (pp. 8–31). Edward Elgar Publishing Limited.

Nilsen, P., & Birken, S. A. (2020). Prologue. In P. Nilsen, & S. A. Birken (Eds.), *Handbook of implementation science* (pp. 1–7). Edward Elgar Publishing Limited.

Nilsen, P., Ingvarsson, S., Hasson, H., von Thiele Schwarz, U., & Augustsson, H. (2020). Theories, models, and frameworks for de-implementation of low-value care: A scoping review of the literature. *Implementation Research and Practice.*

Nott, M. T., Barden, H. L. H., Chapparo, C., & Ranka, J. L. (2020). Evidence based practice knowledge translation: A survey of Australian occupational therapy practice with clients experiencing neurocognitive impairments. *Australian Occupational Therapy Journal, 67*(1), 74–82. https://doi.org/10.1111/1440-1630.12625.

Proctor, E., Silmere, H., Raghavan, R., Hovmand, P., Aarons, G., Bunger, A., Griffey, R., & Hensley, M. (2011). Outcomes for implementation research: Conceptual distinctions, measurement challenges, and research agenda. *Administration and Policy in Mental Health and Mental Health Services Research, 38*, 65–76. https://doi.org/10.1007/s10488-010-0319-7.

Pyatak, E., King, M., Vigen, C. L. P., Salazar, E., Diaz, J., Schepens Niemiec, S. L., & Shukla, J. (2019). Addressing diabetes in primary care: Hybrid effectiveness–implementation study of Lifestyle Redesign® occupational therapy. *American Journal of Occupational Therapy, 73*(5). https://doi.org/10.5014/ajot.2019.037317.

Rapport, F., Clay-Williams, R., Churruca, K., Shih, P., Hogden, A., & Braithwaite, J. (2017). The struggle of translating science into action: Foundational concepts of implementation science. *Journal of Evaluation in Clinical Practice, 24*(1), 117–126. https://doi.org/10.1111/jep.12741.

Research America. (2019). U.S. investments in medical and health research and development 2013-2018. https://www.researchamerica.org/sites/default/files/Publications/InvestmentReport2019_Fnl.pdf.

Restall, G., Diaz, F., & Wittmeier, K. (2020). Why do clinical practice guidelines get stuck during implementation and what can be done: A case study in pediatric rehabilitation. *Physical & Occupational Therapy in Pediatrics, 40*(2), 217–230. https://doi.org/10.1080/01942638.2019.1660447.

Schell, S., Roth, K., & Duchow, H. (2020). Developmental coordination disorder in Alberta: A journey into knowledge translation. *Physical & Occupational Therapy in Pediatrics, 40*(3), 294–310. https://doi.org/10.1080/01942638.2019.1664704.

Slavin, R. (2012). Foreword. In B. Kelly, & D. F. Perkins (Eds.), *Handbook of implementation science for psychology in education* (pp. xv). Cambridge University Press.

Townley, A., Wincentak, J., Kingsnorth, S., & Raffaele, C. (2018). Feeding and swallowing: Aligning knowledge translation, research, and clinical practice to bring evidence to care. *Occupational Therapy Now, 20*(6), 28–30.

van Achterberg, T., Schoonhoven, L., & Grol, R. (2008). Nursing implementation science: How evidence-based nursing requires evidence-based implementation. *Journal of Nursing Scholarship, 40*(4), 302–310. https://doi.org/10.1111/j.1547-5069.2008.00243.x.

Verhagen, E. (2020). Guideline implementation requires a dialogue between research and practice. *International Journal of Therapy and Rehabilitation, 21*(4), 157. https://doi-org.gcu.idm.oclc.org/10.12968/ijtr.2014.21.4.157.

Warner, G., & Stadnyk, R. (2014). What is the evidence and context for implementing family-centered care for older adults? *Physical & Occupational Therapy in Geriatrics, 32*(3), 255–270. https://doi.org/10.3109/02703181.2014.934942.

Warner, G., & Townsend, E. (2012). Applying knowledge translation theories to occupation. *Occupational Therapy Now, 14*(2), 19–21.

White, C., Colquhoun, H., Cramm, H., & Lai, S. (2013). Developing a knowledge translation strategy in occupational therapy. *Occupational Therapy Now, 15*(6), 16–18.

World Health Organization. (2004). World report on knowledge for better health: Strengthening health systems. https://apps.who.int/iris/handle/10665/4305.

Zur, B. (2016). A new opportunity for knowledge translation. CJOT: Evidence for your practice. *Occupational Therapy Now, 18*(3), 8.

Leadership, Supervision, and Management Skills for Practice

14

Improvement Science in Practice

Lianne McInally

HIGHLIGHTS

- Improvement science has been adapted from industry into health care.
- This chapter provides an introduction to what improvement science is, its use within health care in general and within occupational therapy.

- Specific synergies are highlighted between the principles of improvement science and the principles and practice of occupational therapy.
- The chapter provides succinct introductions to a range of improvement science methods.

WHAT IS IMPROVEMENT SCIENCE?

Improvement science is about finding out how to improve and make changes in the most effective way. It is about systematically examining the methods and factors that best work to facilitate quality improvement.
(Health Foundation, 2011).

DEFINING QUALITY

Quality and quality improvement can mean different things to different people. If you think about a product or service you have recently received, then there may be multiple reasons why you thought that you received a quality product or service. These may differ from the thoughts and experiences of someone else.

The World Health Organization (WHO, 2006) describes six dimensions of quality that are often viewed as a universal definition of quality in health care:

1. **Effective:** delivering health care that is adherent to an evidence base and results in improved health outcomes for individuals and communities, based on need
2. **Efficient:** delivering health care in a manner that maximises resource use and avoids waste
3. **Accessible:** delivering health care that is timely, geographically reasonable, and provided in a setting where skills and resources are appropriate to medical need
4. **Acceptable/patient centred:** delivering health care that takes into account the preferences and aspirations of individual service users and the cultures of their communities

5. **Equitable:** delivering health care that does not vary in quality because of personal characteristics such as gender, race, ethnicity, geographic location, or socioeconomic status
6. **Safe:** delivering health care that minimises risks and harm to service users

IMPROVEMENT VERSUS RESEARCH

The World Federation of Occupational Therapists (WFOT, 2021) recognises the importance of promoting the development of research evidence to support responsive, ethical, culturally sensitive, and contextually relevant occupational therapy practice. Graduate programmes for occupational therapists have focused on research methodologies to support practice.

Improvement science approaches also have a role to play in the practice of Occupational Therapy.

There are similarities between research and improvement science as they both involve qualitative and quantitative data. Sometimes the data is collected (e.g. through observations, interviews, measures). Sometimes, the data may already exist and analysed in different ways depending on the type of data.

However, there are also some distinctions between research and improvement science. Research follows rigorous methods, which often have strict guidelines. Research aims to answer specific questions. Research designs vary according to the question being asked, some are specific and hypothesis focused, others consider greater complexity and integrate understanding of context with an evaluation of specific outcomes.

Improvement science differs in its approach to knowledge generation. The focus may be on a specific problem, system or process. The sample size is normally small initially (e.g. one patient, one staff member, one area/ward). Once improvements are noted in one area, larger numbers of people are involved. Improvements can be rapidly adopted, adapted or abandoned depending on the results. In this way, the evidence is built over a series of cycles that are known as plan, do study, act (PDSA) test cycles. These cycles can take place sequentially or in parallel.

QUALITY IMPROVEMENT AND IMPROVEMENT SCIENCE

Quality improvement and the application of improvement science draws on a wide range of methods and tools with a knowledge of the subject matter to develop, test, spread, and implement changes.

Improvement science has been used globally as a focused approach to improve quality within health care systems for many years. However, in 2006, the WHO highlighted that, notwithstanding this effort, there was evidence that quality efforts varied and in some areas the standard of health care delivery remained unchanged. The expected health care improvement outcomes were often not being achieved, particularly in low- and middle-income countries.

In 2018, the WHO, Organisation for Economic Co-operation and Development (OECD), and World Bank highlighted that substandard care wastes significant resources and harms the health of populations, destroying human capital and reducing productivity. These three global institutions recommended a quality call to action and for the provision of universal health coverage by 2030. Their aim is to achieve universal access to high-quality, people-centred health services (WHO et al., 2018).

These institutions recommended actions for governments, health systems, citizens and patients, and health care workers to ensure that the universal health coverage aim is met. Quality improvement and improvement science is threaded through these recommendations. In summary, they recommend that all governments should have a national quality policy and strategy, all health systems should implement evidence-based interventions that demonstrate improvement, all citizens and patients should be empowered to actively engage in care to optimise their health status, and all health care workers should participate in quality measurement and improvement with their patients (WHO et al., 2018). Knowledge about and use of improvement science and quality

improvement is therefore an imperative of good occupational therapy practice.

ORIGINS OF IMPROVEMENT SCIENCE

The science of improvement originated from the work of W. Edwards Deming, an engineer and academic who believed that you could improve all aspects of life and advance prosperity and peace through systems thinking (The W. Edwards Deming Institute, 2020). He spent his lifetime learning and teaching about the application of quality improvement within the areas of science, management, and engineering. In 1982, Deming published a book that outlined 14 key principles for management to follow to significantly improve the effectiveness of a business or organisation. Following this, Deming (1994) encapsulated these 14 principles in a model known as the system of profound knowledge (SoPK).

THE SYSTEM OF PROFOUND KNOWLEDGE

The application of SPoK as the lens for quality improvement (Fig. 14.1) is now viewed as fundamental to the science of improvement. SoPK has four components: appreciation of the system, human behaviour, understanding variation, and theory of knowledge. These components are interrelated, and there is a dependency on ensuring that all aspects of the lens are considered.

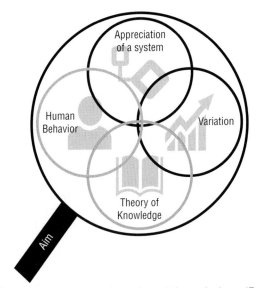

FIG. 14.1 The lens of profound knowledge. (From The Network for Improvement and Innovation. [2020]. Step 4 Understand the problem. College Health. https://collegehealthqi.nyu.edu/.)

- Appreciation of a system: All the elements of a system are united by a common aim. Processes and flow impact on the system. There are connections and interactions across the system.
- Human behaviour: This important element recognises that human beings are not cogs on a machine. Everyone brings individual talents and abilities. Creating an environment where people flourish is important.
- Understanding variation: Data are important. What do current data tell you? What areas are working well? Where do you need to improve?
- Theory of knowledge: Understanding how people think and act based on their predictions underpins the theory of knowledge. Often people see what they want to see based on their own beliefs, rather than what is evidence based. Using PDSA cycles allows individuals to understand whether their predictions result in improvement.

KOTTER EIGHT-STEP CHANGE MODEL

Improving quality within systems involves change. It has been said that "the world is now changing at a rate at which the basic systems, structures and cultures cannot keep up with the demands placed on them" (Kotter, 2014, p. vii).

John Kotter of the Harvard Business School highlighted that 70% of improvement initiatives fail because most organisations do not put in the necessary steps or see the project through to completion. He published an eight-step model to leading change in organisations and advocates that it is even more relevant now than when first published due to the speed at which change continues to increase (Kotter, 2012).

Eight-Step Change Model*

Step 1: Establish a sense of urgency. Complacency in an organisation stifles the ability of people within the organisation to make changes. It can be difficult to create enough power in the system to drive improvements. Establishing a sense of urgency helps to accelerate changes as people are more invested. Understanding the system can help to identify areas of urgency. The Covid-19 pandemic is one example of a crisis that has created the sense of urgency for improvement.

Step 2: Create a guiding coalition. Building a team with the right composition, level of trust, and shared objective supports improvement. There are four key characteristics to the team: having the key players with positions of power and influence, expertise of the team, credibility, and leadership.

Step 3: Develop a vision and strategy. Investing in creating a shared vision and strategy that is owned by everyone involved helps to accelerate the changes that result in improvement.

Step 4: Communicate the vision. The power of a vision is unleashed when communicated and shared. This helps motivate and coordinate the kinds of actions that create transformations.

Step 5: Empower employees for broad-based action. If employees feel powerless, then it is difficult for them to engage in change. Sharing a sense of purpose, making structures compatible with the vision, providing training, aligning information, and confronting blockers are all ways to empower employees and improve motivation for change.

Step 6: Generate short-term wins. Being able to see that your efforts are generating positive results motivates people to continue to take part in change. Short-term wins ensure that you can keep the momentum of change building.

Step 7: Consolidate gains and produce more change. Take time to ensure that the new practices are firmly grounded in the organisation's culture.

Step 8: Anchor new approaches in the culture. Cultural change is the last step and occurs at the end of a transformation process.

HUMAN FACTORS AND ERGONOMICS FOR IMPROVEMENT

Human factors and ergonomics explores a problem by looking at the people within a system, their interactions with each other, and the system and then redesigning the tasks, interfaces, and system (Hignett et al., 2015). Some of the early safety work in the aeroplane industry focused on human factors and ergonomics. More recently this approach has been recommended in health care particularly in relation to medication errors, wrong diagnoses, poor communication, and medical device failure (Chartered Institute of Ergonomics and Human Factors). Human factors and ergonomic theory can be appropriately combined with improvement science methods in health care settings.

IMPROVEMENT SCIENCE AND THE CONNECTION WITH OCCUPATIONAL THERAPY

The knowledge and skills of occupational therapists provide an excellent basis to apply improvement science within their practice and within the organisations in which they work. As with improvement science, occupational therapy practice is focused on the concept of improvement. It works

---

*Adapted from Kotter, J. P. (2012). Leading change. Harvard Business School.

"with people and communities to enhance their ability to engage in the occupations they want to, need to, or are expected to do, or modifying the occupation or the environment to better support their occupational engagement".

Various synergies exist between the conceptual models and frames of reference of occupational therapy practice (Duncan, 2021) and improvement science. Like the WHO (2006) dimensions of quality, occupational therapy practice is set within a person-centred framework (Parker & Sutherland, 2021). Comparisons can be drawn between the person-environment occupation performance (PEOP) model (Baum et al., 2021) and SoPK. Both PEOP and SoPK are based on systems theory and apply this either to an individual or community (in the case of occupational therapy) or an organisation or staff group (in the case of quality improvement). The initial stage of appreciation of a system can be compared with the initial interview process with a person where the occupational therapist begins to understand what matters to the individual. The psychology of human behaviour can be compared to the person's occupations and understanding variation to the performance data that are established with an individual through observation and standardised assessment. The theory of knowledge can be compared to occupational therapy practice where the person's and occupational therapist's perceptions of prediction may influence the outcomes. The intervention process where the tasks are broken down, analysed, and modified to ensure that improvement is made over time are similar to the PDSA process outlined earlier.

The model of human occupation (MOHO) Kielhofner (2008) also links with improvement science. Within MOHO occupational therapists review individuals' readiness for change and volition. This parallels with Kotter's (2012) eight-step change model, where the state of readiness of a team or organisation may influence their ability to establish a sense of urgency and empower employees for broad-based action. There is also a connection to occupational therapy practice and human factors and ergonomics, as occupational therapists have a strong basis in ergonomics through their anatomy, physiology, and activity analysis knowledge (American Association of Occupational Therapists, 2017).

IMPROVEMENT JOURNEY

The improvement journey taken during a quality improvement project or initiative involves drawing on the wide range of methods and tools of improvement science. NHS Education Scotland (2020) has developed an interactive quality improvement zone online that includes free resources to support people with experience at all levels of quality improvement to develop their knowledge. The improvement journey outlined on the NHS Education Scotland website is underpinned by the theories of Deming and Kotter outlined earlier. NHS Education Scotland (2020) recognises that the journey is likely to be more fluid and may move back as well as forward. The improvement journey includes these concepts:

- Build the will and conditions for change
- Understand the current system
- Develop and aim and change theory
- Identify specific change ideas, test and refine using PDSA
- Implement and sustain change where tested
- Share the learning and spread where relevant

Project Charter

A project charter is a plan to record the intended improvement journey from start to finish. A project charter template is normally completed at the start of a project or initiative. It is helpful at the very start of an improvement journey to familiarise yourself with the project charter questions to enable you to think about all the different elements that will be required. It is a fluid document that should change over time depending on the outcomes of PDSA cycles.

The following key questions should be contained in a project charter*:

What are you trying to accomplish (your aim statement)?
Why is this important? (e.g., what is the rationale and business case for your improvement project?)
- What problem will the work address and what is the impact of doing nothing?
- How do you know this is a problem and what is your starting position?
- How big a gap is there between where you are and where you want to be?
- How does your aim fit into the strategic vision of your organisation?
- What is the expected impact (outcomes, benefits, cost)
- Why do you believe the time scale you have set is realistic?

What is the scope of the project?
- Who, specifically, will be affected by the success or failure of this project (children impacted by your services, staff, patients, community, etc.)?
- How many people/how large an area is included in your project?
- Are there any processes/areas of work associated with the problem that won't be included in your project?

*Adapted from NHS Scotland 2020 sample Project Charter Template.

How will you know that a change is an improvement?

What measures will you use to help you monitor progress toward your goal? These should include:

- Outcome: how you will track the progress of your improvement aim
- Process: how you will know whether the parts of the system you are trying to change (to get you to your improvement aim) are performing and the impact of your changes on these
- Balancing: areas you need to keep watch in case your action has an unintended impact on other parts of the system or to see if something unrelated to your project is influencing project success

What changes can you make that will lead to improvement?

- Do you have some initial ideas that your team can test to move toward your goal? What can you change about how your processes and system currently operate to make things better? Tasks and activities are different to change ideas and should not be included here. They are included in the next section.
- Is there evidence about what works?
- What are the subject experts telling you?
- Have you conducted any "as is" analysis (e.g., cause and effect, process mapping) that has generated change ideas?

What initial activities do you have planned?

These are the tasks associated with your project—not to be confused with change ideas (e.g., setting up an improvement team, gathering baseline data, and applying improvement tools to help you understand how things are currently working to help identify change ideas)

Participation (team membership) and leadership support

Who is on your improvement team? People to consider:

- Subject matter expert
- Process owners who can make changes
- Representatives of those impacted by your project (families, young people, patients, customers, etc.)
- Finance representative, if needed
- Sponsor with links to executive level for leadership support

What may risk the success of your project?

- List any risks associated with your project and any action you have planned to monitor or manage these.

The Responsible, Accountable, Consulted, or Informed (RACI) MATRIX

Improvement projects fail when staff do not have ownership or control over the direction of the improvement journey. A RACI matrix (Jacka & Keller, 2009) is a good tool to determine who is responsible, accountable, consulted, or informed about the various aspects of the project. Having clear expectations of each of the key stakeholders enables the people involved to have clarity of roles and responsibilities.

Build the Will and Conditions for Change

The importance of the human side of change should never be underestimated. According to Diniakos and Senn (2011), organisational and individual habits can either support or undermine a healthy, high-performance culture. Habits mean that we do what we have always done. Individuals' own perspectives of a situation will depend on whether they perceive that a change is required. This can lead to resistance if the proposed change is not seen as a benefit. Kotter (2014) advocates that to make change happen, you harness the power of the people and maintain a strong sense of urgency through the big opportunity that the change will create. It is important to build the will and the conditions for change at the start by identifying who the key people are that will be required to make the change happen. This may involve a small group of people initially; however, it is important to consider if the change is to be scaled and spread where this would happen and who may be required to be consulted or informed. It is equally important at this stage to think how you will engage these people in the improvement project. This may be through communication updates or reports that inform them of the progress, or they may be part of a steering group. This will help to eliminate any issues that may arise managing change in the future.

Understand the Current System

To identify changes that are required for improvement, it is important to understand the current system. Similarly to occupational therapy, a holistic appreciation of the system is required, and there are a number of tools that can be utilised to facilitate this. The most common tools are outlined in this section.

Surveys/Feedback

Surveys and feedback are used to gather information and are recognised as a tool to provide the opportunity for improvement (Provost & Murray, 2011). Information can be gathered about aspects of patient care or to collate the views of staff.

Pareto Chart

A Pareto chart is a type of bar graph that plots a number of variables. These are plotted from highest to lowest value. Qualitative data can be transferred into a count (e.g., the number of occurrences of a particular theme of

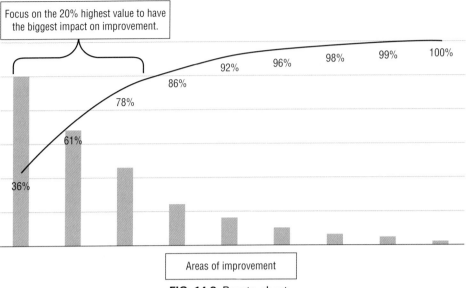

Focus on the 20% highest value to have the biggest impact on improvement.

36% 61% 78% 86% 92% 96% 98% 99% 100%

Areas of improvement

FIG. 14.2 Pareto chart.

complaints). The principle of a Pareto chart (Fig. 14.2) is that 80% of the problems are due to 20% of the reasons for the problem. This is known as the 80-20 rule. If you focus your improvement efforts on the 20% of your problems with the highest value (known as the vital few) then this will lead to improvement (Langley et al., 2009). If we consider how some projects fail because they do not result in improvement, much is due to the time, energy, and effort being focused on the wrong area.

Process Mapping

Understanding the current processes is an important aspect of improvement. There are various approaches to process mapping ranging from flow diagrams, process-outputs-customer diagrams, to value stream mapping (Langley et al., 2009). These can be a simple map or a complex systems map. Mapping normally takes place with a group. Sticky notes are helpful to use to plot a draft process before formalising it. During the process mapping, areas of waste or gaps for improvement may be identified. Sometimes there can be differing opinions on the way particular processes are completed. This highlights the human aspects of improvement where information or processes are interpreted differently. This can help to identify areas where efficiency and effectiveness of processes may be improved.

Fishbone Diagram

A fishbone diagram, also known as a cause-and-effect diagram or Ishikawa diagram, is a tool used to help organise

current knowledge about potential causes of problems or variation. It visually looks like fish bones where the head is the problem and the skeleton is the potential causes or variation (Fig. 14.3). This is often a helpful visual representation to understand where areas of improvement are required.

Forcefield Analysis

Forcefield analysis is a visual tool displaying information on the forces for and against change. The tool may uncover restraining or driving forces that those planning changes are unaware of (Langley et al., 2009). A comparison can be made between the current driving and restraining forces versus the potential driving and restraining forces. This allows you to plan for improvement.

Develop and Aim or Change Theory

The next step in the improvement journey is to develop and aim or change theory. The model for improvement is utilised to support this.

Model for Improvement

The model for improvement (Fig. 14.4) was developed by the Associates in Process Improvement. It is split into two parts often referred to as the thinking part and the doing part. Part 1, the thinking part, asks three key questions:
- What are we trying to accomplish?
- How will we know that a change is an improvement?
- What change can we make that will result in improvement?

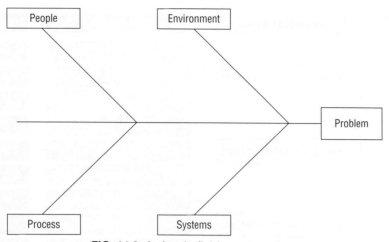

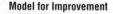

FIG. 14.3 A simple fishbone template.

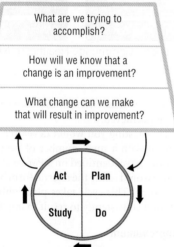

FIG. 14.4 Model for improvement. (From Associates in Process Improvement. [2020].)

These three questions are part of the project charter described earlier. Part 2, the doing part, is the previously referred to PDSA cycle of testing.

Aim Statements

An aim statement describes the vision of the improvement project (e.g., What are we trying to accomplish?). An aim statement should be SMART (specific, measurable, achievable, relevant, and timed). The statement aligns to the goals of the team or organisation. Without a clear aim statement, a team can become side-tracked or focus efforts in the wrong place (Provost & Murray, 2011).

Driver Diagram

A driver diagram is a visual display of the theory for improvement in a project. There are four key components of a driver diagram: aim, primary drivers, secondary drivers, and change ideas.

- Aim: The vision of the improvement project (as outlined in aim statements).
- Primary drivers: factors or improvement areas that must be addressed to achieve the desired outcome
- Secondary drivers: linked to the primary drivers, are specific areas where you plan changes or interventions
- Change ideas: ideas that you plan to test to determine if they will result in improvement

Central London Community Healthcare NHS Trust designed an online driver diagram template to help teams document their improvement projects (NHS Improvement, 2020) (Fig. 14.5).

PDSA Cycle of Testing

Part 2, the doing part of the model for improvement, is the PDSA cycle of testing. Often you will hear staff talking about tests of change. Sometimes in improvement projects people make the mistake of trying to fix the problem by doing before they complete the thinking element of the model for improvement.

The cycle of improvement starts with planning the details of the change idea that you wish to test, conducting the plan and collecting the data, studying the data to determine if the change idea resulted in improvement or if modifications are required, and lastly acting on the changes. There are three questions at this stage: Will you adapt the change (some improvement but not as much as predicted)? Will you adopt the change (as it worked)? Will you abandon the

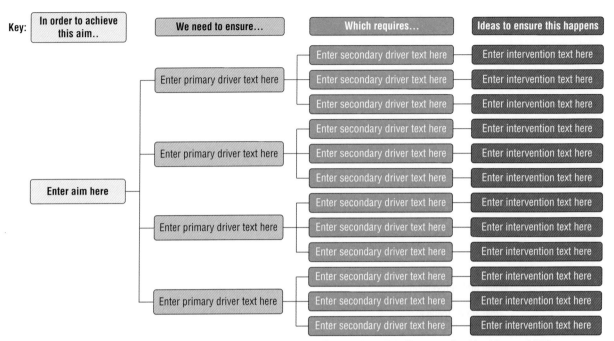

FIG. 14.5 Driver diagram template. (Designed by Central London Community Healthcare NHS Trust.)

efforts (as it failed)? If you decide to adapt the change then another PDSA cycle would take place.

This can be likened to occupational therapy practice where you plan an intervention with an individual or group, try the intervention, measure the result through observation or standardised assessment, and then decide whether to adapt, adopt, or abandon that particular intervention. Once an improvement process has been adopted, it can be determined if it can be scaled or spread to another area. It is important that the test takes place independently so that you know that the factors being tested result in improvement. If you test too many changes at once, it is difficult to determine what change has resulted in improvement. Starting small is important. This means testing with one individual or one area. Sequentially testing and then scaling up allows you to quickly make adjustments and know what is working.

PDSA testing does not mean that you require perfection first time around. Often previous pilot work has introduced new processes where time has been spent on perfecting the design, missed testing, and moved to implementation, normally on a large scale. For example, a new referral process is circulated to everyone referring to occupational therapy. Time is spent on developing a referral form making sure that the content is perfect and then it is sent to everyone who is able to refer to the service. This is known as "spray and pray," where you disseminate an improvement

and hope that it works. Often in this scenario the desired outcome is not achieved.

Using PDSA testing you would develop a draft referral form and try it with a small number of people (often the people who you have identified on a Pareto chart who refer the most). You would refine the referral form based on studying the outcome. This cycle takes place until the referral process is found consistently to result in improvement.

Data for Improvement

Data for improvement is important to help deliver the aim and understand what changes are resulting in improvement. One of the key strategies in improvement is to control variation (Provost & Murray, 2011). Data enable analysis of variation of what is being measured over a period of time. This approach varies from the occupational therapy practice where therapists often review data pre- and postintervention.

When measuring for improvement there are three types of measures that will be collected:
- Outcome: associated with the aim of the project
- Process: processes that must happen reliably to achieve the desired outcomes
- Balancing: measures that determine any unintended consequences of the improvement elsewhere in the system

Normally there is more than one measurement that is gathered to identify improvement.

Displaying Data

In addition to the previously described Pareto charts, two other charts are helpful to understand variation: a run chart and a Shewart chart (also known as a process behaviour chart). These charts are recommended to be completed in real time. A run chart is a simple line graph that reviews data over time. This may be plotted with paper and pen or using an electronic spreadsheet. There are three core questions that Graban (2019) suggests are important to consider when reviewing the data on a run chart:

1. Are we achieving our target or goal?
   a) Occasionally?
   b) Consistently?
2. Are we improving?
   a) Can we predict future performance?
3. How do we improve?
   a) When do we react?
   b) When do we step back and improve the system?
   c) How can we prove we've improved? (p. 23)

Once you have 10 or more data points on a run chart, you should display a median line (Fig. 14.6). The median is the middle number in a sorted (ascending or descending) list of numbers and can be more descriptive of that data set than the average.

There are four run chart rules known as STAR that help to understand a variation in the data (Fig. 14.7):
- **Shift:** 6 or more points all above or below the median

- **Trend:** 5 or more consecutive points all going up or all going down
- **Astronomical:** a data point that lies dramatically outside the other data points. It would appear unusual to anyone looking at a chart. It signals a non-random pattern.
- **Runs:** too many or too few points will tell you whether the data have too few or too many runs (number of times the data cross the median) based on the number of useful observations

A Shewart (process behaviour) chart is a statistical chart that allows you to measure variation caused either by common causes or by special causes. Common cause variation is expected within a system, whereas special cause is unexpected within the system from unusual occurrences. A comparison of both types of variation could be described when baking a cake. The temperature of the oven may vary slightly during baking, which would be common cause variation. On the other hand, if you were to open the oven or changed the temperature dial on the oven, then the temperature would fluctuate. This is special cause variation where there is an attributable cause. There are different types of charts for different types of data.

Implement and Sustain Change Where Tested

Following the adoption of a change it is important to implement and sustain change. There are three forms of implementation (NHS Education Scotland, 2020):

1. Just do it: implement immediately
2. Parallel: run the new change in parallel with the old process and gradually phase out the old process
3. Sequential: build the change in sequence

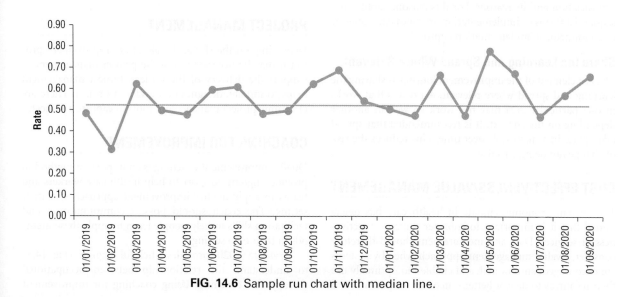

FIG. 14.6 Sample run chart with median line.

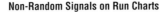

Non-Random Signals on Run Charts

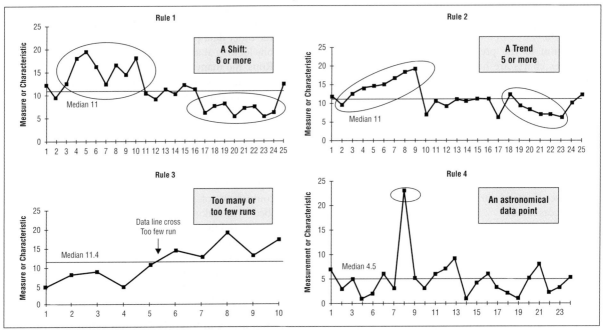

Evidence of a non-random signal if one or more of the circumstances depicted by these four rules are on the run chart. The first three rules are violations of random patterns and are based on a probability of less than 5% chance of occurring just by chance with no change.

FIG. 14.7 Run chart rules. (From Provost, L. P., & Murray, S. K. [2011]. *The health care data guide.* Jossey-Bass.)

Improvement data can support implementation as the impact of implementation can be monitored to identify variation and its reasons. For this reason, parallel and sequential forms of implementation are viewed as superior to an immediate implementation approach.

Share the Learning and Spread Where Relevant

The last element of the improvement journey is sharing the learning and spread where relevant. A process that works in one particular area may not work so well in another depending on the context. It is recommended that spread takes place in a small scale over time. This reduces the risk of change not being effective.

COST EFFECTIVENESS/VALUE MANAGEMENT

The current economic climate in health care has determined that it is important to consider the cost effectiveness of services. Data and measurement should therefore consider a value management approach whereby systems are encouraged, empowered, and enabled to optimally use their resources to deliver better outcomes for patients and

achieve financial sustainability (Institute for Healthcare Improvement, 2020).

PROJECT MANAGEMENT

Depending on the size and scale of an improvement project it may be necessary to utilise project management to support the delivery of the project. Project management helps to initiate, design, and develop a project. There are electronic project management tools to capture a project.

COACHING FOR IMPROVEMENT

Quality improvement coaching is an important method to provide ongoing support to help health care workers and teams to apply quality improvement approaches in their setting. The coach should possess communication and facilitation skills to help people learn to apply these methods in their own setting.

Drysdale (2020) provides a helpful diagram (Fig. 14.8) to understand the relationship between occupational therapy and coaching. Using coaching for improvement

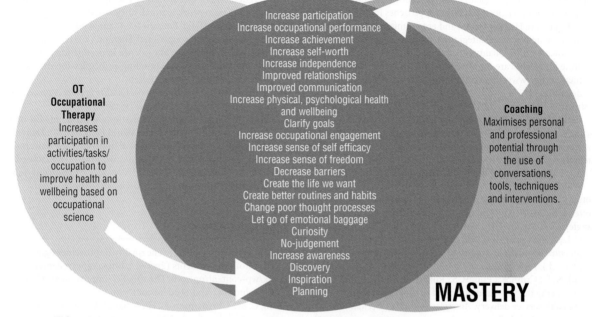

FIG. 14.8 Coaching for improvement. (From Drysdale, B. (2020). The master of doing what is coaching. https://masteryofdoing.com.au/what-is-ot-coaching/.)

creates a powerful motivator and driver of positive change. The outcomes for the individual or the organisation can be a very successful way to enable them to move forward.

SUMMARY

Improvement science is a well-established discipline. It is increasingly used in health care settings across the world and offers a breadth of methods to employ to improve quality in practice. There are many similarities between improvement science and occupational therapy. It is important for occupational therapists to embrace their skill set and harness their abilities to improve outcomes and processes for individuals, groups, and communities.

REFLECTIVE LEARNING

- Where could the principles and practice of improvement science be used in practice situations I know?
- What are the main opportunities and barriers to using improvement science in practice?
- How could I introduce improvement science into a practice area I am familiar with?
- What are the limitations of improvement science when trying to improve practice?

REFERENCES

American Association of Occupational Therapists. (2017). Occupational therapy practitioners and ergonomics. https://www.aota.org/About-Occupational-Therapy/Professionals/WI/Ergonomics.aspx.

Associates in Process Improvement. (2020). http://www.apiweb.org/index.php.

Baum, C. M., Bass, J. D., & Christiansen, C. H. (2021). The person-environment occupation performance model. In E. A. S. Duncan (Ed.), *Foundations for practice in occupational therapy* (6th ed., pp. 87–95). Elsevier.

Deming, W. E. (1982). *Out of the crisis.* Massachusetts Institute of Technology.

Deming, W. E. (1994). In *The new economics for industry, government and education* (2nd ed.). Massachusetts Institute of Technology.

Diniakos, P. R., & Senn, L. (2011). In *The human operating system* (5th ed.). Senn Delaney.

Drysdale, B. (2020). The master of doing what is coaching. https://masteryofdoing.com.au/what-is-ot-coaching/.

Duncan, E. A. S. (Ed.). (2021). *Foundations for practice in occupational therapy* (6th ed.). Elsevier.

Graban, M. (2019). *Measures of success: React less, lead better, improve more.* Constancy.

Health Foundation. (2011). Improvement science. https://www.health.org.uk/publications/improvement-science.

Health Foundation. (2013). *Quality improvement made simple: What everyone should know about healthcare quality improvement.* Author.

Hignett S, Jones Human factors and ergonomics and quality improvement science: integrating approaches for safety in healthcare Human factors and ergonomics and quality improvement science: integrating approaches for safety in healthcare | BMJ Quality & Safety.

Institute for Healthcare Improvement. (2020). Value management. http://www.ihi.org/Topics/QualityCostValue/Pages/default.aspx.

Institute of Medicine. (2001). *Crossing the quality chasm: A new health system for the 21st century*. National Academy Press.

Jacka, M., & Keller, P. (2009). *Business process mapping: Improving customer satisfaction*. John Wiley and Sons.

Kielhofner, G. (2008). Model of Human Occupation: Theory and Application. Fourth Edition. Philadelphia, PA : Lippincott, Williams and Wilkins.

Kotter, J. P. (2012). *Leading change*. Harvard Business School.

Kotter, J. P. (2014). *XLR8 accelerate*. Harvard Business School.

Langley, G. J., Meon, R. D., Nolan, K. M., Nolan, T. W., Normal, C. L., & Provost, L. P. (2009). In *The improvement guide: a practical approach to enhancing organisational performance* (2nd ed.). Jossey-Bass.

Leland, N. E., Crum, K., Phipps, S., Roberts, P., & Gage, B. (2015). Advancing the value and quality of occupational therapy in health service delivery. *American Journal of Occupational Therapy*, *69*(1), 1–7.

Moses, J. (2020). *What's the difference between research and QI?* [video]. http://www.ihi.org/education/IHIOpenSchool/resources/Pages/Activities/Moses-ResearchVsQI.aspx.

NHS Education Scotland. (2020). Implementation. https://learn.nes.nhs.scot/10103/quality-improvement-zone/improvement-journey/implement/implementation.

NHS Improvement. (2018). A model for measuring quality. ACT Academy Online Library of Quality Service Improvement and Redesign Tools. https://webarchive.nationalarchives.gov.uk/20201029174745/ https://improvement.nhs.uk/resources/measuring-quality-care/.

NHS Improvement. (2020). Driver diagrams. https://improvement.nhs.uk/resources/creating-driver-diagrams-for-improvement-projects/.

Parker, D. M., & Sutherland, C. (2021). The person-centred frame of reference. In E. A. S. Duncan (Ed.), *Foundations for practice in occupational therapy* (6th ed., pp. 128–140). Elsevier.

Provost, L. P., & Murray, S. K. (2011). *The health care data guide*. Jossey-Bass.

The Network for Improvement and Innovation. (2020). Step 4 Understand the problem. https://collegehealthqi.nyu.edu/improvement-journey/4-understand-the-problem/.

The W. Edwards Deming Institute. (2020). System of profound knowledge. https://deming.org/explore/sopk/.

World Federation of Occupational Therapists. (2016). Code of ethics. https://www.wfot.org/resources/code-of-ethics.

World Federation of Occupational Therapists. (2018). Quality indicators framework manual. https://www.wfot.org/assets/resources/WFOT-QI-Framework-Manual.pdf.

World Federation of Occupational Therapy. (2021). Guiding principles from the use of evidence in occupational therapy. https://wfot.org/resources/guiding-principles-for-the-use-of-evidence-in-occupational-therapy.

World Health Organisation. (2006). *Quality of care: A process for making strategic choices in health systems*. Author.

World Health Organisation, Organisation for Economic Co-operation and Development, & The World Bank. (2018). Delivering quality health services: A global imperative for universal health coverage. http://documents1.worldbank.org/curated/en/482771530290792652/pdf/127816-REVISED-quality-joint-publication-July2018-Complete-vignettes-ebook-L.pdf.

BIBLIOGRAPHY

1000livesplus Wales. (2012). The quality improvement guide for educators and students (2nd ed.). https://gpexcellencegm.org.uk/wp-content/uploads/The-Quality-Improvement-Guide-for-Educators-and-Students.pdf.

Baum, C. M., Christiansen, C. H., & Bass, J. D. (2015). In *Occupational therapy: Performance, participation, and well-being* (4th ed.). Slack Inc.

Centre for Creative Leadership. (2020). Characteristics of a good leader. https://www.ccl.org/blog/characteristics-good-leader/.

Covey, S. R. (1999). *Principle centred leadership*. Simon & Schuster.

Dixon-Woods, M., McNicol, S., & Martin, G. (2012). *Overcoming challenges to improving quality*. The Health Foundation.

Fresko, A., & Rubenstein, S. (2013). *Taking safety on board: The boards role in patient safety*. The Health Foundation.

Marquet, L. D. (2015). *Turn the ship around a true story of turning followers in to leaders*. Penguin.

Mullins, L. J. (2016). In *Management and organisational behaviour* (11th ed.). Prentice Hall.

Perry, C., Chhatralia, K., Damestick, D., Hobden, S., & Volpe, L. (2015). *Behavioural insights in health care*. The Health Foundation.

Senn, L., & Hart, J. (2010). In *Winning teams, winning cultures* (2nd ed.). Senn Delaney.

Starr, J. (2016). In *The coaching manual: The definitive guide to the process, principles and skills of personal coaching* (4th ed.). Pearson.

Vincent, C., Burnett, S., & Carthey, J. (2013). *The measurement and monitoring of safety*. The Health Foundation.

Vissers, J., & Beech, R. (2005). *Health operations management: Patient flow logistics in health care*. Routledge.

Whetten, D. A., & Cameron, K. S. (2015). In *Developing management skills* (9th ed.). Pearson.

15

Developing Research Skills in Practice

Edward A.S. Duncan

HIGHLIGHTS

- People have various reasons for wanting to "do" research in practice.
- There are increasing opportunities to actively participate in research in practice.
- Research career opportunities are now beginning to unfold. These require a structured and comprehensive research training.

- Deciding what to research requires careful consideration.
- Research collaborations vary in form but are essential for most practice-based research. These require careful consideration in order that you find the best collaborator(s) and clearly articulate your expectations of the collaboration.

INTRODUCTION

The emphasis on research is probably the biggest development in occupational therapy practice in recent years. Whilst research once appeared a very remote issue to most practitioners, today it is central to the reality of their everyday working lives. Developing research in practice, however, is not simple. If it were, there would not be such a dearth of evidence. Doing research is challenging, whether you are a busy practitioner (Vignette 15.1) or a full-time researcher. There are many issues and options to consider if you wish to conduct meaningful studies that can impact on practice.

This chapter is neither a how-to guide to the research process nor to specific research methods; there are myriad of books that already cover this, some of which are written from an occupational therapy perspective and give relevant examples (Depoy & Gitlin, 2015; Taylor, 2017). Instead, this chapter addresses the *why, what,* and *how* questions that practitioners should initially consider when they wish to conduct research in practice. It describes various rationales that people may have for conducting research (the why), explores potential areas of research (the what), and latterly examines different models of conducting research in practice (the how). Once these questions have been answered, practitioners can more meaningfully explore the research process and specific research methods.

The Challenge of Research

On the whole, occupational therapy continues to lack a substantial evidence base to support its practice in a wide variety of areas; however, it is important to note that this situation is not substantially different from many other professions (Scottish Executive Health Department, 2002, 2004). There have been some excellent examples of occupational therapy research in various areas, including falls, stroke rehabilitation, and dementia (Crofton et al., 2020; Garvey et al., 2015; Graff et al., 2006; Walker et al., 1999).

Of course, generating robust evidence to support practice is challenging. Much of practice is difficult to predict, and uncertainty appears to abound in all occupational therapy practice.

Uncertainty

It is true that uncertainty is not all bad. Life would be very boring indeed (and potentially very stressful), if we were able to predict exactly how our day, our career, our family, or our life would unfold. Sometimes it is good not to know what lies ahead in life. In most situations, uncertainty cannot be completely excluded from decisions practitioners make in practice; even in a robust multicentre clinical trial there is still a (low) chance that the crucial finding was due to luck and not causally related to the intervention. But as

VIGNETTE 15.1

Angela was a senior practitioner in a busy social work department where she had worked for the last 7 years. A core part of her job was the assessment of adults' needs at home after they had been discharged from hospital. Usually she assessed her client's needs over one or two visits and then made specific recommendations for adaptive equipment and, if required, environmental alterations (which required more frequent visits). Following this, her service's usual practice was for technical services and support staff to deliver the equipment and carry out the alterations. Angela would then visit her clients at a later date to see how the clients were getting on.

Over the years, Angela had noted that many of the pieces of adaptive equipment she had initially ordered were not being used by her clients when she visited them several weeks after their delivery. As these were usually relatively straightforward appliances Angela felt that their lack of use was not related to a lack of knowledge about how to use them, but she wasn't sure why this occurred.

As a first stage, Angela decided to conduct a longitudinal audit of equipment usage by clients throughout her local authority over time. This audit indicated a marked decline in equipment usage by a large percentage of clients over a 6-month period. As a next stage, Angela decided to conduct a series of semistructured interviews with 10 clients who had received equipment 6 months previously to enquire about their perceptions of the initial assessment and intervention process. She applied for and received appropriate ethical and managerial approval for the study. Following this, Angela decided to pilot a shared decision-making intervention (Légaré et al., 2018; see Chapter 3) with a cohort of clients. This intervention focused on developing partnership working and the development of trust and mutual respect between the therapist and client; explicitly exchanging information about the technical options, social and personal contexts, and values and preferences; deliberating on options by considering both the pros and cons of certain pieces of equipment for a client; and ongoing partnership working in deciding and acting upon the decision reached together, so that the decisions can be revisited if circumstances change. Whilst these were all aspects of therapy that Angela had previously thought she and her colleagues carried out routinely, it had become apparent through her audit and qualitative groundwork that the service's clients did not feel this occurred in practice. Angela wondered whether this more explicit strategy of shared decision making would affect the number of adaptive appliances ordered (with a potential cost saving for equipment that had previously been inappropriately placed in clients' homes) and improve outcomes by increasing the usage of equipment ordered for clients over time.

health care professionals, occupational therapists have an implicit contract with clients to select and guide them to interventions or recommendations that (in general) have a higher chance of being successful or beneficial than not. If this were not the case, then clients would have no reason to see an occupational therapist and would be as well consulting their next-door neighbour instead! Therefore the reality of uncertainty must not stop us from working to limit it in clinical practice. This requires good-quality research to develop a strong evidence base. For some, the difficulty in generating evidence of the effectiveness of occupation for health has led to the conclusion that it is impossible to achieve, not least due to the complex nature of occupational therapy interventions (Cook, 2003; Creek et al., 2005). That it is difficult is unquestionable, but it is not impossible (Duncan et al., 2007; Sweetland, 2007; Wade, 2007), and the previous examples of high-quality controlled trials in occupational therapy clearly evidence this. More recent examinations of complexity in occupational therapy have taken a more optimistic perspective, within which a more contemporary view of occupational therapy was proposed.

This perspective now needs to be understood through more research (Pentland et al., 2018).

The quest to limit or accept unpredictability through research has often polarised the profession, with one camp championing the cause of randomised controlled trials (RCTs) and measurement in general, and the other camp not only rejecting such a position and embracing constructivist epistemologies as an equally valid form of evidence but also suggesting that an embracement of measurement is a betrayal of the profession's core values. Such polarisation of views is unhelpful. Frequently studies would benefit from a mixed methods approach (O'Cathain, 2020), which draws on both quantitative and qualitative methods to answer a study's questions. Moreover, a third epistemologic stance exists, is increasingly recognised as being of value in health care research, and has much to offer occupational therapy: realism.

Critical and Subtle Realism

There are various forms of realist understanding. The largest body of work that relates to research lies in the work of Roy Bhanskar (Archer et al., 2013), who developed the idea of critical realism in the 1970s, and Martyn Hammersley, who developed a variation of subtle realism. Critical realists suggest that what is real does not necessarily equate with what can be observed; thus it is far greater than that. Therefore we can only ever measure parts of that reality, and even that measure can be perceived and understood differently by different people. Our knowledge and our reality therefore will always be imperfect. We need to critically examine what we are interested in, to gain the best possible understanding of what is occurring. Subtle realists recognise that all research involves subjective perceptions and concede that different research methods will produce different pictures. However, this perspective is not taken to the same extent as constructivists. The aim of research from a subtle realist perspective is to "search for knowledge about which one can be reasonably confident" (Murphy et al., 1998). To some this may appear as epistemologic fence sitting. Yet it does bridge the yawning gap between researchers and practitioners who recognise the importance of measurement with others who reject measurement and embrace personal narratives or other qualitative approaches. Subtle realism recognises the reality of uncertainty but upholds that, whilst it can never be completely controlled, it can be and should be significantly diminished. Surely the critical or subtle realist perspective, which lends itself to a mixed methods approach (Maxwell et al., 2015), is the most useful perspective for contemporary occupational therapy research.

It is vital that all practitioners are consumers of research; but we are also asked, and have an ethical obligation (Bannigan & Hughes, 2007; College of Occupational Therapists, 2015), to be research active as well (i.e., to generate new knowledge about what works—and what doesn't!) with the clients with whom we have the privilege to meet (see Chapter 15 where Bannigan highlights the importance of deimplementation).

WHY CONDUCT RESEARCH?

While the importance of undertaking good-quality research that answers clinically relevant questions has been gathering momentum for several years, the opportunities have arguably never been greater than they are currently. Yet relatively few practitioners undertake research. There are many reasons that may motivate someone to undertake research in practice. This chapter considers three (personal curiosity, project-based research, and a research career), but these are neither exclusive nor exhaustive.

Personal Curiosity

Curiosity, or a naturally inquisitive nature, is arguably the most essential capacity for persons to have if they wish to undertake a research study. Everyone can learn the necessary skills and knowledge of how to do research. Without possessing an inquisitive nature, practitioners will lack the internal motivation that frequently underlies the question of why they do it. There are, of course, other reasons for doing research, but for some it relates to personal curiosity alone. Often this arises after a practitioner has worked in an area for some time and notices something about the practice, an intervention or a process, which makes the practitioner question why it happens. There may be little or no external pressure to do research, but such a practitioner wishes to do it anyway to answer the unanswered question.

Project-Based Research

Another reason that a practitioner decides to undertake a research project may be related to a specific personal or collective project (Vignette 15.2). An example of this is the practitioner who decides to undertake a postgraduate degree such as a master's degree. Such degrees can be taught (e.g., MA or MSc) or research based (MPhil), but both contain a research thesis or dissertation of some description. These options are excellent opportunities for practitioners who wish to start conducting research but feel they do not have the required skills or confidence to do so alone and would like to gain some form of formal qualification for their newly acquired knowledge.

A different type of project-based research is to participate in a research study that is led by someone else. Participation may take the form of being a research worker, collecting data, or a clinical collaborator providing the link between the practice and academic settings. Such opportunities are not currently numerous in occupational therapy, but they do exist and will become more common with the increasing development of research in practice.

Research Career

Despite the challenges of an unclear career pathway for an occupational therapy researcher (Bannigan, 2001), undertaking a research career is now a real possibility, and institutions such as the UK National Institute for Health Research provide opportunities to develop a research career through funded fellowships and training programmes. Recent history illustrates how occupational therapists previously had to leave the profession if they wished to pursue a research career. Fay Fransella (1960) published what was probably the first controlled trial of occupational therapy and was later lauded as a groundbreaking researcher (Creek, 2001; IIott & White, 2001). However, an analysis of her career illustrates that while she was groundbreaking there was no research pathway at that time for her to follow and she was left with a choice. Fransella explains it in her own words: "I was at the top of my profession in my early thirties both

---

VIGNETTE 15.2

I worked as a clinical collaborator and data collector whilst working in a high-security psychiatric hospital in Scotland. The department where I was based had formed a collaboration with the UK Centre for Outcomes Research and Evaluation (UKCORE). Part of this collaboration included collecting data for international validation studies of standardised assessments (specifically the Model of Human Occupation Screening Tool [MOHOST; Forsyth et al., 2011]) and developing new versions of existing assessments (specifically the Occupational Circumstances Assessment Interview and Rating Scale [OCAIRS; Forsyth et al., 2005]). These projects provided excellent opportunities to develop my research skills and expertise, collaborate with an international research group, and participate in large international studies. It was more than I could have ever managed to achieve on my own at that stage in my research career. Skills developed during this project, included developing successful research study outlines for the hospital research and development committee, completing and submitting relevant ethics committee documentation, developing local study information leaflets, informing and consenting patients to participate in the study, negotiating with colleagues to act as fellow data collectors and anonymising, cleaning (the process through which you check all the data are there and have been entered correctly), and collating data to be sent back to the study centre in Chicago.

---

in status and in financial terms. The choice was to stay put and know more and more about less and less or do something radical…I chose the latter" (Fransella, 1989, pp. 119–120). She went on to study personal construct psychology and became an international leader in her field (Duncan, 2001)! Undertaking research as a career pathway in occupational therapy is certainly now more achievable; however, this doesn't necessarily make it straightforward or well defined.

Whilst personal curiosity and project-based research can be excellent introductions to doing research, developing a research career demands undertaking a more structured and comprehensive research training. The aim of this training is to prepare a practitioner to undertake larger-scale funded research as a principal investigator. This aim is best met by undertaking a doctorate (i.e., a PhD or clinical doctorate) followed by postdoctoral studies. Undertaking a PhD or postdoctoral research programme is a demanding (but highly rewarding) challenge. Whilst only a few may wish to pursue this option, if you do want to develop a research career it is important to get off to the right start. A helpful position is to consider three factors: you, the research, and the available support (Scottish Executive Health Department & NHS Education for Scotland, 2005).

You

Are you:
- An experienced practitioner? Not essential, but it certainly helps.
- Innovative? You will need to problem solve and spend a lot of your time finding ways around potential hurdles.
- Able to work in a team? Whilst some research may be carried out in isolation, the majority of larger-scale studies require teamwork.

- Focused on improving services? The most pressing research is that which is service focused. Do you want to improve the services in your area of specialism through research?
- Committed? Developing a research career is no mean feat, and there will be plenty of hurdles and obstacles that will need to be overcome. Many individuals undertake a series of temporary appointments before finally being given a permanent research position. Those who remain in practice have the challenge of balancing their clinical duties with their research role.
- Thick-skinned? Are you ready to face up to the highs and lows of applying for, undertaking, and disseminating research? Being a researcher is a real rollercoaster of a professional career. The ups of being awarded grants, undertaking research, and disseminating findings are excellent, but the lows of grant and paper rejections and the struggles to complete some studies can be very challenging and off-putting for some.

Your Research

- Is your research relevant to practice? More important than ever. Consider what the impact of your research could be from the outset.
- Does it fit with the needs of the people with whom you work, and where the research will be based?

Support

- Are your family and friends supportive of what you want to do? A research career is very demanding and will inevitably impact on your family and social life.
- Do you have support from your employer? Make sure the employer understands the rationale and consequences of what you want to do.

• Do you have access to advice from experienced researchers, statisticians, etc. (see later)?

WHAT TO RESEARCH?

Fundamentally the topic of research is up to you, and the subject of your research may have been what spurred you on in the first place. However, there are several issues that you would do well to consider before taking your research plans much further (Vignette 15.3):

• What do the people who use your service consider to be important? Patient priorities have rightly become a key driver in deciding what should be researched. If you can't articulate that the problem you wish to study is a patient priority, you are unlikely to be successful in seeking funding to study it. The James Lind Alliance in the United Kingdom (www.la.nihr.ac.uk) is now internationally recognised for the work they have done in determining priorities for research. They have recently undertaken an exercise to prioritise the top 10 occupational therapy research questions, too (https://www.jla.nihr.ac.uk/priority-setting-partnerships/occupational-therapy/).
• Focus your question on an issue, question, or challenge you are faced with in your everyday professional activity.
• Decide exactly what you want to find out and why it is important to do so.
• Examine the literature to see what is already known about your subject.

• Consult the people with whom you work to see if they agree your subject area is of interest.
• Talk to other people (fellow practitioners and potential collaborators) about your research idea and refine your research question.
• Begin to consider what research method(s) you may use.
• Share or present your ideas in front of an experienced group of researchers and practitioners.
• Consider whether your study requires funding. If yes, how much? Where could you apply for funding for your study?

HOW TO RESEARCH?

Once you have considered why you wish to undertake a research study, it is also important to consider how you wish to conduct the research. Whilst the principal investigator of a study carries the burden of responsibility, and often the work, research is rarely carried out in isolation, and collaboration is the name of the game in the vast majority of successful research projects.

Issues of Scale

Of course the degree of collaboration will largely be dependent on the scale of the research being undertaken. A small research project undertaken in a single site, with low participant numbers, is likely to need considerably less collaboration than a larger-scale multisite RCT or cluster RCT.

VIGNETTE 15.3

Paul had been qualified for 3 years and was employed in a learning disability community day service. He was very interested to learn more about the time use of the clients he worked with and decided to independently carry out a relatively small study exploring the perceptions of 10 clients regarding their time use and then record their actual time use through client self-report. Though the study seemed straightforward, Paul struggled to get his research ethics application approved by the research ethics committee, who repeatedly raised concerns regarding the content of the study information leaflet and the manner in which Paul intended to gain consent. When he eventually managed to negotiate these issues and gained ethical committee approval, he then struggled to recruit clients to his study. Paul hadn't previously discussed the project with the staff of the day service and they did not share his enthusiasm for the importance of the topic he had chosen. This meant

that some of the staff were less than enthusiastic in supporting clients to participate. Eventually Paul managed to interview five clients, three of whom returned their time use data a week later. Though disappointed by this, Paul wrote up the study and submitted it to his national peer-reviewed journal, only for it to be rejected by the peer reviewers who cited the low participant numbers, relative lack of meaningful data, and poor academic presentation of the submitted paper as their reasons. One reviewer suggested that the author (Paul) should consider collaborating with a more experienced researcher/author when next submitting a paper to the journal. Despondently, Paul vowed never to undertake a research project again!

Each of the challenges faced by Paul could have either been avoided or overcome more efficiently and effectively if he had collaborated with a more experienced researcher.

Going it Alone

With small research projects there is always the option of going it alone and foregoing collaboration with others. However, even when it is feasible to do so, it is rarely desirable, especially when you have had little prior experience of conducting research. The research process is like many things in life: relatively straightforward if you know what you are doing, but it can cause real headaches if you don't! Working together with others allows you to learn from their previous experience and knowledge and can save you considerable energy that may otherwise be wasted.

Personal Research Collaborations

Personal research collaborations are partnerships between a practitioner and one or more experienced researchers. Frequently, though not necessarily, the experienced researcher will be based in an academic department of a university. The importance of selecting the right people to collaborate with cannot be underestimated. Often practitioners seek collaborations with academics who had previously lectured them as students and with whom they already have an existing relationship, or alternatively with lecturers in a local university from which they take students on practice placement. Obviously the ease of geographic proximity and previously established relationships are strong bonuses worth considering when looking to form research collaborations, but they may not be the most essential criteria. In the current age of electronic communication (Zoom, MS Teams, email, etc.) the necessity of geographic proximity has become less and less important. Instead, first consider the skills you require from your collaborator, then look for who best fits the criteria. It is important to consider what you are looking for from research collaboration before you look for the best individual(s) to collaborate with, and then negotiate expectations and roles with your collaborators before you agree to work together.

Considering a Research Collaboration

Research collaborations are excellent, and you will often find willing and able individuals with whom you could work. There are, however, some issues worth considering before you contact any potential collaborators. These include:

- At the most basic level: What do you need from your research collaborator(s)? Is it experience of completing ethics applications, navigating the research and development process, writing research grant applications, methodological expertise, statistical know-how, or something else?
- Do you want to be the principal investigator or are you willing to hand that over to your collaborator?

- If you are writing a grant application, where do you want the research funds to be based? There may be good reasons for the funding to be based in your institution, or in the institution of your research collaborator(s).
- What are you willing to offer in return for a potential collaboration? Some people may be happy to collaborate without any quid pro quo or on the basis of negotiated inclusion on a grant proposal and/or research outputs such as publications (see later). Others may ask for you to undertake some visiting lecturing or take a student of theirs for a practice placement in return for their input.

Individual collaborations. Finding such individuals can be challenging, but you may know of someone's specific interest and expertise through their published work, or from hearing them at conferences. Some professional bodies (e.g., Royal College of Occupational Therapists) hold registers for researchers that can be searched for specific criteria. It is also worth searching some key phrases on Twitter to find out who and where active research is in your area. Twitter can be an excellent equaliser as it provides people with access to leading researchers (who are often, though not always, active on Twitter) and lets you ask questions and make approaches about your research ideas. Even if they are unable to get involved themselves, you will often find they are more than happy to direct you to people who may be able to assist.

Research units/research centres. As well as looking for individuals, it may also be worthwhile to look for established research units that are interested in the topic you wish to research. Such units are often very keen to engage with clinical collaborators, as without them they find it very challenging to conduct their research. Research units have a variety of different interests and funding sources, each of which will influence the type and focus of research they conduct. Some research units are interdisciplinary; others have a profession-specific focus. An advantage of collaborating with a well-established research unit/centre is that they often have their own excellent networks and can link you up with experts in specific fields of interest such as statistics or economic evaluation.

Negotiating Collaboration

When developing research collaborations, it is important that you negotiate each other's roles and expectations at an early stage. Time spent doing this at the beginning avoids unnecessary confusion, frustration, and conflict when the research has progressed further down the line. One clear example of where early negotiation pays benefits is in the development of a publication agreement. That is a document that outlines what papers (and other outputs) will be developed from the research, to where they will be submitted (you may have a prioritised list of options here), who will be authors on each publication, and where their name will be listed in each paper. Normally collaborators form part of the author list for papers that are published from their research and contribute to the paper's development. The position of individuals' names on each paper requires agreement; this usually depends on their contribution, both to the research and writing of the paper. Some journals require authors to specify each of their contributions to a submitted paper. If there is more than one paper coming from a study, then negotiation may centre on who is leading on the development of each paper. It can seem a bit strange, and at times awkward, to have such a frank discussion about something that has not yet been completed; however, experience has demonstrated that spending time and effort considering this early on avoids what can be difficult moments and conflicts at a later stage when you discover that you have different ideas about who will be first author, etc. More established researchers, research centres, and academic faculties already have established protocols for developing publishing agreements for precisely this reason.

Service Collaboration

Some services recognise the importance of doing research as part of their professional duties and form specific service collaborations with experienced researchers. These collaborations are therefore at a different organisational level than individual collaborations. Service collaborations take different forms, but there are broadly three types: 1:1, project based, and total service models.

1:1

In this type of service model, whilst the collaboration is at a service level, the experienced researcher engages with individual members of staff on specific individual projects to meet their specific needs. The advantages of this model are that each practitioner is able to receive individual support depending on the need. In one service, where this model successfully functioned, the role of the experienced researcher varied from helping support staff to constructing meaningful clinical notes following sessions with clients to supervising a senior member of staff who was undertaking his PhD part time while based in practice. Staff appreciate this tailored approach to research collaboration, but there are challenges to this approach, too.

The nature of individualised research collaborations means that research outcomes tend to be relatively small scale, to develop in a relatively ad hoc fashion and according to practitioners' interests rather than clinical need (Duncan, 2008). Another interesting challenge that can arise from a 1:1 service model is the perception that such research activities need to be undertaken over and above a practitioner's clinical role. Frequently this can mean that such activities are not given due priority by staff, even when they have direct management support to do so.

Project-Based Service Collaboration

This form of service model typifies the sort of project-based research that academics are on occasion called in to support departments in practice settings. The difference between this model of service collaboration and the following model (total service models) lies with the time frame and the extent of the collaboration. Project-based service collaborations tend to be of a shorter duration than total service models and are more focused in nature.

Total Service Models

An alternative service collaboration approach is for the experienced researcher to collaborate with the service as a whole, not solely individual practitioners, and over a prolonged period of time. One successful model that exemplifies this approach is the scholarship of practice model (Kielhofner, 2005). Hammel et al. (2001) outline the key components of the scholarship of practice model as follows:

- Being committed to carrying out research that directly contributes and impacts on practice
- Working in partnership with individuals and organisations outwith academic settings
- Developing synergies that practice and scholarship simultaneously

An advantage of this approach is that the aims of the research collaboration are central to the practice of individual clinicians and the service as a whole. This means that research activities are more easily integrated into everyday activities and become more relevant to practice. Further, as such collaborations are at a service level, the scale of the research that can be undertaken is significantly increased. Of course these benefits are not without cost, and some practitioners may prefer the individual collaboration and flexibility that is more clearly tangible in a 1:1 model (Duncan, 2008). The scholarship of practice approach has evolved over time, and several versions have been developed (Hammel et al., 2015).

SUMMARY

The opportunities and expectations for occupational therapists to undertake research are greater now than they have ever been. Practitioners conduct research for a variety of reasons, but these can be broadly summarised as personal curiosity, project-based research, and development of a research career. Whatever an individual's motivation for doing research is, it is unlikely to be carried out alone, and close consideration should be given to the type of collaboration that is most suitable for the research and desired by the principal investigator. Forming research collaborations brings together a range of research expertise and can greatly assist in the smooth planning, execution, and dissemination of a research study.

REFLECTIVE LEARNING

- What is my attitude toward research? What has influenced this?
- In what way do I think I could best become involved in developing research within the profession?
- What do I think is the most important piece of research in my clinical area of interest? Why?
- What is the most pressing research question I have in my clinical area of interest?

REFERENCES

Archer, M., Bhaskar, R., Collier, A., Lawson, T., & Norrie, A. (Eds.). (2013). *Critical realism: Essential readings*. Routledge.

Bannigan, K. (2001). Is research valued as a legitimate career pathway in occupational therapy? *British Journal of Occupational Therapy, 64*(9), 425.

Bannigan, K., & Hughes, S. (2007). Research is now every occupational therapist's business. *British Journal of Occupational Therapy, 70*(3), 95.

Cook, S. (2003). What interventions produced the evidence of positive outcomes? *Mental Health Occupational Therapy, 8*(1), 20–23.

Creek, J. (2001). Occupational science as a selected research priority—response [letter]. *British Journal of Occupational Therapy, 64*(8), 420–421.

Creek, J., Illott, I., Cook, S., et al. (2005). Valuing occupational therapy as a complex intervention. *British Journal of Occupational Therapy, 68*(6), 281–284.

Crofton, E., Meredith, P., Gray, P., O'Reilly, S., & Strong, J. (2020). Non-adherence with compression garment wear in adult burns patients: A systematic review and meta-ethnography. *Burns, 46*(2), 472–482.

Depoy, E., & Gitlin, L. N. (2015). In *Introduction to research: Understanding and applying multiple research strategies* (5th ed.). Elsevier.

Duncan, E. A., Paley, J., & Eva, G. (2007). Complex interventions and complex systems in occupational therapy: an alternative perspective. *British Journal of Occupational Therapy, 70*(5), 199-206.

Duncan, E. (2008). Twist and turns: The development of a clinical academic partnership. In E. A. McKay, C. Craik, & K. H. Lim (Eds.), *Advancing occupational therapy in mental health practice*. Blackwell Publishing.

Duncan, E. A. S. (2001). Is research valued as a career pathway? *British Journal of Occupational Therapy, 10*(64), 517–518.

Forsyth, K., Parkinson, S., Kielhofner, G., Kramer, J., Mann, L., & Duncan, E. (2011). The measurement properties of the model of human occupation screening tool and implications for practice. *New Zealand Journal of Occupational Therapy, 58*(2), 5.

Forsyth, K., Walker, K., & Duncan, E. A. S. (2005). Forensic occupational circumstances assessment interview and rating scale. In K. Forsyth, S. Deshpande, & G. Kielhofner (Eds.), *The occupational circumstances assessment interview and rating scale (OCAIRS)*. University of Illinois.

Fransella, F. (1960). The treatment of chronic schizophrenia: Intensive occupational therapy with and without chlorpromazine. *Occupational Therapy, 23*(9), 31–34.

Fransella, F. (1989). A fight for freedom. In W. Dryden, & L. Spurling (Eds.), *On becoming a psychotherapist* (pp. 119–120). Routledge.

Garvey, J., Connolly, D., Boland, F., & Smith, S. M. (2015). OPTI-MAL, an occupational therapy led self-management support programme for people with multimorbidity in primary care: A randomized controlled trial. *BMC Family Practice, 16*(1), 1–11.

Graff, M. J., Vernooij-Dasses, M. J. M., Thijsseen, M., et al. (2006). Community based occupational therapy for patients with dementia and their care givers: Randomised controlled trial. *BMJ, 333*, 1196.

Hammel, J., Finlayson, M., Kielhofner, G., et al. (2001). Educating scholars of practice: An approach to preparing tomorrow's researchers. *Occupational Therapy in Health Care, 15*(1/2), 157–176.

Hammel, J., Magasi, S., Mirza, M. P., Fischer, H., Preissner, K., Peterson, E., & Suarez-Balcazar, Y. (2015). A scholarship of practice revisited: Creating community-engaged occupational therapy practitioners, educators, and scholars. *Occupational Therapy in Health Care, 29*(4), 352–369.

Kielhofner, G. (2005). A scholarship of practice: Creating discourse between theory, research and practice. *Occupational Therapy in Healthcare, 19*(1/2), 7–16.

Maxwell, J. A., & Mittapalli, K. (2015). Realism as a stance for mixed methods research. In T. Abbas, & C. Teddlie (Eds.), *SAGE handbook of mixed methods in social & behavioral research*. Sage.

Légaré, F., Adekpedjou, R., Stacey, D., Turcotte, S., Kryworuchko, J., Graham, I. D., & Donner-Banzhoff, N. (2018). Interventions for increasing the use of shared decision making by healthcare professionals. *Cochrane Database of Systematic Reviews, 7*.

Murphy, E., Dingwall, R., Greatbatch, D., et al. (1998). Qualitative research methods in health technology assessment: A review of the literature. *Health Technology Assessment, 2*(16).

Pentland, D., Kantartzis, S., Clausen, M. G., & Witemyre, K. (2018). *Occupational therapy and complexity: Defining and describing practice*. Royal College of Occupational Therapists.

O'Cathain, A. (2020). Mixed methods research. In C. Pope, & N. Mays (Eds.), *Qualitative research in health care* (4th ed.). Wiley.

Scottish Executive Health Department. (2002). *Choices and challenges: The strategy for research and development in nursing and midwifery in Scotland*. Author.

Scottish Executive Health Department. (2004). *Allied health professions research and development action plan*. Author.

Scottish Executive Health Department & NHS Education for Scotland. (2005). *Making choices facing challenges: Developing your research career in nursing, midwifery and the allied health professions*. Authors.

Sweetland, J. (2007). Guidance in a research journey. *British Journal of Occupational Therapy, 70*(10), 453.

Taylor, R. (2017). *Kielhofner's research in occupational therapy: Methods of inquiry for enhancing practice*. F A Davis.

Wade, D. (2007). Complexity and research. *British Journal of Occupational Therapy, 70*(6), 269.

Walker, M. F., Gladman, J. R., Lincoln, N. B., et al. (1999). Occupational therapy for stroke patients not admitted to hospital: A randomised controlled trial. *Lancet, 354*, 278–280.

16

Presentation and Publication Skills

Edward A.S. Duncan, Alister Landrock, and Ann Landrock

HIGHLIGHTS

- Being able to share your work (i.e., in writing, presenting, and publishing online or in print) is an essential skill for contemporary occupational therapists.
- Be clear in what you want to say.
- Always follow the guidance you are given.

- Seek out a critical friend who can give you honest feedback.
- Don't be disheartened if your first attempts are unsuccessful; effective dissemination is a skill that requires to be developed. Persistence pays dividends.

INTRODUCTION

Occupational therapists are routinely being called upon to share and disseminate their work. University degree programmes now require students to develop good writing skills, design posters, and prepare presentations, yet many are still fearful of broadcasting information more widely when they graduate and start working. Others, on the other hand, did not receive such education during their training. This chapter aims to highlight key skills and issues to help students and therapists overcome the fear factor and/or enhance their existent skills.

Knowledge of publication and presentation skills is essential for all occupational therapists. There are various reasons for this. An understanding of how to communicate in a variety of ways is crucial when developing treatment literature or designing information leaflets for patients and their relatives, colleagues, or students (see Chapter 8), producing health-promotional publications, composing scientific posters, presenting at work or at professional conferences, and submitting your work for publication in a magazine or journal. This chapter focuses on the key skills you require to be successful in disseminating your work.

WRITING AN ABSTRACT

Most formal presentations, be they poster or oral in format, will initially be developed and submitted for consideration as an abstract (i.e., a summary of what the presentation is about). Abstracts are usually submitted to conference organisers who use this information to judge firstly whether to accept your presentation and secondly in which format (e.g., oral presentation, poster, workshop, or seminar). It is vital therefore that the content and presentation of an abstract is accurate, succinct, and appealing. Abstracts are potential presenters' main opportunity to sell their idea initially to conference abstract reviewers and, latterly, if they are successful at that stage, to participants of the conference, who will often decide whether to attend a presentation on the basis of the abstract, which will be published in the conference programme. The format is fairly universal. Krajewska and Vermeulen (2018) emphasise four Cs of good abstract writing: complete (ensure all relevant information), concise (don't waffle), clear (avoid long and complicated sentences), and cohesive (follow abstract guidelines, which generally ask for a variation of introduction, aims and methods, findings, and conclusions). Some research methods have well developed conference abstract guidelines that are useful to follow (e.g., see von Elm et al.'s [2007] guidelines for reporting observational research that includes guidance for conference abstracts).

Guidance

Many people find writing an abstract challenging. Yet most "call for papers" (where organisations request people to submit abstracts for presentations) contain detailed information about the length of the title, the length of the abstract, a rough format of desired content, whether references are desired and if so how many and in what format, and adherence to conference theme, among other specific information. Some "call for papers" go as far as publishing the marking schedule, which gives a fairly detailed idea of the amount of information that is being looked for by reviewers. The first and most important piece of advice that can be given in writing an abstract is to follow the conference organiser's guidance! Failure to do so in a conference that receives a surfeit of abstracts is a sure way to have yours rejected. Reviewers will be looking for easy ways to whittle down the number of abstracts they have to consider, and not following the defined format for an abstract is commonly used by reviewers as being the first and easiest criteria for rejection.

What to Present?

It is often tempting to submit an abstract for a piece of work that is not yet completed but that you expect will be by the time the conference will be held. This is a dangerous strategy (Haigh, 2006), which is best avoided when at all possible. Whilst you may plan for your research to go smoothly, a variety of factors may not be within your control, resulting in delays and an inability to present the paper you have described in your paper; this is not popular with either conference organisers, who have worked hard to develop the programme, or delegates, who may have made a difficult choice between sessions only to be disappointed when they attend your session. Further advantages to submitting abstracts on completed work are that you are then able to include interesting statistics from your study or key theoretical proposals from more conceptual work (Haigh, 2006). Doing so is likely to increase your chances of success further.

Having reinforced the central importance of following the organisers' written guidance and submitting abstracts on completed work, other factors should also be considered to develop an attractive and successful abstract submission: your target audience and clarity of your message (Bannigan, 2005).

Think About Your Audience

Both reviewers and conference delegates are frequently faced with a huge number of abstracts to read and consider when making judgements of whether they should either accept the abstract or attend your session. Your abstract needs to inspire your potential audience (Albarran & Dowling, 2017). You may consider your paper or poster to be fascinating and of vital importance, but if you are not able to communicate this very early on in the abstract (preferably in the title), then you are likely to lose the interest of your reader. So carefully consider your audience. Use words and phrases that are likely to be meaningful to them, and avoid unnecessary jargon. Carefully considering the language you use is important in developing your abstract. Organisations such as the Plain English Campaign and marketing and communication companies exist to help people to communicate well, but these are likely to be expensive and inappropriate for most practitioners' needs. Instead, it can be very helpful to find yourself one or more critical friends, preferably people who have had abstracts accepted for similar events. Asking for their honest feedback and appraisal of your draft abstract can be extremely useful and help create a significantly stronger final work than if you had written it alone. Of course asking for and receiving honest and critical feedback is not always easy, even when it is given in a constructive manner as one would hope it would be. Here, however, lies the necessity to develop another subtle yet vital skill for any practitioners who wish to disseminate their work: the development of a thick skin (Meshack, 2004)! Honest feedback from your critical friends is likely to be at least slightly difficult to accept; after all, if you didn't think it was good you wouldn't have written it like that, would you! However, it is pointless to ignore their comments as you would be as well not soliciting them in the first place if you did that. Therefore careful consideration should be given to all feedback. Even if you do not take on board their suggestions, you should think about ways in which to improve the section(s) they found difficult as you obviously weren't managing to communicate your message there as well as you had hoped. The most helpful attitudes to cultivate when you receive constructive criticism are ones of gratefulness and humility (Meshack, 2004), though this is much easier to suggest than to embrace!

Clarity of Your Message

By their very nature, abstracts are concise: often only 150 to 200 words in length. Use your words wisely and make full use of the number of words you have available (Haigh, 2006). Clear and simple explanations are vital if the abstract is to read well. To achieve this, you first have to have a very good idea of what you want to say; if you don't know, how will you be able to clearly tell other people (Bannigan, 2005)? Ensure that you make your abstract of as wide an interest and relevance as possible. Experience of sitting on the scientific committee of various conferences' organising committees has highlighted that one of the questions that (rightly or wrongly) strongly influences reviewers' opinions of an abstract can be summed up as follows: "Do I give a damn?" Even with the clearest of scoring schedules, if the topic does not grab the reviewer's attention it stands much less chance of acceptance. One way to grab interest is to develop a clear and engaging writing style (Draper, 2012). Use active tense wherever possible because passive tense is naturally disengaging.

CREATING WRITTEN PRESENTATIONS

Although it is important to carefully deliberate over the content within a written document, such as a poster, it is also necessary to be aware of its typographic layout. This advice stands whether the presentation is in person or online. The way that it is composed will add or detract from the reader's understanding. Without order there is chaos, and an awareness of design principles will help organise your information. The principles of good design are long standing. Papanek (1985) stated "design was the conscious and intuitive effort to impose meaningful order" (p. 4); a colleague, Innes (1988) adapted this quote to read, "Design is the conscious and intuitive effort to arrange elements." The elements being arranged would depend on the design work being undertaken, but generally speaking in graphic design these are words, blocks of text, photographs, illustrations, lines, space, and more. If you give careful consideration to layout as well as content, your work will be further enhanced.

All layout is based on the legibility of the message to aid or ease the communication between the written word and the human eye. Anything that impedes this is poor layout. The eye, and to a large extent the mind, is habit formed, and layout is as much to do about what the eye expects to find as with what is easy to read. The eye demands a certain amount of border around a design or a page; too much space tends to compete with and dwarf the work, too little does not allow the work to sit comfortably on the page. Wheildon (1996) stated, "Typography is the art of designing a communication by using the printed word. Typography must be clear. At its very best it is virtually invisible" (p. 23). When the eye is exposed to any image, the brain tries to make sense of it if the image is not readily accessible. You are likely aware of the perceptual illusion drawing of the vase and faces (Fig. 16.1). Viewed one way you will see a vase, viewed another way you will see the profile of two faces. The eye is trying to make sense of the ambiguity of the image. This same ambiguity can also occur on the printed page or website when the unconsidered positioning of type, lines, spaces, and other elements can draw unintended attention away from the message.

The remit of this chapter does not extend to discussing at length the variety of computer programs available to produce finished copy or how to use them. It is enough to state that there are various desktop publishing, word processing, and multimedia (PowerPoint) software packages, which can be used to create a variety of documents. As it would also take too long to discuss how to create the variety of publications that you are likely to produce, this section will focus on designing a scientific poster. Many of the principles for designing a poster also apply to the design of leaflets, newsletters, fact sheets, among other products.

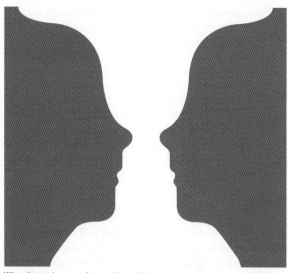

When the eye is exposed to any image the brain tries to make sense of it, if it is not readily accessible. Above is the perceptual illusion drawing of the vase and the faces. Viewed one way you will see a vase, viewed another way, you will see the profile of two faces. The eye is trying to make sense of the ambiguity of the image. The same ambiguity can also occur on the printed page when the unconsidered positioning of type, lines, spaces etc., can draw unintended attention away from the message.

FIG. 16.1 Two faces in conversation.

Scientific Posters

Over recent years there has been a great upsurge in the demand for scientific posters at occupational therapy conferences. This is a healthy sign as it indicates that there are now many involved in research that want to share their knowledge. Increasingly these are often occurring online as well as, or instead of in person. Writing this chapter during the lockdown due to Covid-19 it is hard to imagine that conferences will ever be the same again. Virtual posters may therefore become the norm moving forward. The advice that follows is equally important regardless of the medium in which the information is displayed. A scientific poster can be defined as a recent display of research or educational material on a vertical panel that usually requires the presence of the author to discuss the work. It is important to read a conference's poster presentation instructions before embarking on your design as protocols differ from one conference to the next. It is crucial to know exactly what size the end product should be and understand the explicit layout instructions. Simmonds (1984) suggested that the following questions written by Sir Austin Bradford should be addressed when writing about your research:

- Why did you start?
- What did you do?
- What answers did you get?
- What does it mean?

These answers should then be supported with Dr. Stephen Locks' criteria (see Simmonds, 1984):

- Choose the correct word,
- Choose the familiar rather than the obscure word,
- Prefer the single word to the several,
- Prefer the concrete to the abstract,
- Prefer the short to the long,
- Prefer the word of the Saxon to that of the Roman,
- Write with nouns and verbs not adjectives or adverbs.

For the purposes of presentation the poster can be divided into three main areas: the title, the text or copy, and visual imagery.

The Title

The title is usually written across the top of your poster and is generally the first element that will be read; therefore it should be eye catching, enticing, and perhaps even controversial to engage the reader. Many of the conference delegates who will visit your poster will have read your abstract beforehand and will be sympathetic to your topic. It is imperative that you also try to attract those who may not be particularly interested in your subject matter. One way to do this is to write a short statement or questions that will encourage a wider audience to view your work. We have much to learn from the tabloid press when looking for the short snappy headline that will attract attention. Some conferences will clearly specify the number of words that can be used in the title, but if a limit is not stated, the no more than 10 words would be a good guide to follow. The shorter the title, the larger the type that can be used.

The Text

The vast majority of people prefer reading sitting down, and because posters are generally read standing up (at physical conferences) it is essential to keep posters as visual and concise as possible. A short historical summary followed by the aims of the present study should introduce your content. Simmonds (1984) suggests that one should describe the logical basis for experimentation and mention any limiting factors. Illustrate changes and trends by displaying simplified tables and graphs. Standard deviation, standard errors of the mean, and other details can be given on a handout. Finally discuss the relevance of your work. Transmit a sense of excitement to the observer; state how the results will alter the course of your practice and mention any developments planned for the future. Try to convey all of this in 500 words. You will not be able to present all the data you have collected, so choose the major points you feel communicate the essence of your subject matter. Your contact details will allow those who want to have more information to communicate with you. The text should be written using easily read fonts and only three, at the most, should be used

in your poster; remember that type style (normal, bold, etc.) and point size can alter the appearance of a typeface. Avoid script, calligraphic, or decorative fonts, as these can be difficult to read. Recommended typefaces include Times Roman, New Century Schoolbook, or Palatino, which are serif typefaces, or Arial, Helvetica, or Futura, which are sanserif typefaces. Serifs are lines or curves projecting from the end of a letterform. Sanserif typefaces are also referred to as Gothic and do not have these finishing strokes. A contrasting typeface might be used for actual quotations or within tables, but be sure to assess the overall impact of this before producing the final poster.

Type Size

Harms (1995) advocates the use of a simple calculation, which can help determine the varying point sizes of type to be used throughout the poster:

$$\frac{\text{Viewing distance in mm}}{200} = \text{height of type in mm}$$

$$\frac{2000\ \text{mm}\ (2\ \text{metres})}{200} = 10\ \text{mm high type}$$

Type is measured in points (pts), an old imperial measurement with 72 pts equaling 1 inch or 25.4 mm. The point size of a typeface is determined by measuring from the top of an ascender to the base of a descender. Typefaces that have the same point size will not necessarily have the same height; invariably serif typefaces appear smaller than sanserif typefaces when the same point size is chosen (Fig. 16.2).

Three sizes of type might be used for the title, headings, and text. The title should be at least 72 pts, the section headings 20 to 30 pts, and text 18 to 24 pts; this would depend on the typeface, the type style you employ, and the space available (e.g., bold type might be used for all the headings).

Type Style

There are various type styles that can be adopted to enhance the text:

|Normal **Bold** *Italic* <u>Underline</u> **Outline Shadow**|

Arguably the most easily read of these are normal and bold, but experiment with the typeface styles available to you. Use bold as a contrast to normal type; reading large passages of bold text can be tiring on the eye.

Uppercase (or Capital Letters)

When reading a line of type the eye recognises letters by the shape, specifically of their upper halves. With lowercase letters this is easier because the upper halves of lowercase letters are generally distinctive, framed by white space that

Type is measured in points (pts.)—an old imperial measurement with 72 points equalling an inch (25.4mm). The point size of a typeface is determined by measuring from the top of an ascender to the base of a descender, see below:

Ascender

Abg

10mm (this is known as the "x" height of the typeface)

Descender

Arial

36pt. Arial (10mm) - Sans-serif

Times

40pt. Times New Roman (10mm) - serif

N.B. Typefaces that have the same point size will **not** necessarily have the same height. (see above)

FIG. 16.2 Type measurement.

Capital and lower case letters

RAG BOY BADGER   rag boy badger

When reading a line of type, the eye recognises letters by the shape of their upper halves. With lower case letters this is simple because the top halves of lower case letters are generally distinctive, and, importantly, framed by the white space that surrounds them, permitting easy recognition. If one only uses capital letters the eye is presented with a repeated rectangular shape, and recognising the words becomes a task instead of a natural process (Wheildon 1966).

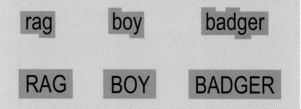

Complete words in capital letters should be used sparingly, if at all, as we recognise words by their shapes as well as sounding out their letters.

FIG. 16.3 Capital and lowercase letters.

surrounds them permitting easy recognition. We also recognise words by their overall shape. If one uses only uppercase letters, then words appear as a series of rectangles, and recognising them becomes a task instead of a natural process (Fig. 16.3 provides some examples).

Use colour to interest the reader within graphs, tables, photographs, and other elements. Coloured lines or bullet points can be added to the poster to enhance a mainly black-on-white page. Use only one or two colours of print within your poster and ensure they do not clash with colours in photographs or illustrations. A contrast between the type and the background is essential, and white or pastel colours are most appropriate. Coloured backgrounds often compete with the various elements in the poster and should be used with care.

Avoid the use of long lines of text as these are tiring to read. The most efficient to read line length in English is around 40 characters long. The best way to achieve this is to use a number of columns to organise your work. Justified line lengths alter the spaces between words to ensure two straight edges to the block of text. This results in larger than usual spaces between the words, which can compromise your writing. Although there is far from universal agreement, evidence suggests that readers find the consistent word spacing found in align left/ragged right text easier to read.

Visual imagery should be positioned in the top half of the poster aligned to the column width. Select your illustration or photographs with care; one good image is much better than three that do not precisely reflect your topic. If using coloured imagery ensure that colour is reflected in the type, lines, and other elements used elsewhere in the poster.

Posters should attract, interest, and inform. To do this, hours must be spent on the typographic layout; the end result will often belie the time and effort expended on the final product (Fig. 16.4).

Visual Presentations

Taking time to address the following guidelines can often further enhance artwork created by clients. A neutral background (black, white, or grey) will be most useful for displaying coloured pieces of artwork to advantage. A coloured background behind a colourful picture will influence what the viewer will be attracted to. When presenting a single piece of work, the borders on the top and sides should be equal. For visual effect the border below should be a little deeper. When displaying several pieces of work on the same presentation either make the top or bottom edges level, also keep the edges of work parallel to the mount, avoid if possible a diagonal arrangement of artwork as this tends to take the eye away from the individual pieces of work. The spaces between the images should be the same; this will

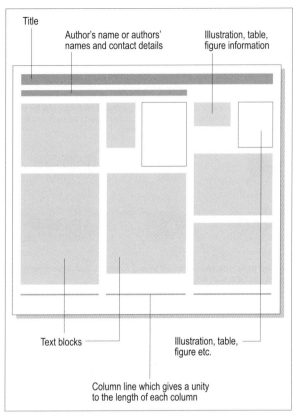

Title

Author's name or authors' names and contact details

Illustration, table, figure information

Text blocks

Illustration, table, figure etc.

Column line which gives a unity to the length of each column

FIG. 16.4 Typographic layout.

bring harmony to the overall arrangement. When displaying circular or irregularly shaped images, consideration should be given to the spacing and balance of the arrangement. Peculiarly shaped spaces created between the images or figures can compete for the eyes' attention. Irregularly shaped work can be most effectively displayed by positioning them on to a rectangular-shaped background before adding them to the overall arrangement. As far as possible keep the background unobtrusive so that all the attention will be focused on the artwork.

ORAL PRESENTATIONS

Delivering an oral presentation to an audience requires many of the skills used by an actor. Your audience wants to know the detail of your presentation but also to be entertained or at least to find it pleasurable and enjoyable to listen to your message. The presentation needs to be prepared, structured, and rehearsed to guarantee a successful performance.

Before embarking on your presentation clearly identify the following:
- What is the purpose of the presentation?
- What facilities will be available to you?
- How much time do you have?
- Who will be in the audience?

The ability to answer these questions will enable you to select an appropriate style of delivery and give structure of your work. The purpose of the presentation will dictate whether a formal or informal approach is chosen. Conferences are usually formal affairs where a chairperson will introduce a speaker, ensure that the time schedule is kept, and oversee the question-and-answer session at the end of your talk. On these occasions formal dress and a formal posture should be considered. For an informal presentation, a more flexible approach can be assumed and a more relaxed posture and dress code selected.

Introduce yourself and your topic to establish credibility with the audience. Then follow the three golden rules of any presentation:
- Say what you are going to say.
- Say it.
- Say what you have just said.

It is also important to remember that an audience's concentration is high at the start, flagging in the middle, and can be distracted towards the end, so use a variety of sensory techniques to keep them alert. Kinder (1973) said that people remember:
- 10% of what they read.
- 20% of what they hear.
- 30% of what they see.
- 50% of what they hear and see.

Therefore a combination of visual images with both oral and written communication will aid the transference of knowledge. The use of visual imagery will also communicate an idea more quickly than words, and it could be argued it will remain longer in the memory than spoken or written words. Photographs, illustrations, and video will all enhance your presentation, but choose the correct image; be cautious especially when using clipart as these computer-generated pictures are often overused and lose their impact when shown repeatedly. Visual aids will also help to engage an audience, but ensure these are positioned or held for all to see.

Presenting

Most people find presenting at least a little nerve wracking. Some will go to great lengths to avoid having to do it; however, the skill of being able to stand up and present your work is invaluable, and the benefits it can bring to you, your service, or your profession are significant. So do not be put off by performance anxiety; stick your neck above the parapet and begin to present your work—initially where you feel most comfortable and then move on to what you may consider to be a more challenging audience.

Nowadays developing presentational skills is a central component to all undergraduate degrees, but the target audience is generally the same (tutorial group, year group, lecturers, etc.). As a practitioner you may be required to present work in a variety of different settings, to large or small groups, to people you do know (such as your clinical team) or do not know (such as at a conference). Each of these different settings requires slightly different skills.

The American psychologist Albert Mehrabian is perhaps best known for his work on nonverbal communication and body language. Mehrabian (1971) examined the impact of the content, voice intonation, and body language on communication and coined the 7%-35%-55% rule. That is, we are more apt to like and accept the presenter if the person manages to convey positive messages with words, tone of voice, and body language; the respective impact of each being 7%-35%-55%, respectively. The importance of having positive body language is therefore clear.

Body Language

Eye contact establishes and maintains rapport with your audience and will help you detect if they understand or are interested in what you are saying. Make eye contact with audience members so they all feel included. If you are in a standing position, then place both feet firmly on the floor, about the same width as your shoulders, and avoid the temptation of trying to balance on one leg! If you are sitting, then keep your legs still and refrain from swinging or twisting your legs as this can be distracting. Gestures should be used in moderation. The use of deliberate hand and arm movements can make you appear more confident and relaxed. Keep hand gestures above waist height so that all the audience can see what you are doing and avoid repetitive hand or arm movement for no apparent reason as this can suggest insecurity or anxiety.

Often we can be unaware of our own idiosyncratic body language when we present. Perhaps you perch on one foot like a stork, or rock back and forth like a Weeble ("Weebles wobble but they don't fall down!"). Alternatively you may use hand gestures more appropriate for conducting the last night of the proms! Whatever it is (and you are likely to have at least some subtle habits) it is quite possible you are unaware of them. Ask colleagues who have seen you present to give you feedback on your body language. Ideally get yourself videoed whilst delivering a presentation and then closely analyse your body language. Few people are completely comfortable watching themselves perform, but it can be an invaluable method of getting feedback and altering your performance.

Using Your Voice

Most presenters get at least a little nervous, and your voice can be one of the tell-tale signs of your nerves to the audience. Anxious presenters often speak much faster than necessary (i.e., a kind of "lets get this over and done with as soon as possible" principle). Unsurprisingly this does not lead to a good presentation, so watch your pace of speech. If you know that you get nervous, then it can be helpful to consciously slow down what you are saying; however, your presentation should flow and not drag. Vary the pace of your presentation and slow down further for important points. Alter the pitch of your voice by using the full range of high and low tones throughout your presentation, to avoid your voice becoming monotonous. Use volume to suit the environment and be prepared to ask the audience if they can all hear you; not only will this ensure that you are speaking loud enough, it will also mean that you are seen as being a considerate speaker. Common sense should prevail, however; if the last three speakers have asked the audience if they can hear them, then don't repeat it because people find this tiresome.

The final word on using your voice must be given not to what you say, but to what you don't: silence and pauses. Pausing, for short periods, during your presentation can be used to excellent effect. It can emphasise a point you have just made or enable your audience to assimilate what you have just said before you move on to your next point.

Presenting Online

While videoconferencing has been growing over the last decade, the onset of Covid-19 catapulted almost everyone into this world. Online presenting has led to the development of therapists using digital video recording to develop and share their skills and knowledge (see discussion of @AHP2mintalks in Chapter 21). Many of us are now also familiar with using platforms such as Zoom, MS Teams, Google Meet, and Skype. Lots of us have also watched with amusement when mistakes have happened while people have used these platforms and the results have gone viral: children appearing uninvited on screen, people leaving funny filters on while in important meetings, people being left on mute or unable to put their camera on (or leaving their camera on when they thought it was off!). The truth is, even if you manage to avoid these faux pas, presenting online can be challenging.

Remembering a few key points can make all the difference to the quality of your online presentation. It is always worth familiarising yourself beforehand with the software so you know how to start sharing your presentation, make sure the sound is on for any videos you may wish to share, work out where the chat function is and if you wish to use it, among other aspects. Practice this before the event so you have checked it all works well. Make sure your Internet connectivity is working and you have a good signal. Try and remove all things that may cause a distraction during your presentation (e.g., your mobile phone, house phone, other people, pets). Check the sound before you go live. Can you hear through your speakers well? Is your microphone clear and loud enough? Think about your background. Too cluttered a background can be a distraction. Virtual backgrounds are available on several videoconferencing platforms. Some people like these, but they can also be a bit distracting in themselves. A simple real background is preferable. Consider your lighting. You should have good light coming directly onto your face. If the background is too light, then you will disappear into a shadow so witch off lights behind you and shut your curtains/blinds if need be. One common error is that online presenters look at the screen to see people's faces or their presentation. This, however, means they are not looking at the camera. Despite being online, you still need to develop good eye contact with your audience, so try as much as you can to look directly into the camera when speaking. It feels a bit off at first, but it makes all the difference when you are on the receiving end. Another challenge with online presentations is maintaining energy. To achieve this, it can be helpful to position yourself so you are seated towards the front edge of your chair with a good posture and your feet flat on the floor. Hand gestures are still useful but need a bit of practice as you have to hold them in front of yourself at a height that can be captured by your camera. Remember your voice intonation and speed can still be very useful when you wish to convey important messages to people in a virtual setting.

Structuring Your Presentation

Think of your presentation like a story. You need to have a beginning, middle, and end. As your audience's concentration is high at the start of your talk, you should try to give an excellent introduction; if you lose them here you will have lost them for good (or at least for the rest of your presentation). So start off strong, introduce yourself, grab their attention with some sort of statement or reflection as to why your presentation is important, and outline what you are going to be talking about.

The middle phase of your presentation is where the majority of your presentation will take place. In effect this is where you tell your story, present your research, etc. Make sure it flows well. For research presentations this is easier as there are tried and tested structures to follow (e.g., background, method, results, discussion); for more discursive presentations there are less traditions, and careful consideration needs to be given to whether what you are saying

makes sense and is easy to follow. Here, too, is an opportunity to use your critical friend.

The last phase of your presentation is the conclusion. This should tie up your presentation, summarising what you have said and neatly bring your audience to realise that you have finished. As your introduction is an excellent opportunity to come in with a high, your conclusion is an excellent opportunity to go out on a high. Leave your audience in no doubt as to the main messages or key points of your presentation. Finally, remember to thank your audience for their attention. It is a simple courtesy and is always well received.

Visual Aids

Your choice of slide-deck (PowerPoint, Keynote, Prezi, etc.) platform will be governed by the programme available to you. Make yourself familiar with whatever you select to use and do not expect technical help to be present on the day. It is always a good idea to have a backup of your presentation too, such as on a different memory stick.

The Fundamental Steps to Presenting Success

Overall, the key to a good presentation is preparation and rehearsal. One of the most highly regarded presentations was when Steve Jobs launched the iPhone to the world. While quite far removed from the subject or sorts of audience where an occupational therapist is likely to speak, the reasons for the wide acclaim of his presentation are equally valuable for therapists to consider when developing their own presentations. (You can watch the presentation at https://www.youtube.com/watch?v=x7qPAY9JqE4; at the time of writing, it has been viewed over 8.5 million times.) Jobs provided excellent context to his presentation: He engaged his audience, told a story, and used well-developed visuals to support what he was saying. What you say is much more important than what people will look at on the screen, which should be used to support what you are saying. So think about your context and how you are going to engage before you go near preparing your slides. Jobs connected with his audience throughout his presentation, and he rehearsed his presentation tirelessly. By the time he came on stage it looked as if he was at ease, but in fact he was performing a very well-rehearsed presentation. If you prepare and practice, then your presentation is much more likely to go well. If you can, present it to a friendly but constructively critical audience(s) before the actual day. While presenting to colleagues or friends is never the same as the real event, it is the closest dress rehearsal you are likely to get. It will quickly show you which parts of your presentation need refined, and they may spot things that you are unaware of.

WRITING FOR PRESENTATION

Writing for publication is another method of disseminating your work. It is an excellent way to share your research or practice. The advantage of having your work published is that it lasts longer and will almost certainly be more widely accessed than if you present your work at a conference. While writing for publication is undoubtedly challenging, it can also be hugely rewarding.

Where to Submit?

The first task is to consider where best to submit your work. Think about who you want to read what you publish: What journals, magazines, websites, or blogs do your desired audience peruse? Could your potential paper fit the format used in one of these publications? Do you want to submit your work to a source, where its inclusion will be accepted or rejected by the editor alone? Or is your work more scholarly or research based and would be suitable to be submitted to a peer-reviewed journal, where it would be independently scrutinised, normally by at least two subject matter experts who would make recommendations to the editor for acceptance or rejection? Such questions will help you make decisions about where to submit your work. Other factors that can be important (typically in considering where to submit a peer-reviewed paper) include whether a journal is indexed in relevant databases (e.g., CINHAL, PsychInfo, Medline) and whether it has an impact factor.

Impact Factors

Impact factors are published in *Journal Citation Reports* by Thomson Scientific (www.isiwebofknowledge.com). An impact factor is a score assigned to a journal based on the number of times that articles published in 1 year were cited in indexed journals the following year, divided by the number of citable items (letters, editorials, and obituaries are not typically counted in this calculation). Considerable controversy exists about the worth and value of impact factors. It is certainly not a perfect system; however, it is the internationally accepted academic measure of a journal's quality. Other types of quality metrics also exist (Brown & Guttman, 2018), though most of these have not built the same traction as index factors, which despite their limitations and criticisms appear to be lasting the test of time. Whatever metrics are considered, potential authors should consider the quality of the journal they wish to publish in, remembering that the ideal one may not be a profession-specific journal and that other journal titles often contain a wider readership and may have great quality recognition (as indicated by their impact factor rating). Some authors, however, may not be so concerned with a journal's impact factor and may be happy to submit a paper based on the target audience alone. Remember, you may be able to submit more than one paper from your work, so there may be opportunities to do both. Indeed it is becoming increasingly important to write for different audiences so that the impact of your work can have the greatest impact.

Developing Papers

Writing for publication is a skill that people develop over time. If you have not written before, and especially if you are aiming to submit a paper to a peer-reviewed publication, then get an experienced coauthor for your paper or at least seek feedback on what you are writing at an early stage. A coauthor's skills and experience will be invaluable for you as a novice author and could avoid some heartache if your paper is rejected fundamentally through lack of writing experience. It is important to note at this stage, however, that an experienced coauthor is certainly no guarantee of acceptance! Even battle-hardened academics face rejection when they submit their work (Chan et al., 2020). The experience of rejection or major article revision is a common experience. Even with experience the emotional pain of rejection can still be difficult (Chan et al., 2020). Trying to remember that it is not a personal attack may also help. So too does the knowledge that just because something is rejected does not mean it does not have value and may be publishable elsewhere. Often (but not always) the feedback can help improve the paper. If you can take on board the reviewers' recommendations, it will help you to get published and develop as a writer.

Journals or magazines normally have advice or author guidelines. As with submitting abstracts, careful attention must be paid to this advice. Failure to comply with it will lead to your paper being rejected. Often the guidance will outline various different categories of submission (e.g., original research, opinion piece, letters to the editor). If you are not sure which would be best, then consider what you are planning to write and have a look through the journal to see if there are any similar publications.

Whether writing with experienced authors or alone it is vital to consider the structure of your paper. Here too it is worth closely examining the guidelines for authors of a journal or magazine, as well as papers that deal with a similar subject or method area. These will often give you an idea of a structure to follow.

Last-Minute Checks

So you have written your paper and chosen a publication for submission. You have probably spent long hours planning, writing, and revising the text, either alone or with coauthor(s). By now, quite frankly, you are probably getting a bit sick of it and just want to send it off! Stop. Before you do, it is wise to spend a little more time checking it and getting someone completely neutral (perhaps your critical friend) to read it and give you honest comments.

Giving your paper to someone for feedback is an excellent way to find out how readable it is. If the paper is unclear to your friend, then it will most likely be unclear to the editor or reviewers. Time spent revising your paper now may significantly enhance its chance of acceptance. Dixon (2001) recommends asking your friend to write down the four or five most important points that they understood from reading your paper; if they are not the same as yours, or are in a different order, then you need to consider the structure and flow of your work. Further things worth carrying out before you submit your paper include checking:

- That (again) you have followed the author guidelines.
- That any statistics included are appropriately presented.
- That (where appropriate) you have included a statement about the ethical issues of your work and, if required, that formal ethical approval was gained.

SUMMARY

Competition for the ever-shrinking attention of people living in a world filled with information is fierce. Understanding when, where, and what to publish or present is important and knowledge of how to publish or present well is paramount. It pays to give attention and time to the details of what you want to communicate and how you plan to do so. Great presentations and publications often belie the time and effort spent on the development, arrangement, and revision undertaken to achieve its perfect result. Writing and presenting, however, can be highly rewarding and are worth the effort they require.

REFLECTIVE LEARNING

- Who have I seen present well? What is it they do that makes their presentations so good?
- Watch a Ted Talk (www.ted.com) or another presentation recorded on YouTube. Analyse the storyline of how it is presented and its delivery. What worked well? What was less effective? Are there any lessons of things you could adopt, or avoid, when you present?
- Read a blog or academic paper from your chosen area of interest. Was it accessible? If not, in what ways would you improve it?
- Give yourself 15 minutes of uninterrupted time. Choose a topic. Now write for 15 minutes about your chosen topic. You will be surprised by how much you get done.
- What presenting opportunities do I have? How could I make the most of them?
- What could I write about relating to my work? What types of publications (blogs, academic journals,

magazines) do the people I am most interested in communicating with read/access?
- What presenting/writing goal can I set for myself for the next 3 months?

REFERENCES

Albarran, J., & Dowling, S. (2017). Writing an effective conference abstract. *British Journal of Cardiac Nursing, 12*(7), 324–328.

Bannigan K. Disseminating research results. *Ment Health Occup Ther* 2005; 10:88–9

Brown, T., & Gutman, S. A. (2018). Impact factor, eigenfactor, article influence, scopus SNIP, and SCImage journal rank of occupational therapy journals. *Scandinavian Journal of Occupational Therapy*, 2019; 26 (7): 475

Chan, H., Mazzucchelli, T. G., & Rees, C. S. (2020). The battle-hardened academic: An exploration of the resilience of university academics in the face of ongoing criticism and rejection of their research. *Higher Education Research & Development*, 1–15.

Dixon, N. (2001). Writing for publication—a guide for new authors. *International Journal for Quality in Health Care, 13*(5), 417–421.

Draper, J. (2012). Writing a conference abstract and paper. In K. Holland, & R. Watson (Eds.), *Writing for publication in nursing and healthcare.* Wiley-Blackwell.

Editorial Board. (2005). Internationalisation and impact factors: A communication from the editorial board. *British Journal of Occupational Therapy, 68*, 97–98.

Fricke, J. (2006). On impacts and other factors. *Australian Occupational Therapy Journal, 53*, 1–2.

Haigh, C. A. (2006). The art of the abstract. *Nurse Education Today, 26*(5), 355–357.

Harms, M. (1995). How to prepare a poster presentation. *Physiotherapy, 81*(5), 276–277.

Innes, G. (1988). Unpublished lecture notes. *Queen Margaret College.*

Krajewska, J., & Vermeulen, L. (2018). Young GI angle: How to write a good conference abstract. *European Gastroenterology Journal United European Gastroenterology Journal, 6*(3), 482–484.

Kinder, J. S. (1973). Using instructional media. *D van Nostrand Co.*

Mehrabian, A. (1971). Silent messages. *Wadsworth.*

Meshack, B. L. (2004). Developing a thick skin: How to accept criticism. *Vision: A Resource for Writers.* http://fmwriters.com/Visionback/Vision24/developingthickskin.htm2004.

Papanek, V. (1985). In *Design for the real world* (2nd ed.). Academy Chicago Publishers.

Simmonds, D. (1984). How to. produce a good poster. *Medical Teacher, 6*(1), 10–13.

von Elm, E., Altman, D. G., Egger, M., Pocock, S. J., Gotzsche, P. C., & Vandenbroucke, J. P. (2007). The strengthening the reporting of observational studies in epidemiology (STROBE) statement: Guidelines for reporting observational studies. *The Lancet, 370*(9596), 1453–1457.

Wheildon, C. (1996). *Type and layout: How typography and design can get your message across—or get in the way.* Strathmoor Press.

17

Self-Care and Self-Management

Katrina Bannigan

HIGHLIGHTS

- As work can provide challenges to health and well-being, occupational therapists need to have strategies for self-care to maintain optimal performance at work.
- A number of strategies, such as taking regular breaks or coaching, can support our ability to self-care.
- Some occupational therapists will need to engage in self-management—the process of learning to manage a health condition on a day-to-day basis—to enable them to continue working with a long-term condition.

- There are challenges that can impinge on our ability to perform well at work, namely a lack of work-life balance, impostor syndrome, and burnout. Self-care strategies can help to ameliorate these.
- Resilience involves the ability to bounce back from difficult experiences; it is not an innate ability and is a skill that can be developed by anyone.

OVERVIEW

Since the last edition of this book, self-care has become a mainstream activity. To perform well at work, individual occupational therapists are expected to take personal responsibility for their self-care. Changes in retirement ages and pension provision mean many occupational therapists will be working for longer. This increases the number of people who will be working with a long-term condition, and so self-management has become more of a consideration in supporting occupational therapists to perform well at work. The key focus of this chapter is looking after ourselves with the overall aim of stimulating thought about how we, as occupational therapists, can take measures to care for ourselves to perform at our best in work. This chapter will explore the following:

- Challenges occupational therapists face in the workplace today
- Concepts of self-care and self-management
- Strategies occupational therapists can use for self-care and self-management
- Challenges of lack of work-life balance, impostor syndrome, and burnout
- Developing resilience

Vignettes, based on the stories of how occupational therapists have managed self-care and self-management, have been included to give a clear description of the reality of achieving self-care and self-management in practice. This chapter has been written in the expectation that you will also make links between its content and the chapters on Clinical Supervision Skills (see Chapter 20) and Leadership Skills (see Chapter 18) because each informs and supports the other.

THE CHALLENGES OF WORKING LIVES TODAY

Occupational therapists extol the virtue of a balanced lifestyle, which includes work-life balance (Westhorp, 2003) and promote it through occupational balance (i.e., "the individual's perception of having the right amount of occupations and the right variation between occupations"; Wagman et al., 2012, p. 322). Wilson and Wilcock (2005) studied the occupational balance of new occupational therapy students, and their findings suggested occupational balance is linked to health and well-being. Much of our everyday work as occupational therapists is dependent on us as people (i.e., our therapeutic use of self; see Chapter 8). Yet how many of us achieve occupational balance, or really look after ourselves? It is very easy for people in caring roles to neglect caring for themselves; hence the aphorism "physician heal thy self." Occupational therapists are a valuable resource and—as we are the main tool we have to do our work—if we do not care for ourselves, we can be prone to a lack of work-life balance, imposter syndrome, or burnout and so undermine our ability to be occupational therapists.

The "Always On" Culture

Self-care at work can be challenging because of the nature of society. Technological developments in particular are changing the way we live our lives. There is a sense that we have an "always on" culture—whereby digital technology is never switched off—creating pressure because if, for example, we receive email alerts outside work hours it can feel like we are never away from work, and there are no boundaries between our personal and professional lives. Another challenge in relation to technology is the number of different generations within the adult working population who have a completely different experience of technology. Whilst we have to take care about stereotyping, thinking about people in terms of a generational cohort—the group of individuals born at a similar time—can be helpful in terms of differences in experience of technology and how they engage with work. The current generations commonly identified in demographic literature are Baby Boomer (1947–1966), Generation X (1965–1981), Generation Y (or Millenials; 1982–1999), Generation Z (2000–2012), and the newest Generation Alpha (the first to be born entirely in the 21st century) (Mahmoud et al., 2020; Perano, 2019; Walker & Lewis, 2010). "The technologies available as a generation matures influence their behaviours, attitudes, and expectations. People internalise the technologies that shape information access and use, as well as the ways they communicate. For each successive generation technology is only technology if it was invented after they were born" (Hartman et al., 2005, para. 4).

As another example of a generational shift, not related to technology, it was a salutary experience for me to realise that many of the students I teach do not know about the UK prime ministers Margaret Thatcher or Tony Blair. Both figures have had a formative impact on my experience but have played no part in the experience of the people I am teaching today. This reinforces the impact of difference generational experiences. These differences contribute to diversity in the workplace and, if well managed, can create a positive work culture (Mahmoud et al., 2020).

Societal Shifts are Reflected in the Nature of Work

Changes in society shape the landscape of work. Technological developments mean, in essence, organisations are no longer defined or shaped by a building in the way they once were (this has been confirmed by the changes to working practices during the Covid-19 pandemic). There has been a shift in the location of work, as well as work not being confined to buildings, and fewer people working in the same place every day of the week. For example, people do not need to leave their home but, if they do, people on the move can receive referrals and update their assessments through handheld devices that update in real time; a check-in to a base may never be needed. Many people who work in an office have to hot-desk if they use office space at all. These developments also mean there is less emphasis on the jobs people have and a greater focus on the tasks and assignments they need to engage in. The significant change that this created for Baby Boomers is mitigated by the fact they are now retiring, and Generation X are becoming the senior managers; this group, whilst technologically savvy in that they use smartphones and social media, has very different communication preferences to the generations coming behind (Mahmoud et al., 2020). For example, people in Generation Z prefer to text rather than email (Mahmoud et al., 2020). This difference in communication indicates that other intergenerational differences will also impact on how the workplace operates. As the workplace changes and adapts in response to technological and other societal changes, the ability of people to be flexible and adaptable over time is a valuable skill.

Working in Health and Social Care

Health and social care settings have not been immune to these changes in the workplace. The nature of modern health and social care services is different from when the Baby Boomers were predominant and could expect cradle-to-grave job security. Many occupational therapists will not work in the National Health Service or social care throughout their careers because many services are now delivered outside the statutory sector, with associated pay and conditions, and (lack of) job security. Some roles might not use the title occupational therapist, especially in nontraditional areas of practice. With the emphasis on tasks and assignments, many occupational therapists will have portfolio careers—careers involving several different roles and/or working patterns over a career or simultaneously—within health and social care; the *BMJ* has recently published an article to explore how medics can do this (Rimmer, 2020). Individual practitioners cannot rely on others to chart their career for them because, with flatter structures, there are fewer managers and they often have a broader portfolio of responsibilities. Moreover there may be no direct professional line management (i.e., by an occupational therapist). It cannot always be assumed that a manager will understand the contribution occupational therapy can make to new agendas.

As well as changes to career pathways, the rate of technological change in health and social care is increasing. This requires occupational therapists to be competent in digital literacy skills—that is, "those capabilities that fit someone for living, learning, working, participating and thriving in a digital society" (Health Education England, n.d., para. 3)—across practice, service delivery, education, and research. This places a wider range of demands on occupational therapists, which means there is a need to take personal responsibility for developing the technological skills needed to function in today's health and social care organisations. To navigate current career pathways as well as keeping abreast of technological developments, self-care should also be a skill occupational therapists want to nurture because it will help us to function optimally. For many occupational therapists it is the number and range of challenges presented by day-to-day work within the context of an "always on" culture that blurs the boundaries between work and personal life. Therefore it is important to be able to identify the warning signs and then do something to rectify the situation if problems arise. The bottom line is self-care has become essential to performing well at work for all occupational therapists.

SELF-CARE

The concept of self-care means different things to different people (Vignettes 17.1, 17.2, and 17.3). Generally, self-care involves taking personal responsibility for maintaining our health and well-being. This can be disconcerting because, whilst we know our health and well-being is at risk if we do not take care of ourselves, we can often feel like we are being selfish if we prioritise our needs. We need to prioritise ourselves and take active steps to care for ourselves, however selfish we may feel that is (Taylor, 2005). This means

we must look after ourselves as well as we can because it will enable us to continue to perform well at work as well as in life generally. How we care for ourselves will depend to a certain extent on our personal interests, needs, and circumstances. For example, someone working full time with young children may have different work-life balance needs compared to another person who is understimulated by work and feels the need to be stretched more. As everyone's needs are different and can change over time (see Vignettes 17.1 and 17.3), we need to monitor ourselves. Self-care is not something that we can address once in our careers and assume all will be well for the duration; we need to revisit the issue every so often to ensure that the measures we put in place are still relevant to our needs. It may be a question we pose for ourselves annually, perhaps at the time of our appraisal, even if it is not a question on the official forms that we have to complete. That is, build in at the very least an annual check-in for ourselves, although we may need more frequent checks such as when were faced with a global pandemic.

If we monitor ourselves regularly, then we should be able to identify warning signs (e.g., we are becoming stressed or anxious about everyday scenarios). By recognising early on that our self-care needs attention we can then take steps to alter the situation before bigger problems arise (see Vignette 17.3) such as burnout, a lack of work-life balance, or succumbing to impostor syndrome, which are discussed later in the chapter. Whilst there can be serious consequences of neglecting our self-care, there are other less serious problems that can also undermine our ability to do our job properly

---

VIGNETTE 17.1   Amy's Story: A Self-Care Routine Is Essential for Managing the Challenges of Life

Self-care is something I feel strongly about. It has helped me through challenging times. Throughout the last 10 years, my roles and responsibilities have changed; however, my self-care prescription has remained the same. I have progressed in my home life from single to a married mother and in my work from a student to an occupational therapist. All my work-life roles have changed considerably, and with each new role comes different challenges. I have been asked on many occasions how I manage it all. The answer for me has been simple, self-care. However, that may look different for others. When there is the right balance of what is meaningful and what is routine, the challenges I have faced in life have not felt as difficult to process.

For me, exercise has been my main self-care activity. In my younger years, that meant going to the gym every

day after studying; however, that level of commitment became impractical when I became a mother. For me, self-care needs to be flexible to be successful. I do not always need to go to high-impact gym sessions. Going for a walk at lunch or a jog around my block is just as beneficial to maintain my well-being. When I exercise I listen to music, which helps me disconnect from the world, my role, and my responsibilities. It gives me time and space to breathe, to think, and to reflect. Although this may sound unappealing to others, it is not the actual activity that is the focus of my self-care, it is how it makes me feel. I feel refreshed and ready to take on my roles once again. Finding something that gives me that feeling has been paramount in preventing burnout and managing my well-being in an ever-demanding world.

VIGNETTE 17.2   Leona's Story: Knowing Myself Is Key to My Self-Care

For me, self-care is doing something that makes me feel grounded. Being a slightly more introverted person, I know that I re-energise best when I have time by myself. This usually means scheduling in time away from friends and family where I can be with my own thoughts, with no to-do lists and where I regain energy and perspective as a result of taking some time out. The key for me is to not put pressure on what I do with this time but to keep it as a priority.

Since moving from a clinical role into academia, I have found an increasing need to be strict with my self-care time as the temptation and pressure to take work physically home (e.g., laptop or books) is prevalent. Now, I love batch cooking at the weekend with my favourite music on. This is not only some enjoyable self-care time, where I can experiment with new recipes, but also provides a grounded feeling that lasts throughout the week when I know I am organised with healthy meals prepped. It also allows me the time to be more consistent with another self-care practice I love: yoga! With a job that is now more office based, incorporating movement and exercise into my self-care routine is essential and what my body craves. But for it to be self-care for me, there has to be no pressure around the exercise. Once there is pressure, then self-care becomes an addition to an already very long to-do list and the value is lost.

VIGNETTE 17.3   Penelope's Story: Getting Stressed Made Me Start to Self-Care

I did not have good self-care, and this came to a head when I was studying for a PhD. I got very stressed and found it hard to sleep, waking up in the night and earlier in the morning. When I woke I would start to work on my PhD, sometimes as early as 4:00 a.m. I also began to experience anxiety, which I had never had before. I recognised that if I did not do something I could become unwell. I was aware, from my interaction with others, that the stress I was experiencing about my PhD was not typical. Other PhD students were not reacting in the same way so I knew I was not coping and that I needed to change. Getting up early to work was not helping; I was not doing my best work.

The change was gradual; self-care is a process that has worked better the more I have engaged it. It started with the decision that I wanted to be successful with my PhD, and to be successful I had to change my approach to the PhD and myself. There was no one thing that made a difference; I made a number of changes over time. I started with making sure that I got enough sleep; I made getting enough sleep a priority. I go to bed between 9.30 and 10.00 p.m., when I am tired, and I do not deviate from this. I like exercise and, whilst I was already exercising, the exercise I did was fast paced. I needed to slow down so I started yoga because it is good for relaxation and used the Headspace app for meditation. I also made a conscious effort to have more balance; I was working too hard because every spare moment was spent working on my PhD. I made a conscious decision to keep my studies in perspective by scheduling time off. I set deadlines, only wrote for specific time periods, and planned time to do something nice as a reward. I also made a conscious decision not to react to situations by choosing not to get involved with the same level of emotion; this way, I have found I can achieve more with a clearer head.

I have learnt that I have to make self-care a priority; it has to be part of my routine, otherwise it is the one thing that gets given up when the pressure is on.

---

such as an inability to prioritise, becoming impatient with colleagues and/or service users, or feeling out of our depth. As self-care has become a mainstream activity, there has been a proliferation of freely available high-quality, evidence-based resources. For example, consider the following:
• "The 10 keys for happier living"
   The 10 keys for happier living are evidence-based precepts that Action for Happiness (n.d.) has found if used will make life happier and more fulfilling, not only for individuals but communities as well. The website has lots of resources to support you in achieving the keys for happier living, such as webinars, action calendars, and news stories (Action for Happiness, n.d.).
• The importance of self-care
   This is a playlist of TED Talks (short digestible podcasts) related to self-care (TED Conferences, LLC., n.d.). It includes talks on topics such as why we all need to practice emotional first aid (Guy Winch), the power of vulnerability (Brené Brown), and one titled "Got a meeting? Take a walk" (Nilofer Merchant).

Self-Care Strategies

There are a number of self-care strategies that we, as occupational therapists, can use to improve our self-care. It is important to remember our differences, as some of the occupational therapists have pointed out in their vignettes (see Vignettes 17.1 and 17.2), and we face different challenges and need to find the strategies that work for us (Vignette 17.4; see also Vignette 17.3). Equally, as well as having different needs, these needs change over time so we should not be afraid to try new strategies if existing strategies are no longer working (see Vignettes 17.3 and 17.4). Self-care strategies include:

- **Assertiveness training:** This involves learning skills, such as active listening and stuck record technique, and building confidence to increase personal effectiveness. This type of training can be helpful if you do not feel like you have any control over your work, such as the inability to say no, which can be very stressful. It is important to deal with this type of stress because it can lead to work spilling into home life and upsetting your work-life balance.

- **Career development planning:** This involves taking responsibility for managing our careers and reflects the fact that, with flatter management structures, the qualifications and gateways required for promotion and development are not uniform or as clear cut as they may once have been. As well as the constantly evolving technological innovations, the changes in organisations that encourage varied and portfolio careers mean we have to manage and map the narrative of our careers. Consequently, career development in occupational therapy may require an alternative approach—an ongoing individualised development programme—for maintaining and extending skills and developing an area of specialism. To do this planning, it may be helpful to work with a life coach or an occupational psychologist. Equally, the Royal College of Occupational Therapists (2021) has developed the Career Development Framework and supporting materials to facilitate career development.

- **Coaching:** This involves working with another person who has formally trained as a coach, to focus on areas of development that may involve a change, a task, or skills and be performance, work, or personal related. The role of the coach is to pass on skills and knowledge, which means your line manager could adopt this role. The agenda is set by the coach and tends to be more directive and short term than mentoring.

- **Creating a positive working environment:** The culture in a work environment can promote or militate against good working behaviours, such as work-life balance. We all have responsibility for our working environment and promoting the behaviours, practices, or ideas that create a positive environment. Is there anything you need to change in your department to promote your health and well-being and that of the people who work in it? If you cannot do it yourself, is this something you could raise in Clinical Supervision Skills (see Chapter 20) or exercise personal Leadership Skills (see Chapter 18) or discuss in a team meeting. Even if there is no appetite for discussing the work environment in your team or organisation, an individual or a small group of individuals

---

VIGNETTE 17.4 Sadie's Story: Using Peer Mentoring for Career Development

I have always recognised that I have responsibility for my career development, and I have worked with others to support it. This has always involved an element of peer mentoring. Examples of this include:

- Using books to structure learning. In the past I wanted to be more focused and felt I had lost some clarity about my work. Following a discussion with a colleague who had similar concerns we agreed to peer mentor each other. The publication of *The 8th Habit* (Covey, 2006) coincided with this discussion, and we decided to use the chapters from this book to structure our peer mentoring discussions. More recently I have worked through *The Gifts of Imperfection* (Brown, 2010) in a similar way. Both times we committed to meeting once a month and to reflect on the reading we had done from the book and current issues from our work. Having a

colleague to work with, who was equally committed to continuing professional development, was a privilege. However, I am not sure if the sessions would have been as effective without the reading to structure it. The reading kept us focused.

- Attending writing groups. Throughout my career I have been part of writing groups whereby a group of colleagues get together regularly to support each other with writing. Women seem to particularly benefit from writing in groups (Schucan Bird, 2014). Generally, we meet for 90 minutes and start by sharing a goal for the session, then write solidly for 60 minutes in silence without any distractions from the internet or mobile phones. Sometimes this has involved longer periods of time—1 day, 3 days, or 1 week—with the day divided into 90-minute blocks with breaks.

can facilitate this through small changes and behaviours (e.g., ensuring you say good morning to everyone no matter how busy you are or engaging in random acts of kindness [https://www.randomactsofkindness.org/]).

- **Developing good habits:** As occupational therapists we understand that our habits—that is, "acquired tendencies to automatically respond and perform in certain consistent ways in familiar environments or situations" (Wook Lee & Kielhofner, 2017, p. 60)—can support or undermine our self-care. The focus on self-care in wider society means we are almost bombarded with suggestions, such as *The Guardian*'s "Ten tips for a better work-life balance" (Box 17.1), about habits we could cultivate to improve our self-care. Other examples of habits we could develop or maintain include developing interests outside of work, asking for help if needed, introducing variety into our daily routines (short term) but also our careers (long term), learning to say no without feeling guilty, and taking frequent breaks.

- **Exercise:** Few, if any, of us will have escaped the message that exercise has an essential role to play in well-being. But how many of us integrate exercise into our everyday routines and habits? The possibilities for incorporating exercise into our working lives are endless. The "How to…Look after your mental health using exercise" is a practical guide that explores the evidence for the impact of physical activity on mental well-being and then provides realistic practical steps for getting started as well as signposting to other resources (Mental Health Foundation, n.d.).

- **Mentoring:** This used to be used exceptionally when the normal support or development structures were not available to individuals, but it has become a more mainstream activity. Although you can engage in peer mentoring (see Vignette 17.4), it is usually a one-to-one relationship with someone who inspires you or is an experienced or trusted adviser. Mentoring is used to support people to manage their learning to maximise their potential, develop their skills, and improve their performance. Mentoring is driven by the mentee, and the mentor may draw upon a number of skills to support their mentee to achieve their aims, including advising, guiding, teaching (this may be by example through being a role model), opening doors for, empathising, challenging, encouraging, promoting, explaining the politics and the subtleties of the job, helping the mentee succeed, being a resource, prompting, supporting (including emotional support), mediating, facilitating, and advocating. It's a long list but this is what makes mentoring so valuable; it is tailored to you (as the mentee) and your needs. A mentor can fulfil a number of roles (Box 17.2). Although the roles of mentor and mentee are clearly defined, mentorship is regarded as a reciprocal relationship from which both benefit.

- **Networking:** A network is a group of people with whom you can exchange information, contacts, and experiences for professional (or social) purposes. Networking operates on several levels and in different ways but is essentially about managing your career. The benefits include information sharing, increasing self-confidence, mutual support, discussion, increased knowledge, and

---

BOX 17.1 Ten Tips for a Better Work-Life Balance (Jeffries, 2014)

1. Step away from email.
2. Just say no: Don't answer instantly to avoid saying yes unthinkingly.
3. Work smarter, not harder: Overworking is not productive.
4. Leave work at work: Even when working at home, we need to close the door on it.
5. Forget about perfection: It may not be perfect, but is it good enough?
6. Don't be a martyr.
7. Ease off the adrenaline: If we are rushing all the time, we will crash.
8. Think about retirement: What will you do when you don't have work, if work is all consuming?
9. Make them wait: We don't need to respond to emails instantly.
10. Set your own rules: Work out what works for you.

BOX 17.2 Skills of a Mentor

1. **Mentor as critical friend**: Enables the mentee to clarify the situation, set goals, and explore options. They provide feedback, which encourages the mentee to find solutions, look for opportunities to practise new skills, and plan action.
2. **Mentor as a sounding board**: Enables the mentee to focus on a real problem and moves the discussion from the problem to searching for alternative solutions by suspending judgement, keeping their own counsel, listening more than talking, and facilitating the individual to understand own motivations and feelings.
3. **Mentor as facilitator**: Enables the mentee get to know relevant parts of a network, facilitates the mentee to map and make better use of an existing networks, and explores with the mentee how to approach contacts and use networking skills.

personal development. The types of activities that can be used for networking are business meetings, email, breakfast meetings, conferences, journeys, events that happen around meetings/conferences (e.g., coffee breaks, workshops, lunch), letter writing, and telephone calls. You may notice that most of these are social-type gatherings, and the predominant skills you need are communication skills. Once you have initiated communication with someone you would like to network with, make sure that you have follow-up strategies in place to establish regular communication.

- **Practice kindness and compassion:** Another big change since the last edition is the increasing recognition that kindness and compassion, including self-compassion, are important components of self-care (Neff, 2011).
- **Rest and sleep:** These are essential components to our physical and mental well-being. As well as making sure we get enough sleep and take time to rest, it is also important to watch our language. This is because sometimes our use of language—constantly referring to how busy we are—reinforces our sense of having little control.
- **Time management:** There are numerous resources on time management skills, but it may be that time management is a misnomer. It may be more helpful to think of time management in terms of self-management (Covey, 2020). This approach acknowledges the challenge is not to manage time but to manage ourselves, and the key to effective self-management is focus— knowing what our priorities are (Covey, 2020)—the three or four things that truly matter most to us. People who have reached the top in their field when asked what was the key determining factor will say focus (i.e., be very clear about what their priorities are) (Covey, 2020). Time management becomes an issue when the things

that are important to us do not receive the care, emphasis, and time we really want to give them. A good self-care technique is to go to work each day with a single priority and make sure whatever else crops up you make significant progress on that task that day.

There has been such an explosion of self-care literature the ideas presented here provide only a flavour of what is available.

SELF-MANAGEMENT

Self-care is important on a day-to-day basis when working as an occupational therapist but, as has already been stated, longer retirement ages and pension provision mean more people are likely to be working with a long-term condition that requires self-management (Vignette 17.5). The concept of self-management, within the context of health and social care, is a model for supporting people with long-term conditions. It is:

The systematic process of learning and practicing skills which enable individuals to manage their health condition on a day-to-day basis, through practicing and adopting specific behaviours which are central to managing their condition, making informed decisions about care, and engaging in healthy behaviours to reduce the physical and emotional impact of their illness, with or without the collaboration of the health care system.
Royal College of Nursing (2020, para. 6)

Just as all occupational therapists are different, there is a huge range of long-term conditions, crossing the panoply of mental and physical health, meaning there is no off-the-shelf self-management plan. There is no one-size-fits-all solution, but there are steps a person can work through to

---

VIGNETTE 17.5   Laura's Story: Self-Management for Living and Working With a Long-Term Condition

Living with endometriosis, self-management is important to allow me to continue working as an occupational therapist despite my chronic pain and fatigue. The most important thing for me was making sure that I was as informed as possible about my condition and possible ways of managing symptoms, such as a modified diet. Making sure I plan time for rest and gentle exercise, such as yoga, helps me to stay well enough for work, but it does take careful planning to carry out my daily tasks and do everything necessary to manage my health. A significant area of growth has been developing my understanding of my limits, particularly at work. This means being able to appreciate when I need to ask for help or when I need to say no, both of which can still be difficult particularly working in a busy service. I have found being open and honest about my symptoms, helps me find support from colleagues when I need it. Sometimes I need to sit down due to pain, and on these days I will modify my duties so I can assist the team with referrals or information gathering rather than working on the wards. I make sure I take my lunch break and try as much as possible to leave on time as I am only able to support service users properly if I am taking care of myself. I have had to learn that self-care is not selfish but is crucial for me to be able to continue in my rewarding work.

develop an individualised self-management plan. Specifically, these steps include:

1. Recognise that you need to care for yourself to maintain optimal performance at work.
2. Take active steps toward caring for yourself, which may involve education to learn more about the condition itself.
3. Self-assess by reflecting on your own needs, systems, and procedures.
4. Identify whether you have any issues impeding your effectiveness at work (e.g., fatigue or diurnal variation in the experience of symptoms).
5. Consider if anything needs to change to enable you to work effectively (e.g., pacing or staggered working hours), and develop solutions tailored to your needs (this may include seeking additional support from your employer if necessary).
6. Implement the strategies.
7. Monitor the impact that the strategies are having on your effectiveness and resilience. If they are having limited impact, then go back to steps 5 and 6 to identify and test alternative solutions.

Being occupational therapists may mean we have knowledge and skills that provide a head start with implementing this, but we can take on the sick role in the same way as others so it does not automatically follow that developing a self-management plan will be easy.

CHALLENGES TO WELL-BEING IN THE WORKPLACE

Having considered the concepts of and strategies to promote self-care and self-management, the particular challenges of a lack of work-life balance, impostor syndrome, and burnout are considered in turn.

A Lack of Work-Life Balance

"Overwork is the curse of our time. Working long hours has become a badge of honour among professional people, whose complaints about overwork are often mixed with a sense of pride in their dedication and importance" (Grosch & Olsen, 1994, p. 101). Overwork is perpetuated through a need for chronic busyness and is prevalent in the helping professions (Grosch & Olsen, 1994). By contrast, work-life balance is about achieving the right balance of focus, energy, and time between your work and other important areas of your life (Lee & King, 2001). It is not easy to achieve because there is no prescription, and everyone has to work it out for themselves, but it is also not about being perfect in all aspects of your life (Lee & King, 2001). Work-life balance helps us to be more effective at work because, for example, single-minded devotion to work is correlated with poor performance (Lee & King, 2001). The benefits of achieving work-life balance will not only be experienced in the work arena but also in our personal lives. Lee and King (2001) suggested five strategies for achieving balance:

- Integrating. Counterintuitively, instead of trying to keep work and life separate through having clear boundaries between the two, we should allow boundaries to be more flexible and allow overlap.
- Narrowing. This involves recognising that there is only so much any one individual can do and so we need to make only those commitments we can keep.
- Moderating. This builds on the maxim "everything in moderation" and means spending the right amount of time in each area of your life, not overdoing things.
- Sequencing. Recognising that we cannot do everything at once so we need to plan and have priorities, and concomitantly some activities may have to fall by the wayside.
- Adding resources. Use additional resources where we can to enable us to get more done.

Impostor Syndrome

Impostor syndrome is the phrase used to describe people who, despite being competent, feel like a fraud in their professional lives; it seems to affect women more than men. It impacts on self-efficacy, and the effects can become crippling over time (Jöstl et al., 2012). Given that occupational therapy is a female-dominated profession, it is likely that impostor syndrome is a challenge faced by occupational therapists whether students, practitioners, managers, teachers, or researchers. People experiencing impostor syndrome play down their successes because they believe their achievements are only through good fortune, and this is likely to exposed at any time. It has been observed that these:

> *vague feelings of self-doubt, intellectual fraudulence and anxiety are so common among people, it's almost an epidemic. The 'impostor syndrome' strikes people everywhere especially high achievers. It makes them discount their success attributing it to luck, not real ability. Along with it comes the fear that anytime they could be found out.*
>
> **Bhargava (2003, para. 4)**

As the experience of impostor syndrome involves an inability to internalise success, strategies for overcoming it are linked to the need to internalise success, such as the following:

- **Recognise the phenomenon exists** and be honest with yourself if you are experiencing it.
- **Accept compliments** to acknowledging the work you do, the experience you have, or the effort you put into achieving the outcome.

- **Become part of a network**. Strong support networks and mentors, particularly ones targeted at women, can diminish imposter syndrome's effects (Jöstl et al., 2012).
- **Challenging the thinking that allows impostor syndrome to flourish** by questioning thoughts such as "I have only got here by luck" or "It's only because I was in the right place at the right time."
- **Developing benchmarks for success** that not only look at future goals but also acknowledge achievements.
- **Focus on and keep track of positive achievements** (e.g., developing a highlights list—a colleague has a "happy folder" to collate these) to help focus on positive achievements and keep them at the forefront of our mind.
- **Keep learning** because asking questions is an important skill for all. We can feel that we should act like we know everything, which means we stop asking questions. We do this because we do not want to admit we do not know, then be found out as an imposter.

Burnout

Burnout is a syndrome, listed in the *International Classification of Diseases*, which results from chronic workplace stress that has not been successfully managed (World Health Organisation, 2019). It is a problem experienced in health and social care settings as much as any other workplace; being a health and social care professional is not a protective factor. Burnout "is characterised by three dimensions:

- feelings of energy depletion or exhaustion;
- increased mental distance from one's job, or feelings of negativism or cynicism related to one's job; and
- reduced professional efficacy." (World Health Organisation, 2019, para. 5)

It is a serious problem because it is not easy to treat; there is no pharmaceutic solution, and the energy depletion that characterises the syndrome leaves a person with little energy to fight it. Taylor (2005) contended that allowing oneself to burnout "is tantamount to negligence as burnout is next to impossible to treat once it is established" (p. 220).

Burnout is a complex problem but, although difficult to treat, it is avoidable. It makes more sense to prevent it rather than treat it (Grosch & Olsen, 1994). As burnout is not caused by any one factor, there are warning signs to be aware of:

- Your energy being used up quicker on a daily basis than you recover it, resulting in experiences such as fatigue, exhaustion, an inability to concentrate, insomnia, and irritability
- Being out of control with demands at work
- Trying to be a hero at work, such as engaging in presenteeism (coming to work when we are ill)

- Lacking the assertiveness skills to say no
- Depression and/or anxiety
- Increased use of alcohol or drugs
- A loss of interest in one's work or personal life
- Seeing patients as problems rather than as people
- A feeling of "just going through the motions" (Taylor, 2005)

Even early in your career you can be vulnerable to burnout: "It takes two years (on average), if the conditions are right, from starting clinical work to burnout" (Taylor, 2005, p. 220).

There are no simplistic formulas to prevent burnout; it is not just about substituting a leisure activity with some of the time you spend at work. Grosch and Olsen (1994) have developed an approach to preventing burnout based on a theory of family origin. However, it is possible to delineate steps to prevent burnout that stand alone from this theoretical perspective:

- **Ongoing self-assessment**: By assessing ourselves regularly we can determine the difference between normal tiredness and early signs of burnout.
- **Understanding our patterns of behaviour**: Recognise the issues that are contributing to burnout (e.g., perfectionism).
- **Breaking behaviour patterns**: Take action to resolve issues identified (e.g., if taking on too many responsibilities is an issue you may need to learn to say no and set firm boundaries).
- **Emotional intelligence**: Develop the capacity to manage strong feelings and impulses in the face of stress and anxiety-provoking situations.

Although maintaining health is required to actively prevent burnout, other issues, such as time management and the control we feel we have over our work, are also relevant. This is why self-care and self-management have a role to play in developing resilience.

DEVELOPING RESILIENCE

Challenges to well-being in the workplace can be prevented by developing resilience. Resilience is our capacity to bounce back from stressful events and situations and is a highly valued skill that anyone can develop (Contu, 2002). Three characteristics of resilient people are the capacity to accept and face reality, the ability to find meaning in some aspects of life, and the ability to improvise (Contu, 2002).

Accepting and Facing Reality

It is often thought that positivity is a prerequisite for personal development and resilience. The challenge with this is it can lead to denial or an overly positive attitude in the face of difficult circumstances (e.g., the death of a colleague or redundancies). It does not promote resilience but can stop an individual facing the reality of the situation and may be regarded as inappropriate by others sharing the same experience. Resilience requires a positive outlook not being so positive you tolerate the intolerable. A positive outlook does not deny the reality of a situation; it is the fundamental belief that, even if the present situation is not good, the future will have a positive outcome. It stems from an optimistic approach to events and situations.

Finding Meaning in Some Aspects of Life

In difficult circumstances many of us take on a victim role revealed in the question, "Why is this happening to me?" The question can equally be posed, "Why not me?" Contu (2002) contends "resilient people devise constructs about their suffering to create some sort of meaning for themselves and others" (para. 10). In this situation, meaning making becomes a coping mechanism (i.e., we cope by making sense of a situation for ourselves by setting it in a context).

The Ability to Improvise

Improvisation is about flexibility. It involves the ability to make do with whatever is at hand particularly during stressful circumstances and traumatic events. It encompasses serendipity; we need to make the best use of opportunities. We cannot always wait for the right time—there is never usually a right time—sometimes we need to seize opportunities. It is recognised that improvisation has not been widely encouraged in health and social care services. We sometimes must take the initiative rather than rely on or expect existing hierarchies or systems to provide the solutions. This is also called adaptive capacity; the ability to transcend adversity and emerge stronger than before (Bennis & Thomas, 2003).

Strategies for Increasing Resilience

Developing resilience is a skill we, as occupational therapists, should want to develop for ourselves, even though it is something our employers want to nurture, because it will help us to function optimally. Inevitably anything individuals do to increase their resilience at work is also likely to have benefits in other aspects of their life. By understanding the characteristics of resilient people we can assess where our personal challenges lie. Strategies to increase resilience include:

- Developing caring and supportive relationships within and outside the family; good social networks increase our resilience
- Increasing our capacity to make realistic plans and take steps to carry them out

- Fostering a positive view of ourselves and confidence in our strengths and abilities (e.g., avoid competitive negativity such as trying to "out busy" everyone else you speak to)
- Increasing communication and problem-solving skills (American Psychological Association, n.d.)

However, as with most things in life, developing resilience requires time, effort, and commitment. It is not a one-off task that can be ticked off a to-do list.

SUMMARY

This chapter has focused on how self-care is an essential element of maintaining optimal work performance in the context of the challenges presented in the current work arena. As more occupational therapists will be working with a long-term condition in the future, self-management was also discussed. The changes in organisations and society and technological advances mean occupational therapists need to take more personal responsibility for their careers, but it also means we can have more control over our careers, including the possibility of having a portfolio career. One of the exciting aspects of working in health and social care today is that we can truly have the careers we want. To achieve this and enjoy the diverse range of work experiences on offer, we need to have the flexibility, adaptability, and resilience required to flourish in an ever-changing work environment.

REFLECTIVE LEARNING

- To what extent do you think your values and beliefs as an occupational therapist require you to be a role model for self-care and/or self-management?
- How would you describe your current self-care? Thinking about your response, could you incorporate any of the strategies outlined in this chapter to develop or enhance it?
- Within the scope of your current role, what could you do to create or promote further a positive working environment?
- Think of a recent challenging event in your life and ask yourself how well you exhibited the three characteristics of resilience.

REFERENCES

Action for Happiness. (n.d.). 10 Keys for happier living. U.K. Action for Happiness. https://www.actionforhappiness.org/10-keys-to-happier-living.

American Psychological Association. (n.d.). The road to resilience. https://www.uis.edu/counselingcenter/wp-content/uploads/sites/87/2013/04/the_road_to_resilience.pdf.

Bennis, W., & Thomas, R.J. (2003). Crucibles of leadership. Harvard Business Review. https://hbr.org/2002/09/crucibles-of-leadership.

Bhargava, S. (2003). The imposter syndrome: Feeling like a fraud. Financial Express. https://www.financialexpress.com/archive/the-imposter-syndrome-feeling-like-a-fraud/76569/.

Brown, B. (2010). *The gifts of imperfection*. Hazeldon Publishing.

Contu, D. (2002). How resilience works. Harvard Business Review. https://hbr.org/2002/05/how-resilience-works.

Covey, S. R. (2006). *The 8th habit: From effectiveness to greatness.* Simon & Schuster.

Covey, S. R. (2020). In *The seven habits of highly effective people* (30th anniversary ed.). Simon & Schuster.

Grosch, W. N., & Olsen, D. C. (1994). *When helping starts to hurt.* WW Norton.

Hartman, J., Moskal, P., & Dziuban, C. (2005). Preparing the academy of today for the learner of tomorrow. In D. G. Oblinger, & J. L. Oblinger (Eds.), *Educating the next generation* (pp. 6.1–6.15). Educause. https://www.educause.edu/research-and-publications/books/educating-net-generation/preparing-academy-today-learner-tomorrow.

Health Education England. (n.d.). Digital literacy of the wider workforce. https://www.hee.nhs.uk/our-work/digital-literacy.

Jeffries, S. (2014). Ten tips for a better work-life balance. The Guardian. https://www.theguardian.com/lifeandstyle/2014/nov/07/ten-tips-for-a-better-work-life-balance.

Jöstl, G., Bergsmann, E., Lüftenegger, M., Schober, B., & Spiel, C. (2012). When will they blow my cover? The impostor phenomenon among Austrian doctoral students. *ZeitschriftfürPsychologie, 220*(2), 109–120. https://doi.org/10.1027/2151-2604/a000102.

Lee, R. J., & King, S. N. (2001). *Discovering the leader in you. A guide to realising your personal leadership potential.* Jossey-Bass.

Mahmoud, A. B., Fuxman, L., Mohr, I., Reisel, W. D., & Grigoriou, N. (2020). "We aren't your reincarnation!" workplace motivation across X, Y and Z generations. *International Journal of Manpower.* https://doi.org/10.1108/IJM-09-2019-0448.

Mental Health Foundation. (n.d.). How to…look after your mental health using exercise. https://www.mentalhealth.org.uk/sites/default/files/How%20to..exercise.pdf.

Neff, K. (2011). *Self compassion*. William Morrow.

Perano, U. (2019). We've had generations X, Y and Z: Meet generation alpha. InklAxios. https://www.inkl.com/news/we-ve-had-generations-x-y-and-z-meet-generation-alpha.

Rimmer, A. (2020). How can I build a portfolio career? *British Medical Journal, 370.* https://doi.org/10.1136/bmj.m3426.

Royal College of Nursing. (2020). Self care. https://www.rcn.org.uk/clinical-topics/public-health/self-care#:~:text=Self%20management%20UK%20defines%20self,condition%2C%20making%20informed%20decisions%20about.

Royal College of Occupational Therapists. (2021). Career development framework: Guiding principles for occupational therapy. 2nd Edition. https://www.rcot.co.uk/publications/career-development-framework.

Schucan Bird, K. (2014). Women's writing groups: Five reasons to start one. The Guardian. https://www.theguardian.com/higher-education-network/blog/2014/jan/24/women-writing-groups-university-research.

Taylor, F. (2005). Will you burn out? *BMJ, 331.* https://doi.org/10.1136/bmj.331.7526.sgp220.

TED Conferences, LLC. (n.d.). The importance of self-care. https://www.ted.com/playlists/299/the_importance_of_self_care.

Wagman, P., Håkansson, C., & Björklund, A. (2012). Occupational balance as used in occupational therapy: A concept analysis. *Scandinavian Journal of Occupational Therapy, 19*(4), 322–327. https://doi.org/10.3109/11038128.2011.596219.

Walker, J. W., & Lewis, L. H. (2010). *Dealing with X, Y, Zs. How to manage the new generations in the workplace.* FTPress Inc.

Westhorp, P. (2003). Exploring balance as a concept in occupational science. *Journal of Occupational Science, 10*(2), 99–106. https://doi.org/10.1080/14427591.2003.9686516.

Wilson, L., & Wilcock, A. (2005). Occupational balance: What tips the scales for new students? *British Journal of Occupational Therapy, 68*(7), 319–323. https://doi.org/10.1177/030802260500800706.

Wook Lee, S., & Kielhofner, G. (2017). Habituation: Patterns of daily occupations. In R. R. Taylor (Ed.), *Kielhofner's model of human occupation* (5th ed., pp. 57–73). Wolters Kluwer.

World Health Organisation. (2019). Burn-out an "occupational phenomenon." International Classification of Diseases. https://www.who.int/news/item/28-05-2019-burn-out-an-occupational-phenomenon-international-classification-of-diseases.

18

Leadership Skills

Charles H. Christiansen

HIGHLIGHTS

- To flourish, all organised groups require some form of leadership.
- Leadership involves influencing people's actions towards specific goals.
- Effective leaders know the difference between management and leadership, and between popularity and effectiveness.

- Levels of leadership equate with circles of influence, beginning with the self.
- The most effective leaders have an attitude of service characterised by trust, courage, empathy, humility, cooperation, and the development of people.
- Occupational therapy prepares practitioners to adopt a service orientation and a systems perspective that is consistent with developing effective leadership skills.

OVERVIEW

Leaders influence people to attain shared goals. Thus, wherever there are groups of people with common goals or aspirations, leaders are needed. In this chapter, key skills for leadership are identified. Knowledge of these skills is applicable to occupational therapists because the ability to influence others also pertains to therapy settings, whether these are applied towards influencing coworkers or clients, either individually or in groups.

Contemporary leadership ideas embrace the principle that becoming a more effective leader starts with becoming a more effective person. Beyond this, specific skills associated with ever-larger circles of influence can be identified, including planning, organising, communicating, and motivating, each of which contributes to the creation of a sense of community based on trust. Effective leadership also requires strategies for organisational and individual performance appraisal. In each case there are multiple parallels between the skills of an effective leader and the skills of an effective therapist.

The chapter also addresses the emergence of virtual groups and meetings, and the growing use of teams. The principles addressed here apply to occupational therapists who function as members of interdisciplinary teams for which they may be asked to provide leadership.

EVOLUTIONARY AND HISTORICAL CONTEXT

According to Harari (2015) primitive humans advanced significantly because they developed the intellect required for language. This enabled them to cooperate and work in groups. Trivers (1971), Dawkins (2016), contend that these cooperative arrangements were key to the survival and advancement of the human species. The idea of groups of people working together for shared benefit and common purpose is key to the idea of organisation. In fact, an appropriate basic definition for the word organisation is a group of people working together to accomplish an overall, common goal or set of goals (McNamara, 2020).

As societies evolved, social groups became larger and more complex. The division of labour in society (Durkheim, 1893/1997), wherein specific work roles are assigned to group members based on tasks necessary to accomplish different purposes, has become commonplace. Nowadays, large organisations may have hundreds or thousands of members, with highly sophisticated structures consisting of many smaller workgroups organised within larger groups, often spread out geographically or even globally.

WHY LEADERSHIP?

Regardless of the nature, size, or structure of an organised group, however, each has in common a need for leadership, whether it requires one person or a group of people. Leadership is necessary to determine the common purposes that will be pursued by the group (i.e., what the group is doing and why?) and to oversee management, or the means or processes for accomplishing those purposes (i.e., determining how work will be done).

Defining Leadership

Leadership has been defined in many ways. Simply put, leadership is setting directions and influencing others to work in pursuit of those directions. The overall direction of an organisation (or an occupational therapy unit) may be spelled out in a mission statement. For example, a recent mission statement of Instagram, a popular but controversial mobile photo-messaging application, is "to capture and share the world's moments" (Mission Statement Academy, 2020). To achieve that purpose, Instagram uses technology supported by employees who maintain its photo-based software platform and features, while others sell advertisements, monitor content, or build algorithms to increase the service's reliability, ease of use, and popularity.

Typically, in many large organisations like Instagram, a group of people (often, a board of directors) determines its overall mission (or purpose for being). Usually only one person, however, is charged to assume overall responsibility for directing and coordinating the actions necessary to attain the mission. This leader, or chief executive officer (CEO), is at the top of the leadership hierarchy.

Operationally, the CEO of a large company sometimes reports to a board of directors and often heads a senior leadership group, the members of which also serve as leaders for their divisions. As organisations or groups become larger, their hierarchies become more complex. These leadership hierarchies are typically depicted in organisational charts. These charts illustrate an important point: Nearly everyone in a leadership role must perform as both an effective leader and an effective follower.

The Art of Leadership in the 21st Century

To begin with, it is vital to understand that effective leaders are developed, not born. The skills necessary for success pertain to knowledge, character, habits, and awareness; yet simply possessing them will not guarantee success. The reason is that good leadership is an art, and becoming a good artist starts with skills but evolves through experience (DePree, 2004). Just as good artists often come from apprentices who learn from masters, so too do most effective leaders learn from excellent mentors who serve as role models for effective action.

The author has been fortunate to have learned from several excellent mentors and role models during his lifetime. Some were supervisors during professional training; others were senior leaders in large organisations. They all provided lessons through example, demonstrating that by paying attention to subtle details important lessons could be learned. Examples include showing respect for everyone in the organisation regardless of position, inviting input and feedback, valuing diverse perspectives, learning the names of colleagues and subordinates, conveying gratitude, and honoring commitments. I recall one leader of a large hospital who impressively sent handwritten notes to those he had learned were celebrating personal accomplishments or grieving family tragedies. Those small gestures made a big impression.

These mentors also demonstrated that there is a difference between popularity and effective leadership. Too often, novice leaders equate the two, assuming that popularity will lead naturally to effectiveness. The reality, however, is that trading lowered expectations for increased popularity is a Faustian bargain. The duty of a leader is to influence people to effectively accomplish a mission. When a leader fails at this, everyone is affected. It is better that a leader earn the respect of coworkers as fair, principled, and kind than to be popular but inconsistent and ineffective. It follows that therapists who strive to relate effectively with their clients not lose sight of the performance objectives paramount in their roles as health care providers.

Leadership Skills, Traits, and Values

The skills necessary for effective leadership vary by situation. Covey (1990) noted that leaders have circles of influence. This idea of ever-increasing circles of influence is a convenient way to think about how the skill requirements of different situations change as the number of individuals being influenced increases. In this model, the first circle of influence is the self. Leaders who are able to manage their own lives effectively through planning, initiative, and self-discipline tend to achieve their goals and earn recognition. Individual success is noticed by others, and this constitutes a second level of influence involving those immediately surrounding a leader.

As groups become larger, different skills are needed because it is difficult to have direct and regular contact with more than a handful of people. Thus a third important set of skills (and the third circle of influence) pertains to being able to organise people, lead meetings, and communicate

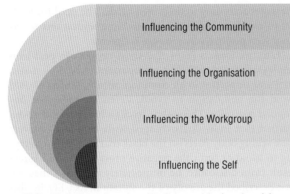

FIG. 18.1 Four levels of influence in leadership.

effectively with larger groups. Finally, the fourth circle of influence involves much larger numbers of people who may only have indirect or occasional contact with the leader but are nonetheless influenced by the person's reputation, results, and observed skills. These fourth-level skills relate to formulating inspiring visions of possibility, planning strategically, and making key decisions in complex situations. Covey noted that the issues of concern by a leader are always larger than the leader's circles of influence. As circles expand, influence requires additional skills. The discussion of leadership skills below is intended to reflect this (Fig. 18.1).

The First Level of Influence: Leading the Self

We have noted that effective leadership begins by having sufficient self-leadership skills or personal habits and characteristics, to be an effective individual and credible role model. The terms *authenticity* and *integrity* are often included in the characteristics necessary for becoming an effective individual. An effective individual enjoys the unqualified respect of others.

Such respect is largely earned through one's interpersonal relationships. It begins acting in a trustworthy manner. A trustworthy person honours commitments and is dependable in other ways, such as through maintaining confidences. We can assert here that the most important characteristic a leader (or effective person) can possess is trustworthiness. It is a basic and essential element of character and leadership temperament.

An effective leader is also responsible. One can interpret the word *responsible* as meaning being able to respond in a capable and dependable manner. When something goes wrong, effective leaders first ask what they could have done differently to influence a different outcome. Because they are attentive, effective leaders are intentional when they act

and clear about the outcomes they desire to achieve. Their achievement, however, is not pursued in a competitive or selfish manner and never at the expense of others. They consistently ask, "How can we achieve our goal according to our values and use the process to develop skills in others?" Here again, one finds parallels between leadership and occupational therapy. Each focuses on goals and developing skills.

Effective leaders are also good managers of personal resources. This pertains to using their resources (money, time, and energy) wisely and efficiently. Effective leaders strive to keep themselves physically healthy through sound nutrition, sleep, exercise, rest, and renewal. They attend to their spiritual needs and recognise the importance of balancing their lives to achieve desired ends. To the experienced occupational therapist, these characteristics may seem closely aligned with concepts of holistic health and life balance. Just as effective therapy cannot be delivered by a therapist who is tired or unwell, neither can effective leadership be provided when personal circumstances interfere with the energy and focus required for competent performance.

An effective leader is also considerate of others. Being considerate means being genuinely concerned with the needs of others and demonstrating such concern with attention and compassion. This requires that leaders listen carefully and sincerely attempt to see matters from others' points of view. This is empathy. A positive attitude is also important. A leader or therapist whose emotional demeanour is gloomy and pessimistic is unlikely to inspire or encourage others.

Closely related to a positive disposition is a good and appropriate sense of humor. By expecting the unexpected and having an attitude of acceptance and equanimity when things go awry, leaders with a sense of humor help to keep things in context and can reduce the tension often associated with errors and setbacks.

Finally, effective leaders, like effective therapists, have a personal orientation that encourages others to succeed. They constantly seek creative solutions that strive to enable everyone to attain their ends. Innovation is the result of a mindset that strives to avoid accepting options that are just good enough and seeks to attain inspired new solutions that avoid creating winners and losers.

The Second Level of Leadership Influence: The Immediate Workgroup or Team

A second set of skills pertains to those necessary for influencing those immediately around us. To be maximally effective, leaders must be knowledgeable, socially involved, enthusiastic, and upbeat. They should strive to conduct their lives in ways that enable them to be perceived as effective role models. This requires living with purpose, kindness, gratitude, and compassion.

To be an effective leader to those around us means having the ability to teach or coach new skills and abilities. Thus, effective leaders are knowledgeable about matters of importance to success in the group and organisation. Successful leaders, like competent practitioners, strive continually to remain current, knowledgeable, and well informed in their fields of endeavor.

Within an immediate workgroup, or team, successful leaders must be able to organise people, facilitate effective meetings, and communicate effectively. Effective organising begins with matching the skills and abilities of people to the tasks needed in a particular workgroup. Occupational therapists are adept at assessing performance skills and selecting challenges that are aligned with skill levels. The effective group leader must likewise fit the task to the appropriate individual or group and ensure that the necessary systems are in place to enable success in performance.

Communicating clear expectations is also vitally important. The expected outcome must be carefully identified along with the time frame for completion and the expected standard of performance, stated in measurable terms. The consequences for failure to the organisation should also be explained because this provides an important connecting link in aligning the workgroup with the enterprise. Provided with this information, a workgroup or team can gain a clear sense of what is expected and why it has importance to achieving an outcome or goal.

Stating clear goals is part of a larger set of communication skills required in an effective leader. People in an organisation, just as occupational therapy clients, need clear information and want to feel valued, connected, and informed. Thus regular communication is a must. The best communication anticipates the information needs of the receiver and provides this in a manner that can be easily understood (i.e., clearly, succinctly, and directly). In today's digital age it is too often the case that communication that should be face to face is handled asynchronously through text messaging or email. Direct voice communication is efficient and effective because it enables quick clarification of uncertainty and ambiguity.

However, caution must be exercised. Communications involving conflict or emotional situations require effective leaders to take the time to respond calmly and thoughtfully; quickly sent messages lacking tact always make difficult situations worse. Second, in situations where the information to be communicated is likely to be unpopular, it is always wise to use direct language that clearly and completely conveys the necessary information. Whenever ambiguity is present, message recipients will interpret messages according to their own needs. The need for leaders to clarify or explain previous communications is seldom seen positively by message recipients.

Effective leaders know that most people can deal with unpleasant truths. While it is important to be diplomatic, civil and respectful in all communications, leaders should avoid the temptation to avoid, soften, or sugarcoat unpopular messages. The author recalls a hospital leader who learned that individuals charged with handling cadavers were selling body parts on the black market. Instead of trying to avoid or limit the negative press that would surely result from disclosure, he immediately released a message that described the gravity of the situation. As CEO, he also assumed responsibility for conducting a full investigation followed by a commitment to sanction those responsible and take steps to ensure such a breach of trust would never happen again. There was negative press, but by being proactive, direct, and transparent, the CEO instilled confidence in others that the matter would be handled appropriately and that the family members would be provided support and just compensation.

Finally, and perhaps most importantly, the orientation or demeanor of an effective leader should be one of service. The most effective occupational therapists can connect with their clients because they communicate humility, authenticity, trustworthiness, and a commitment to others. Just as success in occupational therapy requires providing necessary support systems to enable successful goal attainment, the mission of a workgroup or organisation can only be fully attained if those working towards it have the necessary encouragement, resources, direction, and motivation. Skillful leaders attend to such needs.

Some Important Thoughts About Teams

One distinguishing characteristic of the 21st century workplace involves the prevalence of teams, a popular label for smaller organised workgroups, which may be temporary or permanent. Increasingly, occupational therapists work as members of teams, sometimes as leaders. In practice, despite the common misperception that teams are egalitarian horizontal structures devoid of hierarchy, each team requires leadership. In some cases, leadership rotates, but in nearly all cases the team answers to a responsible individual.

In some situations, teams are colocated geographically and consist of individuals from several organisational units collaborating face to face on a defined project. But work teams may also be virtual, in the sense that they involve individuals who may be geographically dispersed within a region or even globally and do their work electronically.

In cases where a team is virtual, the need for effective coordination and communication is especially important because the reliance on technology can diminish the effectiveness of communication and increase the amount of effort required to establish the levels of trust and collaboration necessary for success. Here, providing support or scaffolding for the team in the form of facilitating work relationships through shared biographies, carefully analysing tasks and goals, and creating a culture where expectations are clear and failed strategies are framed as learning events helps to reduce perceived risk and foster open communication (Edmondson, 2012).

Effective teams include members who are effective leaders and followers, and at different points in the team's progress towards its objectives, different members may assume responsibility for assuming leadership roles. If this is the case, then it is useful for the group to spend time at the beginning of a project communicating expectations and methods for encouraging open communication, productively managing conflict, and facilitating problem solving.

The Third Level of Influence: Organisational Leadership

Third-level leadership competencies add to those previously listed: the ability to effectively organise people, lead meetings, and communicate across teams and larger groups. The organisation or assignment of people into teams or workgroups is both an art and a science. It is an art in the sense that it assembles workgroups based on the tasks and objectives to be accomplished and an alignment of people with the training, experience, and skills best suited to accomplishing those tasks and objectives. Each team or workgroup needs an assigned leader for a particular objective, which may be temporary or ongoing. Just as the effective therapist seeks to match the challenge to the skills of the client, so too do effective leaders exercise care in assigning tasks for people within an organisation or workgroup.

In any organisation, the success of effective workgroups is at least partially dependent on the chemistry of its members. Group chemistry refers to the collective personality of a group, and this may be influenced by traditions, shared values, experience, and other factors. Thus one attempts to best match people and their assigned group leaders based on both objective and subjective criteria. Subjective decision making can be based on intuition and observation as well as a leader's knowledge of the personalities and individual circumstances of coworkers.

Another skill necessary with this third level of leadership competence is the ability to effectively lead meetings. While meetings are a ubiquitous, fundamental, and necessary part of organisational activities, they vary widely in their value and effectiveness based on the skills of their leaders. No meeting should ever be held without thoughtful preparation. Attention should be given to its objectives, the agenda, and the actual conduct of the meeting (Hartman, 2014).

Sometimes agendas are seen as unnecessary formalities. The skillful leader recognises that they are an important tool for attaining focused and productive outcomes. All agenda items should have clear purposes in mind (i.e., information, discussion, action) and, to the extent possible, require some advance preparation from participants (Hartman, 2014).

The final set of skills at this level of influence pertains to spoken communication with larger groups. With larger groups comes the greater probability that one or more persons will misunderstand a message. Therefore clarity and care must be taken in formulating and delivering messages. One cannot become an effective organisational leader without having the skill to speak convincingly and confidently in public arenas and to provide effective impromptu or extemporaneous presentations when these are required.

Level Four: Influencing Communities: Becoming a Strategic Leader

As the responsibilities of a leader increase, so does the complexity of assignments. The leader of a large organisation must contend with the political realities of communities, where other organisations may be competing directly or have interests or objectives that conflict or complicate goal completion. Large organisations also have communities within them because each division or workgroup takes on its own personality and develops its own subculture. When the divisions within the same organisation begin to compete with each other without staying focused on the mission, conflict can result and morale will suffer.

Level four leadership requires the leader to have a systems perspective, recognising that each element is connected to and affects the others. Here again, occupational therapists can easily recognise the importance of this perspective because of their training in systems thinking that conditions them to think of the interconnected elements required for occupational performance. In a similar way, leaders must recognise that organisational components are also interdependent (Senge, 2006).

This interdependence calls to mind the important principle of seeking win-win solutions (Covey, 1989). Here the goal is to resolve problems, challenges, and conflicts in a manner that best enables all parties of interest to achieve their aims. Strategic leadership situations also require careful planning, with an eye towards anticipating key trends and envisioning the future.

The visioning process is key to strategic planning because it must anticipate conditions and create bold possibilities that collectively motivate group members to align themselves in support of an imagined future or end state. Ideally, good vision statements are succinct, one-sentence statements that motivate and inspire (Collins & Porras, 1991).

Consider the nonprofit humanitarian relief organisation Oxfam, established in 1942 by academics in Oxford, UK, who sought to address a famine affecting people in Greece. Today, Oxfam has grown to a large global humanitarian federation with a succinct vision statement: "A just world without poverty" (Oxfam, 2020). This clear statement serves to unify Oxfam's diverse efforts and motivates donors to give towards the elimination of injustices that lead to poverty. Oxfam helps fund its operations and maintain a visible presence by cleverly selling donated and fair trade merchandise through its network of stores (Fig. 18.2). This strategy enables Oxfam to fulfill its mission while simultaneously communicating its vision.

Leadership Contrasted With Management

It might be said that leadership is to vision as management is to mission. Being a leader and being a manager are different organisational roles requiring different skills. A leader focuses on the big picture, determining direction and inspiring and developing people towards an aspirational goal, whereas a manager plans the specific methods for getting there. Thus the strategic focus of leadership focuses on the "why" of an organisation. In contrast, management functions focus on the "how" (i.e., the specific manner in which the work is accomplished). Thus a manager attends to the operational requirements for getting the job done, such as scheduling and coordination, maintaining quality, and budgeting.

Applying these ideas to occupational therapy, it might be suggested that therapists must simultaneously think as leaders and managers. Long-term goal setting for a client requires a vision of the possible, with careful thought about inspiring the client to work towards a long-term goal. On the other hand, the specific therapeutic equipment and methods required for a given intervention or therapy session require competent management skills because these focus on how the job gets done. Mattingly and Fleming (1994), two occupational therapists, studied clinical reasoning by occupational therapists, doing extensive on-the-job interviews. They found that effective reasoning required therapists be able to move between different thinking styles that they labeled "tracks" of the mind (Fleming, 1991). In some ways, those styles reflect the distinctions necessary between thinking as a leader and thinking as a manager.

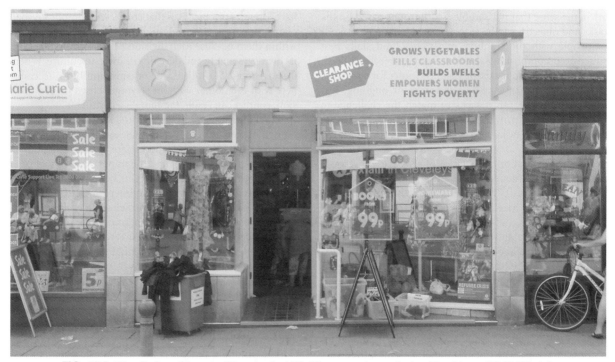

FIG. 18.2 The Oxfam Shop in Cleveley's, UK. (Photograph credit Joe Hawkins - CC BY-SA 4.0, https://commons.wikimedia.org/w/index.php?curid=50695167)

Both leaders and managers value feedback and seek to gather as much information as possible about organisational performance. Organisations typically track their own performance and compare it from year to year, but this information can be more meaningful if supplemented with knowing how an organisation compares to other organisations of its type. Gathering this type of information is sometimes called benchmarking, a process that identifies best practices by answering the question, "How do the leading organisations do this process?" (Wolfram Cox et al., 1997). Benchmarking is a type of knowledge management, a term used to describe the sharing of information throughout an organisation to improve its performance.

Benchmarking encourages thinking about different approaches to attaining a goal. Two types of benchmarking can be described. In competitive benchmarking, data are collected to analyse how an organisation measures up against the competition. In collaborative benchmarking, organisations or groups cooperate to identify performance ranges and share improvements. Any process within an organisation can be benchmarked, and in today's environment it is critical to be aware of the most efficient and effective ways to get the job done (Seabold et al., 2020).

Perhaps Web 2.0 and social media, both of which involve participation, collaboration, and user feedback, best illustrate evolving societal trends that rely upon information from others to assess performance to guide future plans. The prevalence of these feedback systems illustrates the widespread belief that such information is essential if an enterprise is to remain competitive. It is implicit that the consumers of products and services must be considered as credible judges of performance and that successful enterprises should strive to meet the standards expected by those they serve. The idea of enterprises serving others, whether through quality products or services, is consistent with the concept of servant leadership, to which we now turn.

Contemporary Views on Servant Leadership

The idea of benevolent or servant leadership dates back thousands of years and yet remains as viable and germane as it did at that time. Indeed, in the *Tao Te Ching*, a classical Chinese work of virtues and ways of living written 2500 years ago by Lao Tzu, there is a section devoted to benevolent leaders (Le Guin, 1997) (Box 18.1).

Modern ideas of servant leadership are often attributed to an essay by Greenleaf (1991), who emphasised that leaders exist to serve the interests of the organisation and that by adopting an attitude grounded in serving others, leaders become most effective.

Thus servant leadership, like effective occupational therapy, is collaborative rather than hierarchic. Yet, it focuses on the leader as a caretaker of resources, especially individuals

---

BOX 18.1 Wisdom on Leadership Style in the Tao Te Ching*

This English translation of Chapter 17 of the *Tao Te Ching* (Le Guin, 1998) clearly reflects an appreciation for the virtues of effective leaders:

"True leaders are hardly known to their followers.
Next after them are the leaders
The people know and admire;
After them, those that they fear;
After them, those they despise.
To give no trust
Is to get no trust.
When the work's done right,
With no fuss or boasting,
Ordinary people say,
Oh, we did it.

*From Le Guin, U. K. (1998). *The Tao Te Ching: A book about the way and the power of the way* (p. 24). Shambhala Publishing.

---

in an organisation, while also attending to performance and goals so that success in accomplishing the mission is not compromised. The principles of trust, integrity, and ethical practices are paramount in the servant leader approach, which has been adopted by many successful organisations throughout the world. According to Spears (1996), the servant leader has 10 leadership characteristics: listening, empathy, awareness, healing, persuasion, conceptualisation, foresight, stewardship, community, and commitment.

More recently, ideas advanced by social scientist and personality Brené Brown have gained popularity through their emphasis on authentic and transparent attitudes and behaviors of effective leadership. Brown observes that, too often, leaders avoid difficult conversations and unpopular decisions because they feel vulnerable and fear losing social approval. She asserts that the feedback environment created by social media has made it too easy for people to provide anonymous criticism, suggesting that effective leaders should focus on the perspectives of those who are qualified and have a stake in the consequences of actions based on their opinions. Her views align closely with the ideas of servant leadership, with the addition of acknowledging the courage needed to perform as an effective leader.

One practice often used in organisations with servant leader philosophies is 360-degree feedback, sometimes referred to as multisource feedback. This is a type of performance appraisal that differs from the traditional top-down evaluation or even from the process where subordinates evaluate their leaders. In multisource appraisals, these two approaches are combined. Typically, 360-degree feedback processes focus on identifying areas for leadership training (Lepsinger & Lucia, 2005). Reviews of the effectiveness of multisource appraisals have shown mixed results with modest improvements in performance (Smither et al., 2005). However, the effectiveness of the process seems based on the attitudes of the person evaluated, the perceived need for change, and the organisational resources made available to enhance areas of weakness (Hezlett, 2008). Regardless of the method used, leaders should seek objective feedback from those they serve as a means for identifying strengths and weaknesses.

STRATEGIES AND RESOURCES FOR LEADERSHIP DEVELOPMENT

It is clear that one does not become an effective leader after reading a short chapter on leadership. Effective leadership requires skills that are honed over careers, requiring experience, self-development, and feedback. Without objective feedback on how others perceive a leader's skills in the four levels of leadership, one cannot identify areas to focus on further development.

Developing leadership skills requires a willingness to seek feedback from others, to read widely and participate in formal leadership development programmes. Ideally, it involves having a coach or mentor who can provide an honest but supportive context in which self-development is more likely to occur.

Effective coaches and mentors help leaders through recommending useful self-development strategies and through confidential reflective dialogue that enables the aspiring leader to safely and critically analyse their own leadership behaviours. When most effective, coaches and mentors enable leaders to recognise their own weaknesses and identify and practice strategies that are likely to result in more effective performance.

Here again, effective occupational therapists have a commitment to self-development and lifelong learning. While continuing professional development for therapists may be mandated as a requirement for practice in many locations, the most effective therapists, like effective leaders, are motivated by an internal drive towards self-appraisal and continuous improvement.

SUMMARY

Occupational therapy settings, whether facility or community based, are often staffed with large numbers of people and exist as part of larger, complex organisations such as hospitals and systems. But even if they involve only small groups or teams, they require effective leadership. In this chapter we have described four levels of leadership and the skills associated with each level. In describing these

skills, references to the concept of the servant leader have been made, and the traditions of servant leadership and client-centred therapy have been compared. We have also shown similarities between the characteristics of effective leaders and effective therapists. Because of their traditions and training, occupational therapists may be especially well positioned to become effective leaders within therapy units or beyond. Attention to the skills and use of the resources identified in this chapter can be helpful within either context.

REFLECTIVE LEARNING

- Why are vision statements important? How do vision statements differ from mission statements? Sometimes core values are listed. Are core values more related to vision statements or mission statements? Why?
- Vision statements should inspire us and encourage cooperation by providing a clearly understood aspirational goal. In contrast, the mission explains an organisation's everyday purpose and activities in pursuit of the vision. Take some time to review company websites. Note whether they include vision and mission statements. Some companies identify core values. These add to mission and vision statements by providing principles or guidelines for the manner in which employees will pursue their work.

REFERENCES

Brown, B. (2017). *Dare to lead: Brave work. Tough conversations. Whole hearts.* Random House. https://doi.org/2158244013489686.

Collins, J., & Porras, J. (1991). Organizational vision and visionary organizations. *California Management Review, 34*(1), 30–52. https://doi.org/10.2307/41166682.

Covey, S. R. (1989). *The seven habits of highly effective people (rev. ed.). Powerful lessons in personal change.* Simon & Schuster. https://www.simonandschuster.com/books/The-7-Habits-of-Highly-Effective-People-Revised-and-Updated/Stephen-R-Covey/9781982137137.

Covey, S. R. (1990). *Principle centered leadership.* Simon & Schuster. https://www.simonandschuster.com/books/Principle-Centered-Leadership/Stephen-R-Covey/9780671792800.

Dawkins, R. (2016). In *The selfish gene* (4th ed.). Oxford University Press. https://global.oup.com/academic/product/the-selfish-gene-9780198788607?q=the%20selfish%20gene&lang=en&cc=us.

DePree, M. (2004). Leadership is an art. *Penguin Random House.* https://www.penguinrandomhouse.com/books/39634/leadership-is-an-art-by-max-de-pree/.

Durkheim, E. (1893/1997). *The division of labour in society* (trans. W. D. Halls). Free Press. https://openlibrary.org/books/OL7721631M/The_Division_of_Labor_in_Society.

Edmondson, A. C. (2012). *Teaming: How organizations learn, innovate and compete in the knowledge economy.* Wiley. https://www.wiley.com/en-us/Teaming%3A+How+Organizations+Learn%2C+Innovate%2C+and+Compete+in+the+Knowledge+Economy-p-9780787970932.

Ent, M. R., Baumeister, R. F., & Vonasch, A. J. (2012). Power, leadership, and self-regulation. *Social and Personality Psychology Compass, 6*(8), 619–630. https://doi.org/10.1111/j.1751-9004.2012.00446.x.

Fleming, M. (1991). The therapist with the three track mind. *American Journal of Occupational Therapy, 45*(11), 1007–1014. https://doi.org/10.5014/ajot.45.11.1007.

Greenleaf, R.K. (1970/1991). *The servant as leader.* The Robert Greenleaf Center. https://www.greenleaf.org/products-page/the-servant-as-leader/.

Harari, Y. N. (2015). *Sapiens. A brief history of humankind.* Harper Collins. https://www.harpercollins.com/9780062316097/sapiens/.

Hartman, N. (2014). *Seven steps to running the most effective meeting possible.* Forbes. https://www.forbes.com/sites/forbes-leadershipforum/2014/02/05/seven-steps-to-running-the-most-effective-meeting-possible/#fbdd1eb7a613.

Hezlett, S. A. (2008). Using multisource feedback to develop leaders: Applying theory and research to improve practice. *Advances in Developing Human Resources, 10*(5), 703–720. https://doi.org/10.1177/1523422308322271.

Hollins, P. (2017). The science of self-discipline: The willpower, mental toughness, and self-control to resist temptation and achieve your goals. PKCS Media.

Le Guin, U. K. (1997). *Lao Tzu: Tao Te Ching: A book about the way & the power of the way (a translation and commentary).* Shambhala. https://www.shambhala.com/lao-tzu-tao-te-ching.html.

Lepsinger, R., & Lucia, A. D. (2005). In *The art and science of 360 degree feedback* (2nd ed.). Wiley. https://www.wiley.com/en-us/The+Art+and+Science+of+360+Degree+Feedback%2C+2nd+Edition-p-9780470331897.

Mattingly, C., & Fleming, M. (1994). *Clinical reasoning: Forms of inquiry in a therapeutic practice.* F.A. Davis. https://books.google.com/books/about/Clinical_Reasoning.html?id=Vc91PwAACAAJ.

McNamara, C. (2020). *Basic definition of organisation.* Online Integrated Library for Personal, Professional and Organisational Development. https://managementhelp.org/organizations/definition.htm.

Mission Statement Academy. (2020). The mission statement of Instagram. https://mission-statement.com/instagram/.

Oxfam International. (2020). Our history. https://www.oxfam.org/en/our-history.

Seabold, K., Kaufmann, M., & McNett, M. (2020). In *Quality and benchmarking data in health systems. Data for nurses* (pp. 13–29). Academic Press.

Senge, P. (2006). In *The fifth discipline: The art and practice of the learning organization* (2nd ed.). Random House.

Smither, J. W., London, M., & Reilly, R. R. (2005). Does performance improve following multisource feedback? A theoretical model, meta-analysis, and review of empirical findings. *Personnel Psychology, 58*(1), 33–66. https://doi.org/10.1111/j.1744-6570.2005.514_1.x.

Spears, L. (1996). Reflections on Robert K Greenleaf and servant-leadership. *Leadership & Organization Development Journal, 17*(7), 33–35. https://doi.org/10.1108/01437739610148367.

Tomasello, M. (2009). *Why we cooperate.* MIT Press. https://mit-press.mit.edu/books/why-we-cooperate.

Trivers, R. L. (1971). The evolution of reciprocal altruism. *Quarterly Review of Biology, 46*(35), 35–57.

Vohs, K. D., & Baumeister, R. F. (Eds.). (2016). *Handbook of self-regulation: Research, theory, and applications* (3rd ed.). The Guilford Press.

Wolfram Cox, J. R., Mann, L., & Samson, D. (1997). Benchmarking as a mixed metaphor: Disentangling assumptions of competition and collaboration. *Journal of Management Studies, 34*(2), 285–314.

19

Practice Education—Skills for Students and Educators

Stephen Isbel, Thomas Bevitt, Mong-Lin Yu, and Ted Brown

HIGHLIGHTS

- Practice education is a critical component of occupational therapy education where students have the opportunity to apply the skills, knowledge, and attitudes required of an occupational therapist in a structured and supportive environment.
- At a broad level the World Federation of Occupational Therapists is responsible for defining the minimum standards required for the education of occupational

therapists, including practice education. How these standards are enacted is led by national guidelines.
- As the scope of occupational therapy is vast so are the types of placements that students can experience.
- A critical component of a successful practice education placement is the role of supervision. The function and methods of supervision, along with the application of effective feedback, should all be considered.

INTRODUCTION

Several related terms have been used to refer to the practical component of health professionals' education, including *fieldwork, practicums, internships,* and *clinical placements;* however, in this chapter the term *practice education* will be utilised. This chapter covers several areas related to occupational therapy practice education that students complete as part of their entry-to-practice training. A definition of what practice education is, the different types of practice education placements, and professional standards that direct practice education will be presented. The different types of supervision and the formal assessment of students' practice education performance will be reviewed. Finally, establishing the basis for students' success while completing practice education will be discussed. Key points about occupational therapy practice education will be illustrated with the use of two vignettes.

WHAT IS PRACTICE EDUCATION?

All health care professions involve an academic learning component where students are exposed to the foundation knowledge, practice theories and models, intervention skills, and client groups they will interact with. The second key component of a student enrolled in a professional discipline

is practice education where they are exposed to the repertoire of skills needed in real-life workplace contexts. "The purpose of practice education is for students to integrate knowledge, professional reasoning and professional behaviour within practice, and to develop knowledge, skills and attitudes to the level of competence required of qualifying occupational therapists" (World Federation of Occupational Therapists [WFOT], 2016, p. 48). Practice education is described as the "bridge that connects the theoretical didactic classroom instruction to real-world clinical practice" (DeIuliis, 2017, p. 163). Practice education placements provide the environment where students can put into practice the knowledge, psychomotor skills, and theory they have been exposed to in the academic environment.

There are several parties involved in the provision of occupational therapy practice education placements, including the university education programs, academic practice education coordinator, students, practice educators, consumers/service users, site coordinator for practice education, service managers, professional associations, accreditation bodies, and regulatory bodies. University programs will often have a formal agreement with the practice education provider organisations that outlines the policies and procedures as well as roles and responsibilities of each party. The importance of practice education is that it provides the opportunity for students "to apply theoretical and scientific knowledge to address the occupational performance needs of individuals and/or groups in authentic practice settings" (Evensen & Hansen, 2019, p. 1079).

STANDARDS THAT GUIDE PRACTICE EDUCATION

The WFOT Revised Minimum Standards for the Education of Occupational Therapists (2016) specifies that all occupational therapy students are expected to complete at least 1000 hours of practice education over the duration of their course. Students must also exhibit the required practice competencies under the supervision of a qualified occupational therapist who has a minimum of 1 year of professional experience postgraduation. Relative to the country or jurisdiction of the university where a student occupational therapist is enrolled and intends to work once qualified, the practice education requirements for an entry-to-practice course must also meet the national registration and accreditation requirements. The WFOT Standards (2016) do not prescribe the length of what practice education placements need to be, but should be of "sufficient duration to allow integration of theory to practice" (p. 49).

Given that occupational therapy education programs around the world are accredited by a range of different organisations, there are a range of standards that guide practice education internationally. For example, in the United Kingdom the Royal College of Occupational Therapists (2019) is responsible for the registration of educational providers by applying learning and development standards, including in practice-based learning. The Canadian Association of Occupational Therapists (CAOT) has an Academic Credentialing Council (ACC) whose responsibility is to accredit the entry-level occupational therapy courses in Canada. Alongside the CAOT and its ACC, there is the Association of Canadian Occupational Therapy University Programs (ACOTUP) and the Committee on University Fieldwork Education (CUFE; 2011). The College of Occupational Therapists of Ontario published a document titled, *Essential Competencies of Practice for Occupational Therapists in Canada* (ECPOTC), which describes the major functions of the occupational therapist: (i) assumes professional responsibility, (ii) thinks critically, (iii) demonstrates practice knowledge, (iv) utilises an occupational therapy process to enable occupation, (v) communicates and collaborates effectively, (vi) engages in professional development, and (vii) manages own practice and advocates within systems.

In Australia, again there are several organisations involved in the practice education sphere including Occupational Therapy Council of Australia Ltd (OTC) that

accredits education programs according to the *Accreditation of Entry-Level Occupational Therapy Education Programs Guidelines for Education Providers* (OTC, 2018). The Occupational Therapy Board of Australia, Australian and New Zealand Occupational Therapy Fieldwork Academic Group (ANZOTFA), and Australian and New Zealand Council of Occupational Therapy Educators also influence the delivery of practice education in Australia (Farnworth & Kennedy-Jones, 2017). A linked document is the *Australian Occupational Therapy Competency Standards* (AOTCS) (Occupational Therapy Board of Australia, 2018) that outlines the expected standards for professional practice of Australian occupational therapists under four broad standard areas: (i) professionalism, (ii) knowledge and learning, (iii) occupational therapy process and practice, and (iv) communication.

Likewise, in the United States, the Accreditation Council for Occupational Therapy Education (ACOTE) is responsible for the accreditation of occupational therapy education programs. ACOTE is an Associated Advisory Council of the Executive Board of the American Occupational Therapy Association (AOTA; Nastasi, 2017). Students need to have graduated from an ACOTE-accredited program to be eligible to write the National Board for Certification in Occupational Therapy examination. These accreditation bodies and related organisations have standards that influence occupational therapy practice education. The Fieldwork Performance Evaluation for the Occupational Therapy Student (AOTA 2022) is used to assess students' practice education performance in the United States. It covers the following competency areas: fundamentals of practice, basic tenets evaluation/screening, intervention, management of occupational therapy services, communication, and professional behaviour. AOTA (2015) has published the *Standards for Continuing Competence* (SCC) that specifies the "knowledge, performance skills, interpersonal abilities, critical reasoning, and ethical reasoning skills necessary to perform current and future roles and responsibilities within the profession" (p. 1).

In summary, the standards that guide occupational therapy practice education are overseen by several agencies whose influence originates at different levels. At the broad international level, the WFOT has stated that all occupational therapy students must complete a minimum of 1000 hours but has not prescribed the format or makeup of those 1000 hours. At the country level, professional associations, advisory committees, and regulatory bodies have established practice education standards. These can take several forms, including specific committees (such as the CUFE, ACOTUP, ANZOTFA, ANZOTFA, or ACOTE), education program accreditation bodies (such as the RCOT, ACC, OTC, or ACOTE), practice education assessments used with students (see assessment section), and competency standard statements (such as AOTCS, ECPOTC, or SCC). All influence occupational therapy practice education standards directly or indirectly.

TYPES OF PLACEMENTS

Occupational therapy has a broad scope of practice, working with individuals, families, carers, groups, organisations, communities, and populations across a wide range of clinical and community settings (WFOT, 2018). New practice areas with emerging needs for occupational therapy services have continued to increase. In response to these, various types of placements have been developed and used in contemporary occupational therapy practice education. These include but are not limited to clinical placements, project placements, participatory community placements, university supported placements, experiential placements, simulations, student-led interprofessional placements, and international placements (Table 19.1). Occupational therapy programs use a combination of placement types across the recommended 1000 hours of practice education and are usually completed in placement blocks (WFOT, 2018). This ensures that students graduate with fundamental professional competencies required for existing as well as emerging practice settings.

Historically, students complete a placement in one practice context, within a specific practice field throughout one placement period. However, as the profession has developed this model is no longer always possible or favoured. Split placements are now widely used to structure occupational therapy placements and may involve students working across multiple sites with different caseloads, cosupervised by professionals with different practice expertise, and experience more than one type of placement within a placement block. For example, a placement can be split into acute and subacute settings; or a clinical placement in a hospital can be provided in conjunction with a short period of project placement or University-supported placement in a community setting. This further diversifies the types of placements currently provided for occupational therapy practice education. The diversity of placement options in occupational therapy serves the profession well by offering students experience in a range of practice areas and also when adjusting to unforseen events such as the COVID-19 pandemic of 2020. See Vignette 19.1 for an example of a diverse placement model.

WHAT IS SUPERVISION?

There is no one accepted definition of the term *supervision* in the allied health and medical literature. Indeed, the term, concepts, and processes underpinning supervision in the health professions often overlap when mentoring, coaching, and preceptorship are described. *Clinical supervision* is the term often used in the medical, psychological, and counseling literature, whereas *preceptorship* is often described in nursing. In occupation therapy the definition, concepts, and processes of supervision need to be flexible enough to account for the variety of practice areas also acknowledging the profession that engages with individuals, groups, and communities.

In this chapter supervision is defined as:

> *A relationship-based activity which enables practitioners to reflect upon the connection between task and process within their work. It provides a supportive, administrative and development context within which responsiveness to clients and accountable decision making can be sustained.*
>
> *Davies, 2000, p. 204*

The Function of Supervision

Martin and colleagues (2016) provide a useful description of the functions of supervision that can be applied to occupational therapy and fits nicely with the definition by Davies (2000). That is, supervision is comprised of three domains:

Normative: This occurs when the supervision focuses on the administrative requirements of a role such as adherence to policies and procedures or discussions dealing with professional questions around ethics.

Formative: This function of supervision focuses on the educational aspect of the role such as developing specific skills, knowledge, and attitudes related to a role.

Restorative: This is the supportive function of supervision where the emotional demands of the role are addressed.

An important aspect of supervision is the role of feedback in the process. Feedback is defined as "a process through which learners make sense of information from various sources and use it to enhance their work or learning strategies" (Carless & Boud, 2018, p. 1316).

Boud and Molloy (2013) argue that too often information if given to students as feedback, but often the feedback loop is not closed, meaning students do not get the chance to use the information given to change their behaviour. Therefore, if information is given to students even if done incidentally, informally, or spontaneously, there should be a mechanism whereby they can show they have changed their behaviour, learned a new skill, or otherwise enhanced their work or learning.

Methods of Supervision

The delivery of student supervision will depend on several factors, including the practice setting, work demands, and supervisor and supervisee characteristics. Common forms

TABLE 19.1	Types of Placements in Contemporary Occupational Therapy Practice Education
Type of Placement	**Description**
Clinical placement	Clinical placement refers to any placement arrangements in institutional or community settings (e.g., hospitals, community rehabilitation centre) where students are involved in direct observations of, interactions with, and interventions with an individual. Students receive onsite supervision from qualified occupational therapist(s) employed by the placement provider. Clinical placements are generally the places where students experience interprofessional collaboration and learn the role of other disciplines in health care (Brewer & Stewart-Wynne, 2013).
Project placements	Project placements generally ask students to work towards a defined output developed in collaboration with the host organisation and often are community or population centred. These placements may not have an onsite occupational therapist so student supervision can be shared with an offsite occupational therapist (usually a university academic staff member) and an onsite staff member. Students can work individually or in groups and have opportunities to experience all or part of the project management stages: information gathering, outcomes and operational planning, and implementation and evaluation (Knightbridge & Gilbert-Hunt, 2017).
Role emerging placements	Role emerging placements take place in organisations or services without occupational therapists but where potential for occupational therapy services has been identified (Wood, 2005). During the placement, the student applies an occupational perspective in the practice setting showing how an occupational therapist could be beneficial. Students usually attend in pairs or small groups, and receive occupational therapy professional supervision from a qualified occupational therapy employed by universities. Occupational therapy professional supervision can be provided in multiple ways, such as onsite supervision, phone calls, emails, and teleconferences. Students also receive onsite supervision from the host organisation staff. Tutorials, placement workbooks, online resources, and activities developed and provided by university are increasingly used to support student learning when completing role emerging placements.
Experiential placements	Experiential placements occur when students are placed in a setting, to observe aspects of a workplace or service (Knecht-Sabres, 2010). While it is desirable for students to be directly involved in service delivery there are some workplaces where this is not possible but observing practice is possible. Students completing an experiential placement are required to link what they have observed and experienced with the skills and knowledge they have gained at University (Knightbridge, 2014). For example, students may be required to identify and explain the existing role of the occupational therapists and/or potential future contributions occupational therapy can make in the service.
University Health Clinics (UHC)	UHCs are usually clinic-based health services situated on a University campus and/or associated with a University. Services are often offered at a subsidised rate with a focus on student education, health care, community engagement, and research (Moore et al., 2018). Services at UHC can involve student-led clinics that are supervised by health professionals employed by the clinic and/or academics associated with the University.
International placement	International placement refers to placements arranged in countries other than their study country. International placements provide students with opportunities to immerse in a new culture, develop cultural sensitivity and competence, and understand international health systems and issues (Shimmell et al., 2016).
Simulation	Simulation recreates all or part of a placement in a real workplace practice context, in which the practice system, "the environment, people, materials, activities and processes of work are simulated to create a facsimile of occupational therapy practice" (Imms et al., 2017, p. 2). Simulation usually constitutes an aggregate of carefully planned activities, such as written case-based scenarios, standardised patients, video case studies, computer-based virtual reality cases, role play, and mannequins and part-task trainer (Bennet et al., 2017). Simulation has been found to be as effective as block clinical placements in meeting the learning outcomes of practice education (Imms et al., 2018).

VIGNETTE 19.1

Justine and Matthew are on a role emerging placement at a small nongovernment organisation offering community-based support services to people with arthritis. The managing director of the organisation heard that occupational therapy could be useful for people with arthritis and approached the University occupational therapy department for advice. The University department practice education coordinator suggested a student role emerging placement and Justine and Matthew were allocated the placement. Initially Justine and Matthew were apprehensive about the placement because they thought having a nurse (Jenny) as a site supervisor was not ideal but mainly because of their assumption they would not be learning "core authentic occupational therapy skills." The practice education coordinator at the University department had arranged the placement so there were two distinct deliverables of the placement. The first was the production of a business case document to the managing director proposing and justifying the employment of an occupational therapist. The second was a clinical component, whereby the students would provide occupational therapy services to 10 clients of the service, including from an initial assessment, home environmental assessment, workstation ergonomics assessment, and equipment needs assessment to discharge from the service. The practice education coordinator asked Jenny to attend one of the supervisor workshops that were run on a regular basis by the University department where she learned about occupational therapy practice education, including aspects dealing with feedback, supervision, and assessment. During the placement the clinical component was supported by Jenny with specific questions related to occupational therapy being answered by the practice education coordinator either in person when required or via videoconferencing. The end result was an experience for the students that involved learning new business-related skills as well as applying an occupational therapy process to individuals.

of supervision reported in the literature are day-to-day supervision, one-on-one structured supervision, group supervision, and peer supervision (Health Education and Training Institute [HETI], 2012). Day-to-day supervision occurs in real time, often when occupational therapy services are being delivered in a hands-on type of arrangement when the supervisee is building confidence in delivering the skills of occupational therapy. This type of supervision is often done incidentally, informally, or spontaneously. Often this type of supervision is referred to as feedback.

One-on-one structured supervision is a formal process that is often guided by discipline-specific guidelines such as AOTA (2014) or regulatory requirements such as the Australian Commission on Safety and Quality in Health Care (ACSQHC; 2012). This type of supervision is characterised by individualised learning and development plans containing goals and expectations and evidence of reflective practice. Likewise, group supervision is usually led by a senior colleague with the aim of generating group discussion around a specific scenario or challenge. The generation of multiple views and opinions can often lead to robust discussion that may not always occur in individual supervision sessions. Group supervision can be done face to face but is often done remotely if multiple practice contexts are involved.

Peer supervision is a collaborative form of supervision involving two or more clinicians or students. Peer supervision is characterised by each member seeking advice and consultation from a colleague to facilitate reflective practice and practice reasoning (Murphy-Hagan & Milton, 2019). This form of supervision often compliments other formal supervision methods and should be conducted in a way that is respectful of the skills and knowledge of each peer.

What Makes an Effective Supervisor?

Being an effective student supervisor involves a range of different considerations, including understanding the practice context and using interpersonal and supervisory skills appropriately. Understanding the practice context in which occupational therapy is delivered is important to be an effective supervisor. For example, different countries will have different legislative and regulatory requirements around supervision. For example, AOTA (2014) and Occupational Therapy Australia (2019) have published guidelines around the roles and responsibilities of supervision, and many countries such as Australia have regulatory requirements around clinical supervision (ACSQHC, 2012). In addition to these overarching discipline guidelines and regulatory requirements, supervisors need to be aware of local policies and procedures that influence practice that often operationalise the format, duration, and context in which formal supervision takes place.

HETI (2012) suggests that good student supervisors are available, are aware of the supervisory needs of the supervisee, and are organised, meaning that planned sessions take place with a set agenda and clear goals are articulated. Supervisors also need to display appropriate personal skills during supervision. This includes being

VIGNETTE 19.2

Anna is a first-year occupational therapy student completing her first 2-week placement. Anna worked with a number of professionals over the first week of placement and felt that she was demonstrating her professional and communication skills well as she consistently received positive feedback from all her professional colleagues. However, on the Tuesday of the second week during formal supervision, Anna received a number of comments on behaviours that were seen as unprofessional by other staff members and put her at risk of failing the placement. Anna contacted the University occupational therapy department as she was confused by the mixed feedback and interpreted it as a personality clash. Following discussions by the University department practice coordinator, practice educator, and Anna, it was established that the behaviours that were seen as unprofessional had not been communicated to Anna at any stage prior to the second week of placement. Once the feedback was given, explicitly describing the behaviours in question and specifying what behaviours were expected, Anna was able to then modify her behaviour accordingly. Through these discussions by providing clear illustrative feedback and Anna then incorporating the feedback using active reflective practice activities completed in the process, she developed a clearer understanding of how her unintended actions and behaviours could be interpreted in the workplace. This meant that Anna could also apply the same reflective processes when on subsequent placements and continue to monitor and refine her communication skills.

empathic, respecting the diversity and experience that a supervisee brings, having clear expectations around the outcomes of supervision, maintaining confidentiality, being able to reflect on practice, and using feedback effectively (HETI, 2012). See Vignette 19.2 for an example of effective supervision involving student, practice educator and university.

ASSESSMENT

Practice education assessment is completed in different ways internationally. Countries such as Australia, Canada, and United States have developed national standardised assessment tools (Table 19.2) providing national guidelines to assess student practice placement performance. Countries without national assessment forms, such as the United Kingdom, will have individual program practice education assessment forms that address the guiding principles for competency for occupational therapist identified by WFOT (2022).

As our understanding of competency development has occurred, assessment models and processes have also developed beyond practice educator–led standardised assessment. For example, student-led assessments are emerging innovative assessment models. Student-led assessment asks students to self-rate their placement performance prior to the assessment discussion with the practice educator. Student-led assessments support learners to be active agents in their own learning and development, to understanding their competency development as well as initiating the construction of their own solutions. The practice educator's role in this process is to support, guide, and coach (Molloy, 2009). Further research specific to occupational therapy is required to formally investigate if and how this process is assisting with demonstrating competence (Roberts et al., 2015).

Documenting evidence of developing competency in occupational therapy practice education can take multiple forms. For example, the 360-degree assessment approach gains multiple sources of feedback and evidence of competency development in conjunction with standardised assessments. This includes professional reflections, e-portfolios, competency presentations, and consumer feedback.

Reflection is the process where students review their experiences, actions, and responses, and link this to their feelings. Then they interpret and analyse them to learn through this process (Nicol & Dosser, 2016). Students may write daily or weekly reflective journals, a reflective summary or statement at the end of a placement or a course to self-evaluate whether they have attained the learning objectives or required professional competencies and identify further learning needs.

An e-portfolio is an electronic or online resource or document that records students' ongoing professional and personal development and achievements. It is used as an ongoing or final assessment for students to reflect, evaluate, and prove that they have met the learning objectives, or required competencies to graduate. Competency presentation is often used as a final assessment where students are given the opportunity to present evidence that addresses an occupational therapy competency standard. Evidence from practice education or coursework can be presented through a portfolio of practice and/or in a final presentation to demonstrate their readiness to practice.

TABLE 19.2   Occupational Therapy Practice Education Assessments

Country	Assessment	Competency/ Performance Assessed	Rating Scale	Pass/Fail
Australia	Student Practice Evaluation Form - Revised (Second Edition) (School of Health and Rehabilitation Sciences, 2020)	"Professional behaviour, self-management skills, coworker communication, communication skills, documentation, information gathering, service provision, and services evaluation/ reflection"	5-point scale: 1: Performs unacceptably (failing) 2: Performs marginally (experiencing difficulty) 3: Performs adequately (passing) 4: Performs proficiently (passing) 5: Performs with distinction (passing) Not applicable (N/A), and insufficient observation (I/O) N/A or I/O = a rating of 3	Evaluation points: halfway and final A pass to an item is a rating of ≥3 Students need to pass the sets of minimum required items pertaining to all competencies at the final evaluation.
United States	Fieldwork Performance Evaluation for the Occupational Therapy Student (AOTA 2020)	Fundamentals of practice, basic tenets, screening and evaluation, intervention, management of occupational therapy services, and communication and professional behaviours.	4-point scale: 1: Unsatisfactory 2: Emerging 3: Proficient 4: Exemplary There are 42 items each worth 4 points: 4 × 42 = 168	Evaluation points: midterm and final Midterm: satisfactory score = ≥90 Final pass score = ≥111
Canada	Competency Based Fieldwork Evaluation (CBFE) (Miller et al., 2001)	Practice knowledge, clinical reasoning, facilitating change, professional interactions, communication, professional development, performance management	Three stages of professional competencies: 1: Knowledge application 2: Translation 3: Consolidation 8-point numeric rating scale: 1: Low stage 1 competencies 2: Rudimentary stage 1 competencies 3: Mastery of stage 1 competencies; transition to stage 2 4: Rudimentary stage 2 competencies 5: Intermediate stage 2 competencies 6: Mastery of stage 2 competencies; transition to stage 3 7: Rudimentary stage 3 competencies 8: Mastery of stage 3 competencies; ready to enter clinical practice	Midterm and final assessment completed Graded expectations are outlined according to level of placement (1, 2, or 3) Students must meet expected ratings at the final assessment to pass the placement.

(Continued)

Country	Assessment	Competency/ Performance Assessed	Rating Scale	Pass/Fail
United Kingdom	There are no universally used assessment processes or forms. Individual Universities administer their own assessments that have common features.	Common areas assessed: professional behaviours, communication skills, occupational therapy process, practice reasoning, service delivery	This varies from formative assessment, summative assessment using grades (A+ to F) or criteria (outstanding to fail)	Common approaches are midterm formative evaluation with a summative pass/fail based on grades or specified criteria.

TABLE 19.2   Occupational Therapy Practice Education Assessmen (*Cont.*)

Peer assessment uses peer(s) to observe a student's practice, grade, or evaluate the student's practice performance, and provide feedback. Peer assessment is often used for enhancing peer collaborative learning. Consumer involvement in student occupational therapy student evaluation is in its infancy. Other professions such as nursing have used a national consumer feedback process to assist with the evaluation of student performance while on practice education (Masters & Forrest, 2010). In occupational therapy, consumer involvement in student assessment is variable which offers the profession an opportunity to develop this increasingly important aspect of student assessment.

SETTING UP PRACTICE EDUCATION PLACEMENTS FOR SUCCESS

Establishing successful practice education placements is a four-way responsibility between the student, the University/academic department, the placement site, and practice educator(s). Practice education is often a time of significant professional growth for both the student and the practice educator. Students are often eager to impress; however, they are processing large amounts of information in short periods of time. Practice educators are eager to provide ideal learning experiences; however, they are limited in time because of many competing priorities. Preparing, setting expectations, and consistently clear communication can assist with setting up and maintaining a successful placement.

PREPARATION

Placements are ideally allocated early to enable preparation time for the university, the student, and the placement site. Many universities complete preplacement workshops with the students to assist them with preparing for placement. Preplacement workshops often include education and practice around giving and receiving feedback, working in different models of placements, integrating theory into practice, and reflective practice processes. Universities are also responsible for ensuring that the students have completed all the legal and medical requirements contained in agreements and contracts with the placement site prior to starting the placement.

Universities often develop general practice education information handbooks to assist both the student and practice educator to understand the course and placement requirements. Practice handbooks typically include course information; experiences student have completed prior to the placement; roles of the student, practice educator, and university; specific rules and processes to assist with seeking assistance; as well as what is required for the student to demonstrate the learning outcomes for the specific placement. It is both the student's and practice educator's responsibility to become familiar with the information in the handbook. The information assists all involved to understand the expectations of the placement as well as the processes about who and how to seek assistance as required.

Prior to starting placement, students are encouraged to review any placement site online material as well as reviewing lecture material associated with the type of placement they are completing. Students will often contact the placement site and educator prior to the start of placement to assist with their preparation, which often comes in the form of an introductory letter and draft learning contract. The letter and learning contracts are the beginning of forming a professional relationship and setting expectations. Students often ask for additional advice to assist them with preparing for placement, such as key readings, assessment tools, and interventions that are used on placement.

The following strategies are reported to assist with preparing for placement (Rodger et al., 2011):

Student:

- Familiarise yourself with the University placement handbooks.
- Review practice site online materials.
- Review lecture and workshop materials (specific assessment, intervention, etc.).
- Familiarise yourself with addition preparation materials sent to you by the practice educators.

Practice educator:

- Familiarise yourself with the University placement handbooks, especially assessment.
- Develop orientation to workplace.
- Develop week 1 timetable of activities; blank spaces are encouraged to assist with refection time, project development, and to provide flexibility for unexpected opportunities.
- Develop quality improvement project outline that the student can work on during the placement period.

University:

- Complete preplacement workshops.
- Ensure students are compliant with placement agreements.
- Work with practice educators to assist with setting expectations, placement design, and developing potential projects.

SETTING EXPECTATIONS

Students and practice educators should constantly review their mutual expectations during the placement as this can be a key source of apprehension. Setting expectations around professional and workplace behaviours, tasks and duties the student will complete, supervision and mentoring—all are important. What professionalism is and looks like in one practice context will be vastly different to another practice context (Dart et al., 2018) so this is particularly important to communicate to students. What may be common knowledge for the practice educator may not be for the student so consider what implicit or unwritten workplace expectations exist. For example, is it expected that the student eats lunch with professional colleagues? When is it acceptable to use mobile devices? Discuss what key terms within learning outcomes look like in the practice context such as quantifying the amount and type of supervision. Importantly it is critical that a process is in place to assist students who are struggling on placement and their supervisors. This usually involves early identification of challenges, clear communication of expectations and outcomes, and clear communication about the support the University can provide.

SUMMARY

Practice education is a critical part of occupational therapy education as it allows students to apply skills and knowledge learned at University to a real-world situation under structured conditions and scaffolded support over time. It allows students to engage in a variety of experiences varying from traditional occupational therapy practice to role emerging placements, meaning the full scope and power of occupation focused practice can be appreciated. Practice education is delivered in a variety of different ways around the world with varying methods of assessment but with most following prescribed guidelines and assessment protocols. Successful practice education requires good planning, preparation, and support for the student, the site supervisor, and the site. This should include education around mutual expectations, supervision, communication, delivering feedback, and troubleshooting when challenges arise. As the scope and breadth of practice education increases in occupation therapy so should the scholarship around the development, application, and evaluation of it.

REFLECTIVE LEARNING

- Reflect on how you, as a practice education supervisor, provide constructive feedback to students completing a fieldwork placement. How do you ensure the feedback is effective in regard to how and when it is delivered? Importantly, how do you close the feedback loop for your students?
- How do students add value to your workplace?
- Name three things you might do to change your placement experience that could enhance the student experience. Think about the types of placements your agency could offer that could change the student experience.
- Is there anything you would change around the preparation you do for a placement or request your partnering University to change?

REFERENCES

American Occupational Therapy Association. (2014). Guidelines for supervision, roles, and responsibilities during the delivery of occupational therapy services. *American Journal of Occupational Therapy*, 68(3), S16–22. https:doi.org/10.5014/ajot.2014.686S03.

American Occupational Therapy Association. (2015). Standards for continuing competence. *American Journal of Occupational Therapy*, 69(3), 1–3. https://doi.org/10.5014/ajot.2015.696S16.

Australian Commission on Safety and Quality in Health Care. (2012). National safety and quality health service standards. Australian Commission on Safety and Quality in Health Care.

American Occupational Therapy Association. (2020). *Fieldwork performance evaluation for occupational therapy students.* Author.

Bennet, S., Rodger, S., Fitzgerald, C., & Gibson, L. (2017). Simulation in occupational therapy curricula: A literature review. *Australian Occupational Therapy Journal, 64*(4), 314–327. https://doi.org/10.1111/1440-1630.12372.

Brewer, M., & Stewart-Wynne, E. G. (2013). An Australian hospital-based student training ward delivering safe, client-centred care while developing students' interprofessional practice capabilities. *Journal of Interprofessional Care, 27*(6), 482–488. https://doi.org/10.3109/13561820.2013.811639.

Boud, D., & Molloy, E. (2013). Rethinking models of feedback for learning: The challenge of design. *Assessment & Evaluation in Higher Education, 38*(6), 698–712. https://doi.org/10.1080/02602938.2012.691462.

Carless, D., & Boud, D. (2018). The development of student feedback literacy: Enabling uptake of feedback. *Assessment and Evaluation in Higher Education, 42*(8), 1315–1325. https://doi.org/10.1080/02602938.2018.1463354.

Committee on University Fieldwork Education & Association of Canadian Occupational Therapy University Programs. (2011). Canadian guidelines for fieldwork education in occupational therapy (CGFEOT): Guiding principles, responsibilities and continuous quality improvement process. https://www.acotup-acpue.ca/PDFs/2012%20CGFEOT%20-%20English.pdf.

Dart, J., McCall, L., Ash, S., Blair, M., Twohig, C., & Palermo, C. (2018). Towards a global definition of professionalism for dietetic education: A systematic review of the literature. *Journal of the Academy of Nutrition and Dietetics, 119*(6), 957–971. https://doi.org/10.1016/j.jand.2019.01.007.

Davies, M. (2000). *The Blackwell encyclopaedia of social work.* Blackwell Publishing.

DeIuliis, E. D. (2017). What is fieldwork education? In E. D. DeIuliis (Ed.), *Professionalism across occupational therapy practice* (pp. 163–199). Slack Incorporated.

Evensen, M. E., & Hansen, D. J. (2019). Fieldwork, practice education, and professional entry. In B. A. Boyt Schell, & G. Gillen (Eds.), *Willard and Spackman's occupational therapy* (13th ed., pp. 1078–1099). Wolters Kluwer.

Farnworth, L., & Kennedy-Jones, M. (2017). The education of occupational therapists in Australia: Academic and practice education. In T. Brown, H. Bourke-Taylor, S. Isbel, & R. Cordier (Eds.), *Occupational therapy in Australia: Professional and practice issues* (pp. 129–139). Allen & Unwin.

Health Education and Training Institute. (2012). *The superguide: A handbook for supervising allied health professionals.* Author. https://www.heti.nsw.gov.au/education-and-training/our-focus-areas/allied-health/clinical-supervision.

Imms, C., Chu, E., Guinea, S., Sheppard, L., Froude, E., Carter, R., & Symmons, M. (2017). Effectiveness and cost effectiveness of embedded simulation in occupational therapy clinical practice education: Study protocol for a randomised controlled trial. *Trials, 18*(345), 1–16. https://doi.org/10.1186/s13063-017-2087-0.

Imms, C., Froude, E., Chu, E., Sheppard, L., Darzins, S., Guinea, S., & Mathieu, E. (2018). Simulated versus traditional oc-cupational therapy placements: A randomised controlled trial. *Australian Occupational Therapy Journal, 65*(6), 556–564. https://doi.org/10.1111/1440-1630.12513.

Knecht-Sabres, L. J. (2010). The use of experiential learning in an occupational therapy program: Can it foster skills for clinical practice? *Occupational Therapy in Health Care, 24*(4), 320–334. https://doi.org/10.3109/07380577.2010.514382.

Knightbridge, L. (2014). Experiential learning as an alternative practice education placement: Student reflections on entry-level competency, personal growth, and future practice. *British Journal of Occupational Therapy, 77*(9), 438–446. https://doi.org/10.4276/030802214X14098207540956.

Knightbridge, L., & Gilbert-Hunt, S. (2017). Population-centred occupational therapy practice and project management in Australian settings. In T. Brown, H. Bourke-Taylor, S. Isbel, & R. Cordier (Eds.), *Occupational therapy in Australia: Professional and practice issues* (pp. 339–351). Allen & Unwin.

Martin, P., Kumar, S., Lizarondo, L., & Tyack, Z. (2016). Factors influencing the perceived quality of clinical supervision of occupational therapists in a large Australian state. *Australian Occupational Therapy Journal, 63*(5), 338–346. https://doi.org/10.1111/1440-1630.12314.

Masters, H., & Forrest, S. (2010). How did I do? An analysis of service user feedback on mental health student nurses' practice in acute inpatient mental health placements. *The Journal of Mental Health Training, Education and Practice, 5*(1), 11–19. https://doi.org/10.5042/jmhtep.2010.0215.

Miller, L. T., Bossers, A. M., Polatajko, H. J., & Hartley, M. (2001). Development of the competency based fieldwork evaluation (CBFE). *Occupational Therapy International, 8*(4), 244–262. https://doi.org/10.1002/oti.149.

Molloy, E. (2009). Time to pause: Giving and receiving feedback in clinical education. In C. Delany, & E. Molloy (Eds.), *Clinical education in the health professions* (pp. 128–146). Churchill Livingstone/Elsevier.

Moore, K., Bacon, R., Bevitt, T., Bialocerkowski, A., Ciccone, N., Haworth, N., & Wells, C. (2018). The university health clinic: Definition, educational practices and outcomes. *Focus on Health Professional Education, 19*(2), 1–13. https://doi.org/10.11157/fohpe.v19i2.213.

Murphy-Hagan, A., & Milton, L. E. (2019). Towards identifying peer supervision competencies for graduate-level occupational therapy students: A scoping review. *Journal of Occupational Therapy Education, 3*(1). Article 4. https://doi.org/10.26681/jote.2019.030104.

Nastasi, J. A. (2017). Fieldwork education. In K. Jacobs, & N. MacRae (Eds.), *Occupational therapy essentials for clinical competence* (3rd ed., pp. 635–643). Slack Incorporated.

Nicol, J. S., & Dosser, I. (2016). Understanding reflective practice. *Nursing Standard, 30*(36), 34–42. https://doi.org/10.7748/ns.30.36.34.s44.

Occupational Therapy Australia. (2019). Professional supervision framework. https://otaus.com.au/publicassets/2e35a9f6-b890-e911-a2c3-9b7af2531dd2/ProfessionalSupervisionFramework2019.pdf.

Occupational Therapy Board of Australia. (2018). Australian occupational therapy competency standards 2018.

https://www.occupationaltherapyboard.gov.au/Codes-Guidelines/Competencies.aspx.

Occupational Therapy Council of Australia Ltd. (2018). *Accreditation of entry-level occupational therapy education programs guidelines for education providers.* Author.

Roberts, M. E., Hooper, B. R., Wood, W. H., & King, R. M. (2015). An international systematic mapping review of fieldwork education in occupational therapy. *Canadian Journal of Occupational Therapy, 82*(2), 106–118. https://doi.org/10.1177/0008417414552187.

Rodger, S., Fitzgerald, C., Davila, W., Millar, F., & Allison, H. (2011). What makes a quality occupational therapy practice placement? Students' and practice educators' perspectives. *Australian Occupational Therapy Journal, 58*(3), 195–202. https://doi.org/10.1111/j.1440-1630.2010.00903.x.

Royal College of Occupational Therapists. (2019). *Learning and development standards for pre-registration education.* Author. https://www.rcot.co.uk/node/2263/.

School of Health and Rehabilitation Sciences. 2020. Student practice evaluation form - Revised (second edition). In Student practice evaluation form - reviewed (second edition) package. The University of Queensland.

Shimmell, L., Al-Helo, H., Demille, K., Kandel-Lieberman, D., Kremenovic, M., Roorda, K., & Baptiste, S. (2016). Targeting the global, internationalisation in occupational therapy education. *World Federation of Occupational Therapists Bulletin, 72*(1), 16–23. https://doi.org/10.1080/14473828.2016.1149980.

Wood, A. (2005). Student practice contexts: Changing face, changing place. *British Journal of Occupational Therapy, 68*(8), 375–378. https://doi.org/10.1177/030802260506800806.

World Federation of Occupational Therapists. (2016). Minimum standards for the education of occupational therapists revised 2016. https://www.wfot.org/assets/resources/COPY-RIGHTED-World-Federation-of-Occupational-Therapists-Minimum-Standards-for-the-Education-of-Occupational-Therapists-2016a.pdf.

World Federation of Occupational Therapists. (2018). Definition of occupational therapy. https://www.wfot.org/resources/definitions-of-occupational-therapy-from-member-organisations.

Occupational Therapists. (2022). Guiding principles for competency in occupational therapy. https://www.wfot.org/resources.

20

Clinical Supervision Skills

Jenny Strong and Amy McKenzie

HIGHLIGHTS

- Professional or clinical supervision is an essential part of practice for occupational therapists.
- Supervision provides the therapist with the opportunity to reflect on, refine, and enhance one's skills while ensuring the practice standards of the organisation are met,
- Effective supervision encourages both the supervisor and the supervisee to utilise appropriate models of practice to describe and reflect on clinical reasoning.

- Occupational therapists are urged to make use of supervisory agreements, agendas, and to keep records of supervision sessions.
- A variety of learning methods are recommended for supervisions sessions, including case review and discussion, appropriate observation of practice, reading, and scenario role-plays.

INTRODUCTION

Over a century ago, the great French essayist Marcel Proust (1899) wrote, "The real voyage of discovery consists not in seeking new landscapes but in having new eyes." It is our contention that good clinical supervision is a process and experience that offers occupational therapists new eyes with which to see their skills and daily clinical practices. In supervision, clinicians have both the benefits of distance and the expertise of the supervisor with which to relook at their practice (Yasky et al., 2019). Such reflection and acquisition of self-knowledge can then be used by occupational therapists to refine, enhance, and modify their future practice. What a useful discovery voyage this can be for occupational therapists!

Professional or clinical supervision is now regarded as an essential professional practice for occupational therapists working across the world; such supervision is typically mandated in national professional standards for occupational therapists. For example, Standard 9.8 of the Royal College of Occupational Therapists (2017) Professional Standards for Occupational Therapy practice states, "As a practitioner, you will receive regular professional supervision and appraisal, where you use critical reflection to review your practice" (p. 15). In Scotland, all allied health practitioners are required to have access to supervision and to make use of this supervision (National Health Service

[NHS] Education for Scotland, 2018). In the Australian jurisdiction, the Australian Occupational Therapy Competency Standard 1.12 states the practitioner "identifies and uses relevant professional and operational support and supervision" (Occupational Therapy Board of Australia, 2018). Similarly, the Occupational Therapy Board of New Zealand (2020) mandates the need for all practicing occupational therapists to undertake professional supervision. Thus clinical supervision is regarded as a vital part of clinical governance, with the bottom line being the delivery of safe and high value care to patients, clients, and consumers (Australian Council on Safety and Quality in Health Care, 2017; Leggat et al., 2016).

The intent of this chapter is to provide occupational therapists with ideas to ensure that their supervisory experience is a pleasant and productive voyage of discovery and they have the tools to ensure the three important functions of supervision are met in supervision. Supervision has been defined as a "working alliance between two or more professional members where the intention of the interaction is to enhance the knowledge, skills and attitudes of at least one staff member" (Spence et al., 2001, p. 136). The three important functions of supervision were articulated by Proctor (1994) as (1) normative, which deals with service delivery according to professional and legislative standards; (2) formative, which deals with the professional development of the supervisee, and (3) restorative, which is concerned with supporting the supervisee who manages the stressors of practice. Or as summarised by Spence et al. (2001), clinical practice issues, administrative/organisational issues, and personal support issues are all worked on in supervision.

The chapter begins by reviewing three contemporary models of clinical supervision that have been found useful across a variety of clinical settings and professional groupings. It then synthesises key aspects from the models to offer a useful working model to assist the occupational therapist. Strategies considered to be best practice in supervision are then enumerated. Vignettes are used to illustrate benefits of supervision and the requisite skills practitioners can incorporate as they manage themselves in their occupational therapy practice.

In addition to formal supervision relationships, informal supervision and peer supervision will be briefly considered.

SUPERVISION MODELS

Having a model that underpins the supervision process is useful for both the supervisee and supervisor to gain clarity about the process. It assists everyone to have a clear understanding about purpose, content, and the rights and responsibilities of all parties. Concurrent with an acceptable model of supervision there needs to be a policy and workplace attitude that supports this use of staff time to promote positive outcomes for patients or clients and the ongoing professional development of staff. A model of supervision should be built on a belief that supervision is a desirable and valued activity that enhances the quality of clinical practice, improves client outcomes, and supports staff who may be working in difficult circumstances.

There is a plethora of models of clinical supervision. It is interesting, or perhaps alarming, to note some of the findings in the recent paper by Hardy et al. (2017), who working in the mental health field identified 52 different models of clinical supervision. They then reviewed the content of each of the models and found that most of these models focused on the professional development and learning of the supervisee—the formative function of supervision. Meanwhile, just over half focused on the management and ethical responsibilities—the normative function of supervision. The restorative function of supervision, dealing with the emotional effects of the supervisee's work, was a focus in over half of the models, as was the writing-up supervision sessions and using recorded therapy session transcripts. Less than half of the models reported focusing on clients. As Hardy et al. (2017) stated, "Therefore, one of the starkest findings of this review is the lack of focus on the patient in supervision, challenging the widely held

assumption that supervision ensures positive patient outcomes" (p. 1242). Furthermore, none of the models had been empirically tested to determine if they were effective. Nonetheless, we, like others such as Leggat et al. (2016), believe that good clinical supervision is essential for ensuring quality patient or client care and the professional development of the occupational therapist.

Here, we first report on the flexible working alliance model of clinical supervision, which was presented in the first edition of this book. This model was built on our supervision research work with 272 allied health staff in one Australian mental health service (Kavanagh et al., 2003, 2008; Spence et al., 2001; Strong et al., 2003; Wilson et al., 2001).

The flexible working alliance model posits three important players in the supervisory relationship: the supervisee, the supervisor, and the patient or client (Fig. 20.1). The supervisor must not only facilitate and support the supervisee's professional development but also must focus on the supervisee's individual work with patients and manage service delivery within the work team. This model is quite explicit about role of the supervisor in the supervisory process (Vignette 20.1).

The supervisor has three important functions in the process:
1. The supervisor will ensure that organisation policies are implemented, that the quality and quantity of the supervisee's work is meeting standards, and prioritising that service delivery is optimised.
2. The supervisor will focus on the supervisee's work through a detailed consideration of individual pieces of work. This individual will instruct or advise the therapist about appropriate strategies, model professional behaviour and practice, consult in the context of solving clinical and ethical problems, evaluate the effectiveness of particular approaches based on observation, record interviews and discussion, and provide support.
3. The supervisor will facilitate the supervisee's professional development and learning and assist the supervisee to fit into the workplace.

At all times, the supervisor needs to be mindful of the focus upon the needs of the client, the needs of the supervisee, and the needs of the organisation. For example, if the supervisor focuses exclusively on only a few pieces of the supervisee's work, the supervisor may neglect to ensure that the needs of all clients are being met and an assessment of the worker's professional development needs may be inaccurate. The model highlights how different aspects of the work are linked and may be in tension with each other. This tension may manifest itself as conflict (e.g., asking an underprepared therapist to take on tasks because of a high demand for services).

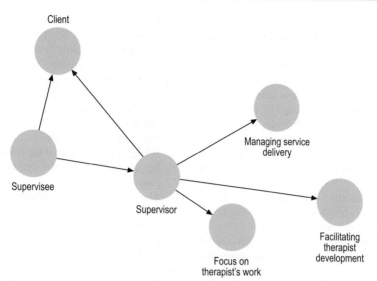

FIG. 20.1 A model of supervision, highlighting the importance of the client, the supervisee, and the supervisor, in addition to the supervisor's responsibilities in managing service delivery, focusing on the therapist's work, and facilitating the therapist's professional development.

VIGNETTE 20.1

Liz is an occupational therapist in her second year of practice, working in a busy public mental health service. Whilst there are a number of other occupational therapists within the service, Liz is the only occupational therapist working within her caseload (adolescent mental health). Her supervisor is Kate, the operational manager of the occupational therapists. Kate works within the community mental health team but provides professional support and supervision to all occupational therapists within the mental health service.

To form an effective supervisory relationship, Kate encouraged Liz to develop some goals for supervision around three core priorities of the organisation and service delivery, the needs of her caseload, and her own professional development. In this way, time each session is devoted to ensuring the three competing priorities are addressed. Although Kate does not work directly within the same caseload as Liz, this focus ensures the Liz seeks feedback from the adolescent mental health team to review if the needs to the client and the organisation are being met, or if Liz can support Kate to extend her skill set in this area.

The model identified the need for the supervisor to adapt personal responses and the use of other resources depending on the following:

- Supervisee's personal goals, current work challenges, abilities, and learning styles
- Quality of the relationship between the supervisee and the supervisor
- Characteristics of individual clients and clients as a group
- Organisational structure of the team
- Availability of resources of time and money
- Supervisor's abilities and professional background and current organisational priorities

Supervisors need to have the following core skills (Strong, 2009):

- Capacity to form effective relationships with people
- Well-developed problem-solving, negotiation, advocacy, and conflict resolution skills
- Ability to clearly articulate the approach to practice
- Capacity for self-reflective practice
- Capacity to form evidence-based assessments of the other's practice and to use this assessment to inform future decisions.

The flexible working alliance model's strengths are in its focus on the supervisor's roles and functions, especially in relation to service delivery and client care. A randomised controlled trial of the outcomes of supervision training based on this model, however, found only limited impact in terms of long-term adoption of potentially beneficial supervisory methods by supervisors (Kavanagh et al., 2008).

Fitzpatrick et al. (2015) developed the allied health key dimensions model of clinical supervision. The model was derived from their qualitative work with 113 allied health professionals in the state of New South Wales in Australia. They identified four important dimensions necessary for a successful supervision experience, as perceived by the supervisee, and adopted into their concentric supervision model:

1. At the centre of the model is the supervisee's needs. Fitzpatrick et al. (2015) identified the supervisee's needs for "reflection, support, confidence, and learning" (p. 7).
2. This is followed by the need to clarify the purpose of supervision, its structure, and the roles of the supervisor and supervisee.
3. The next aspect of the model is the quality of the relationship between the supervisee and supervisor.
4. The final requirement of the model is for accessibility of regular supervision.

By using this model, a therapist is encouraged to enter the supervisory relationship with self-awareness of abilities and areas that need further development. This can help to focus the content of the supervision to maximise the therapist's learning and skill development. Strengths of the allied health key dimensions model include its detailed focus upon the needs of the supervisee. Use of this model is illustrated in Vignette 20.2.

The Scottish clinical supervision model for midwives has been recently published (Key et al., 2019). This model consists of five cyclic steps:

1. It begins with writing a supervision contract that specifies purpose, frequency, expectations, boundaries, and responsibilities.
2. The second step is maintaining focus and is concerned with the content of the supervision sessions: the setting of priorities for discussion, the preparations to be made prior to supervisory meetings, and the methods to be used such as different reflective tools and case note reviews.
3. The third step is knowing the importance of space and deals with setting both the physical and relational environment to enable deep reflection on practice. The supervisor has a key role in establishing a safe space so the supervisee is comfortable to honestly and frankly explore the events, actions, and thoughts/emotions surrounding the clinical scenarios.

VIGNETTE 20.2

Robert is an occupational therapist with 3 years of clinical experience in community-based practice. He regards himself as skilled in working with his clients to determine occupation-focused goals and keeping people independent in the community. He recently commenced a rotational position in a major metropolitan hospital. His only previous hospital experience was a 7-week student placement in the third year of his course. Prior to his first supervision session, Robert reflects on his skills and areas where he lacks confidence. He comes up with the following list:

Strengths	Weaknesses
Initial assessments	Limited experience with cognitive screening
Developing client rapport	Minimal experience in pressure injury prevention and management
Trained in functional independence measure (FIM) assessments	Somewhat basic splinting skills
Subjective, objective, assessment, and plan (SOAP) documentation skills	Minimal experience in cognitive assessment
Assistive technology prescription	

Robert is then able to use this list to discuss his learning needs when he meets with his supervisor Jane. Jane, who is a busy senior occupational therapist with eight other junior therapists on her team, is pleased that Robert has identified what he believes to be his training needs. This makes it so much easier for her to help Robert. Jane talks with Robert about the frequency of supervision, her expectations, and documentation requirements. Together, they complete their supervision agreement and then plan the professional development and training program they will implement for Robert over the next 3 months, in addition to the mandatory training program that all therapists undertake annually.

4. The fourth step in the model is building a bridge, which is a metaphor for the next steps the supervisee and supervisor will take after the supervision session ends. What goals do they identify? What information has been shared? What is the action plan going forward?
5. The fifth step is the review, whereby the supervisee provides views on what has been helpful in supervision and if objectives from past sessions have been met.

The strength of the Scottish clinical supervision model is its focus on the content of the supervision session. The NHS Education for Scotland (2018) has a useful suite of supervision learning modules and accompanying resources that expand on this model and can support supervision practices.

Vignette 20.3 illustrates how the supervisor has created a safe space for a new graduate occupational therapist to discuss a client case where she felt ineffective as a therapist.

It is suggested that aspects of each of these three clinical supervision models can be extracted to guide best practice. Focusing on the supervisor's roles and functions, the supervisee's needs and the supervision session itself have many benefits. In the next section, additional key strategies and processes that have been described in the literature as best practices in clinical supervision will be described.

BEST PRACTICES IN CLINICAL SUPERVISION

The American Association for Counselor Education and Supervision (ACES) published its *Supervision Best Practice Guidelines* in 2011 (Borders et al., 2014). This document identifies 12 areas needed for best practice. Many of these aspects are covered in the three supervision models identified earlier; however, the framework used in these guidelines is useful and is presented here:

1. Initiating supervision: Here, the supervisor will provide the supervisee with information about the experience on supervision and the supervision style. A written supervision agreement or contract, which will cover the expectations of supervision, the limits of confidentiality, and the practical aspects of supervision (e.g., its frequency, location, and responsibilities), will be developed in this session. The informed consent of the supervisee is obtained. It is useful to discuss with the supervisee any previous supervisory experiences and learning styles.
2. Goal setting: The supervisor and the supervisee work together to identify goals that will ensure effectiveness of service delivery, and the supervisee's learning needs in the context of the clinical setting. These goals are

VIGNETTE 20.3

Sally is in the first 6 months of her first job as an occupational therapist working in a child and youth facility. Her caseload includes a number of children aged 7 to 12 years who are school avoidant and who are falling behind in their schoolwork. Her supervisor, Sharon, has been working in the facility for the past 8 years and is very experienced. Sally always valued her supervision sessions with Sharon. She felt that Sharon had been providing her with lots of encouragement.

In the past month she had begun work with a new client, Stu, who comes to therapy with his mother, Rachel. Sally dreads these therapy sessions because each time Stu and his mother end up screaming at each other, after which he sits stony faced for the rest of the session. This has happened for 3 weeks now, and Sally doesn't know what to do.

Sally brings this case to her next supervision session. Her supervisor asks her to describe what happens when the session starts. What was the triggering event for the screaming? Instead of being overwhelmed, Sally begins to see the clinical encounter more clearly. She thinks she can see how Stu would have felt disempowered and got frustrated.

Sally identifies that her goals for Stu are to assist him to improve his school performance and to get on better with Mum. As she talks it through with her supervisor, Sally sees how she can better structure the therapy sessions, so she works alone with Stu on his performance skills. She also schedules time to meet with Mum, to explain the things she's doing with Stu and to reinforce Mum's efforts to support and encourage Stu.

At the next supervision session, Sharon asks Sally how her client is getting on. Sally describes how her work with Stu is going well, and his Mum reports that things are much better for him at school. She's glad she raised the case in supervision and had the opportunity to look at the case with clearer eyes. Since she felt supported by her supervisor, she knew she could trust her to not be judgemental about a lack of skills. This enabled her to reflect and learn and be a better therapist for her client.

From 1 January 2007 – 30 June 2007

Agreed goals of supervision:

1 To gain experience in working with individuals with chronic pain
2 To become competent in using a variety of different assessment tools
3 To become competent in formulating occupationally focused treatment goals
4 To develop expertise in working with so called difficult patients

Structure of supervision:

1 To occur once per month, on third Thursday from 2-3pm, in interview room 2
2 Resources required will be the interview room, the 60 minute time period, video player and screen on occasion, support to enrol in next scientific meeting on pain
3 Preparation as mutually agreed to occur
4 Preparatory agenda to be set up at the conclusion of each monthly session, it can be modified by mutual agreement
5 Supervisor will be available between sessions if required
6 Discussions/case materials to remain confidential between 2 parties, except in situation where supervisor has concerns about the safety of patients or supervisee. If this occurs, the supervisor will advise the supervisee of his need to disclose
7 A variety of methods to be used in supervision, including verbal discussion, listening to audio-tapes or watching video-tapes of client sessions, use of direct observation, role play and article review

Records:

1 Monthly notes, as per Figure 20.3 to be kept
2 Both supervisor and supervisee to keep a copy of these notes
3 These records to be used for personal use, and for review at end of supervision period
4 Records to be stored in the supervisor's filing cabinet for a 12 month period

Evaluation of supervision:

1 Preferred process will involve review of original goals and progress made from perspectives, with comparison between supervisor and supervisee
2 To occur in month 5, or sooner if either supervisor or supervisee request a review

Signed by: AJ Supervisor and AT Supervisee on 08 August 2006

FIG. 20.2 Supervision practice agreement.

seen as important for enhancing the therapeutic relationship between the supervisee and the patient or client. These goals are written into the supervisory agreement. In each subsequent supervision session, at least one of the goals will be addressed.

Fig. 20.2 provides an example of a completed supervisory agreement that clearly articulates the practical arrangements for supervision and the goals for supervision.

3. Giving feedback: The supervisor will provide a balance of both supportive and challenging feedback, which will be based on both the supervisee's self-report and additional direct observations of the supervisee's performance. This feedback will be constructive and descriptive.

4. Conducting supervision: Supervision is provided in accordance with the relevant professional and legislative standards. The supervisor will be sure to provide a safe and supportive supervision environment. This aspect was nicely articulated in the Scottish model of clinical supervision for midwives referred to earlier. The supervisor will use a variety of methods in the supervision, including review of case notes, discussion of theory, review of transcripts, and observation.

5. The supervisory relationship: The supervisor works to ensure a productive supervisory relationship with mutual trust.

6. Diversity and advocacy considerations: There is a recognition of the influence of the various cultural factors that may influence the supervisory relationship and experience. These include (but are not limited to) factors such as gender, sexual identity, race, religion, spirituality, socioeconomic status, and privilege.

7. Ethical considerations: It is the supervisor's role to ensure the supervisee, and oneself, adhere to all relevant ethical codes. The supervisor will be aware of one's own level of competence as a supervisor, engage in own professional development as a supervisor, and seek supervision of the supervisory practice.

8. Documentation: The requirements for documentation were well explained in the aforementioned supervision models.

   Fig. 20.3 provides an example of a supervision session documentation.

9. Evaluation: The supervisor understands and is committed to the importance of both formative and summative evaluation methods. When evaluating performance, information should be sought from a variety of sources, and the supervisor should take care to highlight areas of strength and provide opportunity for growth.

10. Supervision format: This may take the form of individual, peer, or group supervision.

11. The supervisor: The responsibilities of supervisors have been well described in the models section.

12. Supervisor preparation: We contend that supervisors should complete supervision training prior to commencing supervision; however, as alluded to earlier, we are aware that there is limited evidence of the efficacy of such training (see Hardy et al., 2017; Kavanagh et al., 2008).

SITUATIONS THAT MAY ARISE IN SUPERVISION

There are times when the best laid plans "of mice and [wo]men" come unstuck in supervision. Some supervisory relationships proceed without a hitch, and the agreed goals of assisting the supervisee to become a more competent practitioner are realised. In other cases, situations arise in supervision that challenge either the supervisor or the supervisee. A special issue of *The Clinical Supervisor* was devoted to the theme of harmful clinical supervision (Ellis, 2017; Ellis et al., 2017). Some of the matters raised in a series of personal narratives on harmful supervision dealt with boundary issues; a lack of respect for cultural, sexual, and racial differences; and power issues. Referring back to the model that underpins supervision can provide a working solution to problems that arise.

Let us consider one example of what might occur in supervision, as described in Vignette 20.4.

Between AJ Supervisor and AT Supervisee

Date: 10 August 2006
Topic: Working with difficult patients, especially angry, hostile patients, when seen both individually and in a group

Discussion revolved around the reasons why some patients present as difficult, and its impact on therapy.

Discussion about possible antecedents to patient anger, including being unjustly hurt, being misled, violation of norms, attacks on ego integrity, or being unjustly treated.

Discussed use of of a process approach, which develops rapport using active listening, a thorough assessment and developing a therapeutic alliance with the patient.

Role played use of process approach with 'an angry patient'

Agreed action: Supervisee to read chapters by Large et al (2002) and DeGood & Dane (1996) and article by Fernandez and Turk (1995)

Agenda items for next session: the patient who somatisizes
Preparation required: Supervisee to consider examples from patient load, and outcomes of therapy

Signed by ....and...
Date: 10 August 2006

FIG. 20.3 Sample of monthly supervision notes and agenda planning.

VIGNETTE 20.4

Anna has been schooled in attachment informed approaches to working with patients with chronic health conditions (see Hunter & Maunder, 2016; Meredith & Strong, 2019). Anna's supervisor has a different theoretical orientation, being a strong advocate of cognitive-behavioural–based therapy. Rather than argue over which approach is superior, in supervision the supervisor reframed the questions to consider what was in the best interests of the client, Ramilla. Anna explained how she felt Ramilla was so anxious and distressed that she was unable to even begin to think about or use any cognitive strategies. She needed first to develop a level of trust and comfort.

SUMMARY

In this chapter we have articulated what we believe are the necessary and sufficient steps to ensure clinical supervision meets its important but lofty goals of supporting the clinician, the organisation, and the patient or client to whom occupational therapy services are delivered. We have provided some tools and strategies that can be used and have used vignettes to illustrate strategies that can enhance the supervisory experience.

REFLECTIVE LEARNING

- Effective supervision requires active planning and engagement from both the supervisee and supervisor.
- When approaching supervision, it is helpful for the supervisee to have an informed view of one's own strengths and learning needs.
- The supervisee has a major responsibility in ensuring supervision supports the supervisee, meets the organisational needs of the facility, and contributes to quality and safe services to patients and clients.

REFERENCES

American Association for Counselor Education and Supervision. (2011). Best practices in clinical supervision. https://aces-online.net/knowledge-base/aces-best-practices-in-clinical-supervision-2011/.

Australian Council on Safety and Quality in Health Care. (2017). *National safety and quality health service standards* (2nd ed). https://www.safetyandquality.gov.au/standards/nsqhs-standards www.safetyandquality.gov.au.

Borders, L. D., Glosoff, H. L., Welfare, L. E., Hays, D. G., DeKruyf, L., Fernando, D. M., & Page, B. (2014). Best practices in clinical supervision: Evolution of a counselling specialty. *The Clinical Supervisor, 33*, 26–44. https://doi.org.ezproxy.library.uq.edu.ay/10.1080/07325223.2014.905225.

Ellis, M. V. (2017). Narratives of harmful supervision. *The Clinical Supervisor, 36*, 20–87. https://doi.ezproxy.library.uq.edu.au/10.1080/07325223.2017.1297752.

Ellis, M. V., Corp, D. A., Taylor, E. J., & Kangos, K. A. (Eds.). (2017). Narratives of harmful clinical supervision: An unacknowledged truth. *The Clinical Supervisor, 36.* [special issue].

Fitzpatrick, S., Smith, M., & Wilding, C. (2015). Clinical supervision in allied health in Australia: A model of allied health clinical supervision based on practitioner experience. *Internet Journal of Allied Health Sciences and Practice, 13*(4). Article 13.

Hardy, G. E., Simpson-Southward, C., & Waller, G. (2017). How do we know what makes for 'best practice" in clinical supervision for psychological therapists? A content analysis of supervisory models and approaches. *Clinical Psychology Psychotherapy, 24*, 1228–1245. https://doi.org/10.1002/cpp.2084.

Hunter, J., & Maunder, R. (Eds.). (2016). *Improving patient treatment with attachment theory. A guide for primary care practitioners and specialists.* Springer.

Kavanagh, D. J., Spence, S., Strong, J., Wilson, J., Sturk, H., & Crow, N. (2003). Supervision practices in allied mental health:. *A staff survey. Mental Health Services Research, 5*, 187–195.

Kavanagh, D. J., Spence, S., Sturk, H., Strong, J., Wilson, J., Worrall, L., Crow, N., & Skerrett, R. (2008). Outcomes of training in supervision: Randomised controlled trial. *Australian Psychologist, 43*, 96–104. https://doi.org/10.1080/0050060802056534.

Key, S., Marshall, H., & Hollins Martin, C. H. (2019). The Scottish clinical supervision model for midwives. *British Journal of Midwifery, 27*, 655–663.

Leggat, S. G., Phillips, B., Pearce, P., Dawson, M., Schultz, D., & Smith, J. (2016). Clinical supervision for allied health: Necessary but not sufficient. *Australian Health Review, 40*, 431–437. http://dx.doi.org/10.1071/AH15080.

Meredith, P. J., & Strong, J. (2019). Attachment and chronic illness. *Current Opinions in* Psychology. 25, 132–138. https://doi.org/10.1016/j.copsyc.2018.04.018.

NHS Education for Scotland. (2018). Scotland's position statement on supervision for allied health professionals. https://learn.nes.nhs.scot.

Occupational Therapy Board of Australia. (2018). *Australian occupational therapy competency standards.* Author.

Occupational Therapy Board of New Zealand. (2020). Supervision requirements for occupational therapists.

https://www.otboard.org.nz/document/4786/Supervision-Requirements-for-Occupational-Therapists.pdf.

Proctor, B. (1994). Supervision: Competence, confidence, accountability. *British Journal of Guidance & Counselling, 22,* 309–318.

Proust, M. (1899). *The remembrance of things past.* Faber & Faber.

Royal College of Occupational Therapists. (2017). *Professional standards for occupational therapy practice.* www.rcot.co.uk.

Spence, S. H., Wilson, J., Kavanagh, D., Strong, J., Murdoch, B., & Krasny, J. (2001). Clinical supervision in four mental health professions: A review of the evidence. *Behaviour Change, 18,* 135–155.

Strong, J. (2009). Clinical supervision skills. In E. A. S. Duncan (Ed.), *Skills for practice in occupational therapy* (pp. 338–348). Elsevier.

Strong, J., Wilson, J., Kavanagh, D., Spence, S., Worrall, L., Crow, N. (2003). Supervision practice within a large allied mental health workforce: Exploring the phenomenon. *The Clinical Supervisor, 22,* 191–210.

Wilson, J., Kavanagh, D., Worrall, L., Spence, S., Strong, J., Skerrett, R., Sturk, H., & Crow, N. (2001). *A research evaluation of professional supervision and mentoring of allied health professionals in the mental health services. Report 4. A model of allied health professional supervision in mental health in Queensland.* Queensland Health.

Yasky, J., King, R., & O'Brien, T. (2019). The peer supervision group as clinical research device: Analysis of a group experience. *British Journal of Psychotherapy, 35,* 305–321.

21

Professional Use of Social Media

Edward A.S. Duncan

HIGHLIGHTS

- Social media is a largely unavoidable component of contemporary society in the Global North.
- Social media presents occupational therapists with wide-ranging opportunities to develop and communicate as professionals.

- There are several potential pitfalls to engaging in social media; these relate to both personal and professional accounts.
- Careful and conscious engagement with social media platforms following the advice set out in this chapter will enable you to safely optimise your impact.

INTRODUCTION

Without doubt one of the biggest changes that has happened both professionally to society since the publication of the last edition of this book, a little over 10 years ago, has been the explosion of social media. The earliest social media platform, called Bolt, was founded in 1996. In the last 10 to 15 years, social media has become a mainstream component of the lives of many in our society. In little more than a decade the use of social media platforms such as Twitter (founded in 2006), Facebook (founded in 2004), YouTube (founded in 2005), and a host of other platforms has changed the way we interact as individuals, professionals, and society. In 2020 alone it is estimated that there are more than 3.81 billion global users of social media. Within the United Kingdom, 66% of the population is estimated to engage in social media in one way or another, with 77% of people aged over 13 years actively involved in social media. Similar statistics are present across the rest of the Global North, where on average 63% of the population aged over 13 years is active on social media (Dean, 2020). Such widespread usage can easily cover the increasing digital divide that exists in the United Kingdom and other nations. Indeed, the importance of being able to access and use the Internet and social media is an indicator of progress in the United Nations Sustainable Development Goals (United Nations, n.d.). So while social media is a powerful tool and the focus of this chapter, it is important to remember that it is not available to everyone. In 2018, there were still 5.3 million adults in the United Kingdom (10% of the adult population) who had either never used the Internet or not used it in the last 3 months (Serafino, 2019).

Since the birth of social media, occupational therapists have embraced its possibilities and potential for networking, continuing professional development, engaging in conferences, and developing formal and informal communities of practice (BJOT & #OTalk, 2016). Social media has also been found to be supportive to individual occupational therapists who are working in nontraditional settings or remote working environments. Despite the clear professional opportunities and advantages that social media can bring, there are clear ethical and professional challenges and limitations. Professional boundaries must be clearly adhered to in order to maintain working within professional context and in keeping professional guidance. This chapter provides an introduction to the use of social media by occupational therapists. While the chapter is written with occupational therapists in mind, its key concepts are relevant for other allied health professions, nurses, and health care professionals. The chapter mentions specific social media platforms, but there are a large and growing number of social media platforms, each with particular audiences and demographics. It is therefore important to apply the general principles outlined in this chapter across whatever social media platform you use.

THE BENEFITS OF SOCIAL MEDIA

The UK Health and Care Professions Council (HCPC; 2017) outlines four key benefits to using social media in the professional context. Within an occupational therapy–specific context these can be translated as follows: (1) developing and sharing skills and knowledge, (2) helping the public understand what an occupational therapist is, (3) networking with other occupational therapists nationally and internationally, and (4) raising the profile of occupational therapy. It has also been suggested that social media has the potential to influence health organisations and government(s) on policy matters (Royal College of Occupational Therapists [RCOT], 2019). Another benefit of social media is that it is intrinsically egalitarian. Well-known individuals, prolific academics, leading politicians, and celebrities who previously would have been hard to reach are now a simple message away. At times these people can provide a means to answer a question you may have or promote your work to a much wider audience than you yourself could achieve.

One of the earliest digital means that occupational therapists used to develop and share skills and knowledge were online discussion groups. These early forms of social media enabled occupational therapists who worked in similar settings to network with each other and share good practice. One example of this is a forensic occupational therapy discussion group set up using the social media services of Yahoo! Inc. Over 8 years this group received contributions from 20 countries and was used for purposes such as seeking and giving advice, networking, requesting and sharing materials and resources, service development, helping to define the role of occupational therapy within this challenging setting, and supported student learning. As with other groups, the forensic occupational therapy discussion group was found to be particularly useful for professionals who were working in a rare relatively specialised area and often isolated from other occupational therapists working within the same specialism (Dieleman & Duncan, 2013). Groups such as the Forensic Occupational Therapy discussion group, however, could be justifiably critiqued for reflecting tribal online behaviours (Rolls et al., 2016). While membership was not explicitly restricted to forensic occupational therapists, its very specific focus limited the potential for wider professional group involvement. As technology developed and other social media platforms became available, the popularity of such discussion groups declined. More easily accessible social media platforms became available and therapists like the rest of society transferred their focus and usage of social media to these emerging platforms.

In recent years more contemporary social media platforms have become the go-to online locations to share skills and knowledge, and have widened participation. One highly successful example is the Twitter chat #OTalk (www.otalk.co.uk). OTalk was founded in 2011 with the first Twitter-chat session happened in October of that year. It continues to take place each Tuesday evening between 8:00 and 9:00 p.m. GMT. Each week different chat topics are suggested and facilitated by guest hosts who are supported by a core team. This weekly social media event has become a highly popular and successful means for occupational therapists to develop and share their skills and knowledge. The @OTalk Twitter account has over 20,000 followers (as of November 2020) and individual chats have a very wide reach, with some gaining over 2 million impressions and involving over 100 participants. Other professional Twitter groups are also highly successful. For instance, @WeAHPs brings together allied health professionals in a single group in which they can learn and share examples of how they can improve their care across professional boundaries. They hold monthly Tweetchats and have a following of almost 24,000 Twitter account users.

In 2018, capitalising on allied health professionals' online presence, two UK allied health professionals (a dietitian and the speech-language therapist) developed the idea of developing #AHPsDay. AHPsDay (https://www.england.nhs.uk/ahp/ahps-day/) is an online social movement developed to focus on and highlight the contribution of allied health professionals to health and social care practice. This event helps improve public understanding of the diverse roles of the individual allied health professions and raises their profile within health care in society. Originating within the United Kingdom, #AHPsDay is now a global phenomenon, with colleagues in Australia and elsewhere joining this social movement.

Of course, social media is not restricted to text-based interactions. The use of video and podcasting has come to the fore as a means for occupational therapists and others to develop and share their skills and knowledge. An excellent example of this is the Twitter group @AHP2mintalks. This group, founded in Scotland in 2019, is a global community run by allied health professionals for allied health professionals. It aims to overcome the research into practice gap and to make research findings easily understood and implemented. AHP2mintalksis a simple concept. People wishing to post to the group provide a 2-minute video of themselves in which they summarise a piece of published research that they have either been involved in or read and been inspired by. There is no need for complex technology as most videos are recorded using a smartphone. The idea for the group emerged from a research project to develop novel ways of making research useful for practice. The brief and engaging format created by @AHP2mintalks team provides an easy and digestible means of summarising recent research and keeping up to date with evidence in a way that suits many people. The group welcomes videos that comply with their format and simply asks that such videos are uploaded to Twitter including the handle @AHP2mintalks. Their only stipulation is that videos are under 2 minutes long and that each video focuses on research that is of relevance to allied health professionals.

PROFESSIONAL AND ETHICAL CONSIDERATIONS FOR ENGAGING IN SOCIAL MEDIA

While social media undoubtedly offers a range of benefits and opportunities for occupational therapists and others, it is an environment that requires careful and considered use. It is worth remembering that an online presence can be hard to erase, and a digital footprint of what you post often remains indefinitely. I am certainly grateful that previous generations' social faux pas were rarely known outwith their immediate social circle and their memory faded with time. The same is not true today. A quick Instagram photo during a night out where you get a bit carried away can swiftly make it to the screens of thousands of people and remain findable for years to come (Vignette 21.1).

Professional organisations and registration bodies such as HCPC (2017), RCOT (2019), and Australia's Occupational Therapy Board Aphra (2019), among others, provide guidance on how to adhere to strict professional guidelines while engaging in social media activities. Keeping some key concepts and rules in mind can avoid occupational therapists from breaking these professional codes of conduct.

KEY CONCEPTS AND RULES FOR ENGAGING IN SOCIAL MEDIA

Setting Up a Social Media Profile

As has been discussed there are many advantages to setting up and maintaining a social media profile as an occupational therapist. Among other reasons social media can help you keep up to date with news, provide an opportunity for continuing professional development and learning, as well as sharing and engaging good practice with others. Before you get started it's a good idea to consider which of the social media platforms most likely meet your requirements. If you are not already engaged in that platform it is worth spending a bit of time looking at the accounts of key and well-respected individuals who you wish to follow. It is likely that their accounts will lead you to other accounts that are available and would be beneficial to your career. Using this snowballing method you can rapidly develop a list of key individuals to follow. It is rarely of value to follow an account that does not post at least semiregularly. Attention also needs to be given to accounts that are fake or computer generated. These are usually easy to identify by looking at their name, description, and posting history. Developing a social media presence takes time, commitment, and perseverance. Few individuals are interested in following an account that does not engage with others. So it is best to be an active user and not a lurker (someone who looks at other people's accounts but does not post anything). Some people are concerned that social media is too time consuming and that they do not have time or space in their life for it. It is certainly true that social media platforms can become a drain on time. However, as with many things, with efficient time management social media platforms can become a highly valuable resource and need not take you away from other valuable activities. I find some of the best times to catch up on social media activity are the periods of the day in which I find myself waiting for a task to complete (e.g., waiting for the kettle to boil). In this way engaging in social media need not necessarily become an onerous task. When posting to social media, however, I usually take a bit more time to reflect on what I am posting, how I am sharing the information, and what my aim for posting the content is.

VIGNETTE 21.1

During her third year of occupational therapy studies Grace was out for a night with her friends. They had been to a few bars and then went clubbing. Having had a few too many drinks Grace found herself in the toilet throwing up. While one of her friends held up her hair, another "friend" thought it would be funny to take a picture and post it on Instagram. The next day Grace saw the picture and was furious at her friend. But the damage was done and she soon forgot about it. Three years later Grace was working in her first postqualification job. She was an occupational therapist in an inpatient acute into health ward. Several of the patients admitted to the ward had problems with alcohol, either as a primary reason for admission or secondary to another condition. While working with the group of patients who had problems with alcohol, one of them approached Grace with the picture from that night out on his phone. He had found it by simply looking her up in a search engine and following some url links. This image directly conflicted with the health messaging Grace was promoting at work.

Maintaining Boundaries

It is important that in everything we do as professionals we maintain boundaries. This is especially important within social media where the boundaries between the professional and personal can often be blurred. Some people prefer to keep separate social media accounts for personal and professional use. This can help maintain boundaries, but it is not a straightforward or fool-proof solution. It can be useful to present aspects of your personal life even within a professional account to make it more accessible to a user. In this way others feel they are getting to know a person and not just a bland user profile. Furthermore, keeping separate social media profiles can become hard to maintain and therefore are less likely to be used consistently. However, if you do decide to keep a single social media account you must be even more careful to maintain sufficient professionalism in all that you post or react to (like/favourite).

For some it may be that separate social media platforms are used for separate purposes. For instance, I have a Twitter account (@easduncan), which I use predominantly for work purposes. I have found it an invaluable way to network with others, disseminate my research, and keep up to date with the research and practice activities of people from across the globe.

From time to time I will post a picture on Twitter that is not directly work related or make a comment on a particular social issue that I feel strongly about. I find this a useful way to present a wider picture of myself to those who follow my account. However, I avoid using this account for personal or family matters. Instead, I have a private Facebook account, which I try to keep as separate as possible from my work life. Inevitably there are some overlaps between the two. For instance, I have colleagues at work who are friends and friends who are on Twitter that will spontaneously follow me there (though I can only imagine they are fairly bemused by my work postings!). This means that even for my Facebook account, which I consider to be private, I have to think carefully before I post anything and be mindful of my direct and indirect audience (HCPC, 2017) (Vignette 21.2).

It is certainly important not to mix professional and service user relationships in social media settings. Occasionally you may receive an invitation from a service user to become a "friend" or follow the service user's account. Alternatively, such people may request to become your "friend" on a social media platform (Vignette 21.3). Where social media settings require permission to be given, you should politely refuse such requests. It can be helpful to explain to the person that you are not allowed to mix social and professional relationships, and that doing this would likely break your organisation social policy.

If you have a professional profile on a social media account, it can be helpful to describe the type of setting in which you work (e.g., occupational therapist in a stroke rehabilitation unit). However, if you wish to identify your employer you should make sure you're aware of the employers' social media policy. Some people also provide statements to the effect of "all opinions in this account are my own and not that of my employer." Such statements, however, do not provide you with immunity. It is safer therefore to think carefully about everything that you see before posting (RCOT, 2019).

Always Respecting Confidentiality

Treat social media as you would any other area of your professional practice. In essence, posting something on a social media account is like standing in the middle of a large public square and shouting it out to everyone that's passing by. Think therefore before you post anything. As professionals we are bound by our ethical code of conduct and professional standards to maintain confidentiality with all the service users with whom we work. This remains true within social media settings. Occupational therapists should never post information about a service user on any social media platform unless they have given you explicit

---

VIGNETTE 21.2

Jane worked in a social work department. She didn't have a professional social media account, but did have a personal Facebook account. Jane was very careful about who she accepted to be her friends on Facebook. She had only one or two friends that she had previously worked with, and she had only accepted them both when they left the department for other positions. For some time at work, Jane had found sharing an office with a colleague highly challenging. We'll call the colleague Brian. It was a small room and the ventilation was not good. Jane found the smell of some of the food that Brian regularly brought in unpleasant.

He would often eat his lunch at his desk. She never addressed this directly with Brian. One evening, after a particularly smelly lunchtime experience, Jane posted what she thought was a funny story relating the pungent pickle she found herself in on her Facebook page. One of her ex-colleague friends "liked" Jane's post with a laughing emoticon. That friend was also friends with Brian, and the action of liking that post resulted in it also appearing on Brian's Facebook page. The following day Brian was clearly upset and complained to Jane about what she had said about him. Brian reported her behaviour to his line manager.

VIGNETTE 21.3

David was on his final practice placement, working in a homeless shelter. The placement was challenging as the clients had multiple complex needs. However, after several weeks of getting to know the individuals, David felt he had finally managed to develop good therapeutic relationships with several of the shelter's frequent attenders. One afternoon he received an Instagram friend request from one of the shelter's clients that he had been working with. As he didn't wish to upset the individual, and without thinking about it too much, he accepted the request. Several weeks after he had left his placement, he received a message from the same individual on his account. It was late at night. The individual said that he was feeling very low and was actively planning to kill himself. David was incredibly concerned but wasn't sure what to do. After quickly discussing the situation with one of his fellow occupational therapy students, David phoned the homeless shelter and explained what had happened. The duty manager remembered David and thanked him for phoning. He reassured David that he would immediately follow up the client who was well known to the shelter, check that he was safe, and assess if any further intervention was required. The manager reminded David that had he read the organisation's social media policy in his induction pack he should not have accepted the friend request. The manager asked David to immediately remove the individual from his Instagram account. The duty manager stated he would inform the client on David's behalf that this was the organisation's policy.

and written consent. This includes any information about them as a person, their health or life circumstances, or the work that you undertake with them as a therapist. Even if you think you have not directly identified them, you may post sufficient information for others to realise who or what you are talking about. Equally important in this context is the importance of not posting any images or recordings relating to individuals you work with. If you have any questions or doubts about whether you should post something, refrain from doing so and ask for a trusted colleague's opinion. In all instances err on the side of caution.

Engaging With Others

Social media provides excellent opportunities to engage in a wide range of topics with people who have similar or vastly different views from your own. Like so many aspects of social media this can be a double-edged sword. Many topics (e.g., current affairs, religion, sport) attract a wide range of views. You are of course free to engage in discussions such as these, many of which can help form opinions and understanding about a range of issues. But here, too, the mantra "think before you post" applies. Unfortunately there are many trolls (people whose purpose is to cause disagreement or to inflame a situation) and people who engage aggressively on social media platforms. There are many reasons why people behave like this. Some do it to seek attention because they're bored or find such behaviour amusing. Others may participate in such behaviour due to their own personal insecurity. Trolls' behaviours are unacceptable because they can impact on the receivers' own mental health. Engaging with these individuals is rarely productive. It can lead to frustrating, aggressive, and rude exchanges. As with other social media posts, your responses

to trolls remain for posterity and rarely cast the person who posts a response in a positive light. The best advice in this situation is: "Do not feed the troll!" If you find yourself in a social media exchange with somebody who is aggressive, rude, or insulting, then you should cease your interaction. If necessary, block these people and report them from using the platform's mechanisms. If you are tempted to respond to such behaviour when you see it online, I understand. I often find myself frustrated by what someone else has posted online. My advice (which I am still trying to master) is to pause, consider what your response will constructively add, and on most occasions just let it pass.

Social Media and the Truth

In the Internet era where information and misinformation can travel globally in a matter of hours, all occupational therapists should ensure that the health information they share is evidence based and comes from credible sources. The Covid-19 pandemic is an excellent example of how information and misinformation can rapidly emerge and spread to the general public. Think carefully before you quote or spread information, especially health-related information that you have read online. Use your critical appraisal skills (see Chapter 12) to judge if the information you are sharing is objective and sound. If in doubt, do not post or repost.

SUMMARY

Social media has exploded into most people's lives over the last 10 to 15 years. There are clear professional advantages for occupational therapists to engage in social media. Social media can provide opportunities to network, learn, and share about the latest evidence for practice, raise the profile of the profession within society, lobby organisations and governments to develop effective policies, and engage with people who you otherwise would have no way of reaching. Social media, however, presents a range of potential pitfalls. These pitfalls require occupational therapists to engage with social media in a conscious manner, actively considering the aims, impact, and consequences of their interactions.

REFLECTIVE LEARNING

- What is your social media presence like?
- How much self-disclosure do you think is the right amount for your social media accounts?
- What image do your social media accounts portray of you as a person?
- How do you think your current social media presence could affect your work and career?
- How could you make better use of social media for professional development?

REFERENCES

BJOT & #OTalk (2016). Social media: Creating communities of research and practice. *British Journal of Occupational Therapy, 79*(4), 195–196.

Dean, B. (2020). Social network usage & growth statistics: How many people use social media in 2020? *Backlinko.* https://backlinko.com/social-media-users.

Dieleman, C., & Duncan, E. A. (2013). Investigating the purpose of an online discussion group for health professionals: A case example from forensic occupational therapy. *BMC Health Services Research, 13*(1), 1–8.

Health and Care Professions Council. (2017). *Guidance on social media. Information for registrants.* Author.

Occupational Therapy Board Ahpra. (2019). Social media. *How to meet your obligations under national law.* https://www.ahpra.gov.au/Publications/Advertising-resources/Social-media-guidance.aspx.

Rolls, K., Hansen, M., Jackson, D., & Elliott, D. (2016). How health care professionals use social media to create virtual communities: an integrative review. *Journal of medical Internet research, 18*(6), e5312.

Royal College of Occupational Therapists. (2019). Introduction to social media. https://www.rcot.co.uk/promoting-occupational-therapy/using-social-media.

Serafino, P. (2019). Exploring the UK's digital divide. Office for National Statistics. https://www.ons.gov.uk/peoplepopulationandcommunity/householdcharacteristics/homein%20ternetandsocialmediausage/articles/exploringtheuksdigitaldivide/2019-03-04.

United Nations. (n.d.). Sustainable development goals. 17 goals to transform our world. https://www.un.org/sustainabledevelopment/.

INDEX

Note: Page numbers followed by "f" indicate figures, "t" indicate tables, and "b" indicate boxes.